ECG and INTRACARDIAC TRACINGS

A Toolkit Approach for Analyzing Arrhythmias

ECG and INTRACARDIAC TRACINGS

A Toolkit Approach for Analyzing Arrhythmias

George J. Klein, MD, FRCPC

Professor of Medicine
Division of Cardiology
Western University
London, Ontario, Canada

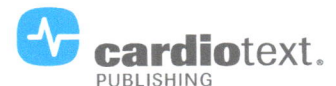

cardiotext.
PUBLISHING

Cardiotext Publishing, LLC
750 2nd St NE Suite 102
Hopkins, MN 55343 USA

https://cardiotextpublishing.com

Any updates to this book may be found at https://bit.ly/KleinToolKit

Comments, inquiries, and requests for bulk sales can be directed to the publisher at: info@cardiotextpublishing.com.

This book is intended for educational purposes and to further general scientific and medical knowledge, research, and understanding of the conditions and associated treatments discussed herein. This book is not intended to serve as and should not be relied upon as recommending or promoting any specific diagnosis or method of treatment for a particular condition or a particular patient. It is the reader's responsibility to determine the proper steps for diagnosis and the proper course of treatment for any condition or patient, including suitable and appropriate tests, medications or medical devices to be used for or in conjunction with any diagnosis or treatment.

Due to ongoing research, discoveries, modifications to medicines, equipment and devices, and changes in government regulations, the information contained in this book may not reflect the latest standards, developments, guidelines, regulations, products or devices in the field. Readers are responsible for keeping up to date with the latest developments and are urged to review the latest instructions and warnings for any medicine, equipment or medical device. Readers should consult with a specialist or contact the vendor of any medicine or medical device where appropriate.

Library of Congress Control Number: 2018959387

ISBN: 978-1-942909-25-5

eISBN: 978-1-942909-32-3

Printed in the United States of America

For an example of a digital caliper program, see PixelStick (Mac only) at https://plumamazing.com/product/pixelstick.

4 5 6 7 8

Table of Contents

Preface

With considerable gratitude to him, I dedicate this book encapsulating an approach to the analysis of ECG and EGM tracings to my old friend and colleague Mark E. Josephson (1943–2017). He is, of course, universally known for his role in bringing the exciting but largely theoretical field of electrophysiology to clinical application, and his book of electrophysiology, *Clinical Cardiac Electrophysiology: Techniques and Interpretation*, is widely acknowledged to be the "bible" of electrophysiology.

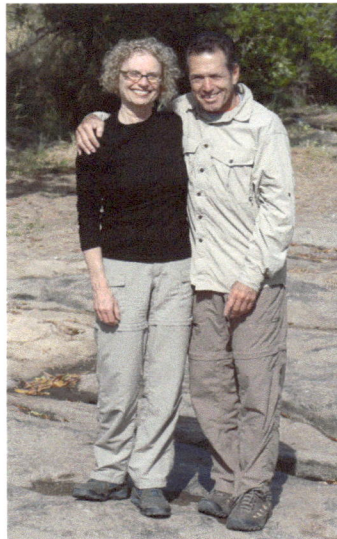

However, I don't think I would get too much disagreement from generations of trainees and students in saying that his major love was teaching, be it one-on-one with his trainees or in front of a large audience come to learn during one of his courses. What always impressed me was his unbridled and infectious enthusiasm, especially for the interesting tracing. This could be intimidating to some of his students initially, but it was guaranteed to get them involved in the issue at hand.

It is with considerable humility that I have tried to capture some of the deductive thinking and problem solving that he was so good at. Rarely at a loss for words and very quick, Mark would be a very difficult act to follow for most of us. Hopefully, a methodical approach using what I call the "tools" of analysis can bring us a little closer to his excellence.

I have included one of my favorite pictures of Mark during happy times with his wife Joan, his lifelong best friend and soulmate.

AF	atrial fibrillation		**CL**	cycle length
AFl	atrial flutter		**CS**	coronary sinus
AP	accessory pathway		**CSM**	carotid sinus massage
AT	atrial tachycardia			
AV	atrioventricular		**ECG**	electrocardiogram
AVCS	atrioventricular conduction system		**EGM**	electrogram
AVN	atrioventricular node		**EP**	electrophysiology
AVNRT	atrioventricular node reentrant tachycardia		**ERP**	effective refractory pathway
AVRT	atrioventricular reentrant tachycardia			
			FP	fast pathway (generally in reference to AVN)
BB	bundle branch			
BBB	bundle branch block		**HB**	His bundle
BBR	bundle branch reentry		**HBE**	His bundle electrogram
BBT	bundle branch reentrant tachycardia		**HP**	His-Purkinje (system)
BPM	beats per minute		**HRA**	high right atrium

IVCD	intraventricular conduction disturbance		**PR**	interval from onset of P to onset of QRS
			PSVT	paroxysmal supraventricular tachycardia
JT	junctional tachycardia		**PVC**	premature ventricular complex depolarization
			Px	preexcited
LA	left atrium			
LAF	left anterior fascicle		**RA**	right atrium
LAFB	left anterior fascicular block		**RB**	right bundle branch
LBBB	left bundle branch block		**RBBB**	right bundle branch block
LPF	left posterior fascicle		**RV**	right ventricle
LPFB	left posterior fascicular block			
LV	left ventricle		**SHD**	structural heart disease
			SP	slow pathway (generally in reference to AVN)
ms	millisecond		**SR**	sinus rhythm
			ST	sinus tachycardia
NCT	narrow complex tachycardia		**St-A**	stimulus-atrial
NF	nodofascicular		**SVT**	supraventricular tachycardia
NFRT	nodofascicular reentrant tachycardia			
NSR	normal sinus rhythm		**TCL**	tachycardia cycle length
NV	nodoventricular			
NVRT	nodoventricular reentrant tachycardia		**VA**	ventriculo-atrial
			VT	ventricular tachycardia
Os	ostium			
			WC	wide complex
PAC	premature atrial depolarization		**WCT**	wide complex tachycardia
PJRT	permanent junctional reciprocating tachycardia		**WPW**	Wolff-Parkinson-White
PPI	post-pacing interval			

Chapter 1

Choosing Cognitive Tools: The Essence of ECG and Electrogram Tracing Diagnosis

Clinical electrophysiology has undergone tremendous evolution since the era of electrocardiogram (ECG) diagnosis in the initial half of the 20th century and the introduction of intracardiac recordings for clinical diagnosis in the 1960s. Exciting and innovative tools encompassing ablation, imaging, mapping, and others continue to dominate our attention, literature, and training programs. It is nonetheless difficult to minimize the importance of ECG and electrogram (EGM) analysis as the portal of entry of patients to our area and the cornerstone of everything we subsequently do in electrophysiology.

ECG and intracardiac tracings are inseparable. One can consider that the intracardiacs provide only additional ECG leads or, conversely, the ECG lead is essentially just another intracardiac channel to look at, albeit providing a more global or "far-field" look. Since they are frequently inseparable and involve the same fundamental analysis principles and knowledge base, I thought it logical and convenient to consider them together in this book.

The traditional approach to teaching arrhythmia has been to organize by *arrhythmia entities* such as atrioventricular (AV) node reentry, Wolff–Parkinson–White syndrome (WPW), or ischemic ventricular tachycardia (VT). While this is useful, it does not teach the learner a strategy or "plan of attack" for an unknown tracing. As in my previous books, I have tried to emphasize the *approach* to the tracings. It seemed reasonable, then, to organize this book on that basis, organizing around the thought process to tackle the problem and not necessarily the arrhythmia entity. That is, not just provide an "answer" but explore how I solved the problem. What physical and mental tools were used, consciously or subconsciously?

This book is intended for those who have looked at a complicated tracing and drawn a blank, not recognizing a pattern from their personal experience or venturing a guess with variable confidence, without a good idea of how to proceed. My goals in this book are to highlight the mental and physical strategies that I have found useful; these are virtually identical for ECG and intracardiac tracings, and they will both be used as examples in "**toolkit**" problem solving. The emphasis is on having strategies for looking at a complicated tracing, be it ECG or EGM. Of course, knowledge of electrophysiology is an essential tool, since there is not much point in strategies if the basic "rules" for our puzzles are not understood.

Whether an ECG or EGM tracing or both, the process begins by an "overview" at the tracing, the highlights being atrial activation sequence, ventricular activation sequence, AV relationship, and the His bundle EGM position. The interpretation of most tracings will be readily obvious, but the more challenging ones are greatly facilitated by having a strategy or approach.

Specific "tools" (cognitive and other) are essentially reflected in the Table of Contents, but include:

1. Careful measurement, optimally on a digital record, using electronic calipers with enlargement of the area of interest where appropriate, is especially valuable for P-wave identification on an ECG.

2. The concept of "framing the problem" provides a focal point for creating explanatory hypotheses. Tables of differential diagnosis for various phenomena can be useful after the problem is framed. A common "frame" in our discipline is determining the mechanism of a wide QRS complex tachycardia (WCT). This can only be explained by a finite group of mechanisms, the "usual suspects," with each tested in a tracing for "goodness of fit" with the observations. I have provided a set of lists describing some of these observations in Chapter 8, and the interested reader will add to these lists by creating their own.

3. It is vital to take a systematic approach to a complicated tracing. I find that dividing the tracings into segments or zones helpful. There is no reason to start at the beginning of the tracing. Starting with a part that is easier to comprehend allows for a solid base to build on for the rest of the tracing.

4. A specific "checklist" for any tachycardia is necessary to define:
   - Ventricular activation sequence using ECG QRS morphology and available intracardiac ventricular EGMs;
   - Atrial activation using P-wave morphology and intracardiac atrial EGMs;
   - The relationship of atrial activation to ventricular activation; and
   - The presence of His bundle activation and its position in the cardiac cycle.

5. Long runs of tachycardia with unchanging landscape often are not diagnostically productive. More informative are what I have called "transition zones" or "change zones," the most valuable of which is the onset of tachycardia. Other important zones are the termination of tachycardia, changes in cycle length, the influence of ectopic beats, and the change of one apparent tachycardia to another.

6. It can be diagnostically useful to examine the parts of the tracing that seem peripheral to the main tachycardia or the "attention-getting" part of the tracing. These might include an available sinus beat or the drive beat during extrastimulus testing. I like to think of this as "paying attention to the sidelines" of the action.

The sample case I highlight in this first chapter is not simple but illustrates these principles. The "answer" was not immediately apparent to me (nor my colleagues), and I needed to work it through. I will try to share with you what I was thinking to accomplish this. If you understand this example, the rest of the book falls easily into place.

All the tracings in this chapter are taken from the same patient followed from original presentation to resolution by catheter ablation. The patient is a young man referred for assessment of WCT, a sample of which is presented as **Figure 1.1A**.

Figure 1.1A

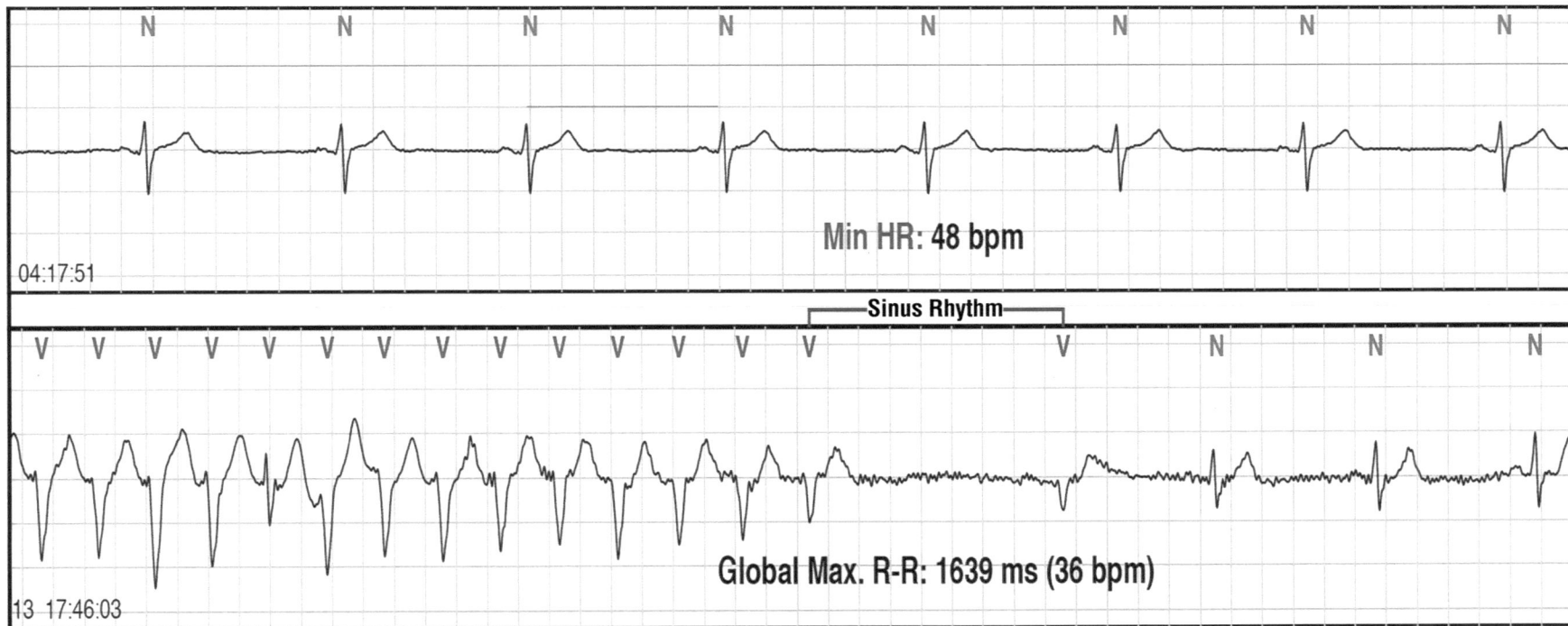

All of us would naturally look at this and try to "short cut" a diagnosis. In this particular example, we have several important "tools" to use to help us. The first is the presence of sinus rhythm shortly before the episode. The second is a spontaneous termination, although this was not helpful here. Finally, we have a "transition" or "change," in this case, a normal beat that interrupts the uniform flow of the WCT.

When we run our calipers across the WCT (**Figure 1.1B**), we notice that the tachycardia is quite regular. The single, narrow beat is right on time and the subsequent WCT beat is similarly right on time. This realistically can only result if the narrow beat is a tachycardia beat and not an ectopic beat. A capture beat would generally alter the WCT timing. Additionally, the QRS is virtually identical to the sinus rhythm—clearly not fused, as would be expected if the capture beat arrived simultaneously with a VT beat. *One can thus confidently rule out VT and conclude that the supraventricular tachycardia (SVT) has bundle branch block aberration (statistically most likely) or that the SVT is associated with a "bystander" accessory pathway (AP), statistically less likely.*

Finally, one carefully compares the single, narrow beat of the tachycardia with the sinus rhythm QRS "on the sidelines" (**annotated Figure 1.1B**, **red arrow**). This indicates a little deflection at the end of the normal QRS during tachycardia (absent during sinus rhythm), which suggests a retrograde P wave during tachycardia and supports the diagnosis of atrioventricular nodal reentrant tachycardia (AVNRT). This is supported further by another example (**Figure 1.1C**), which shows longer transitions between wide and narrow tachycardia and verifies the presence of the terminal QRS deflection present during narrow QRS tachycardia beats but not sinus beats. This tracing also shows some variability of the QRS in WCT, which we can come back to later after the final diagnosis.

Figure 1.1B

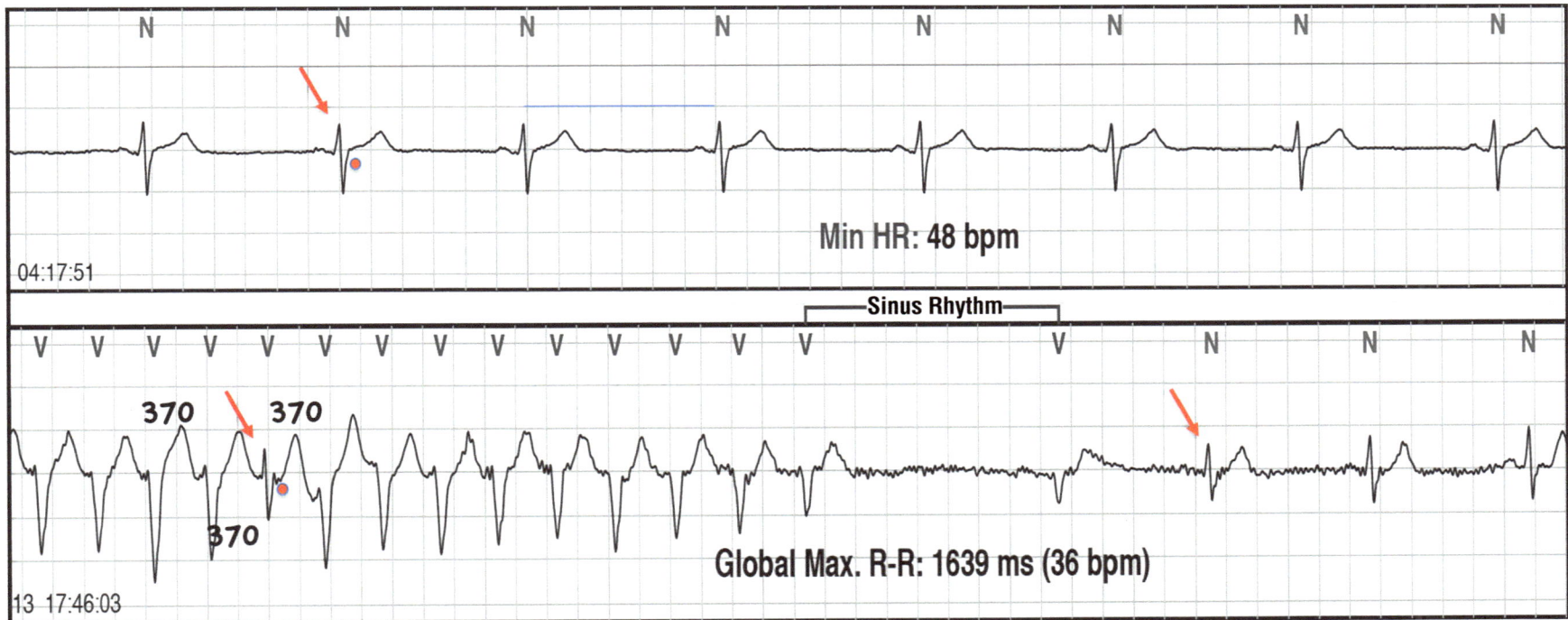

Figure 1.1C

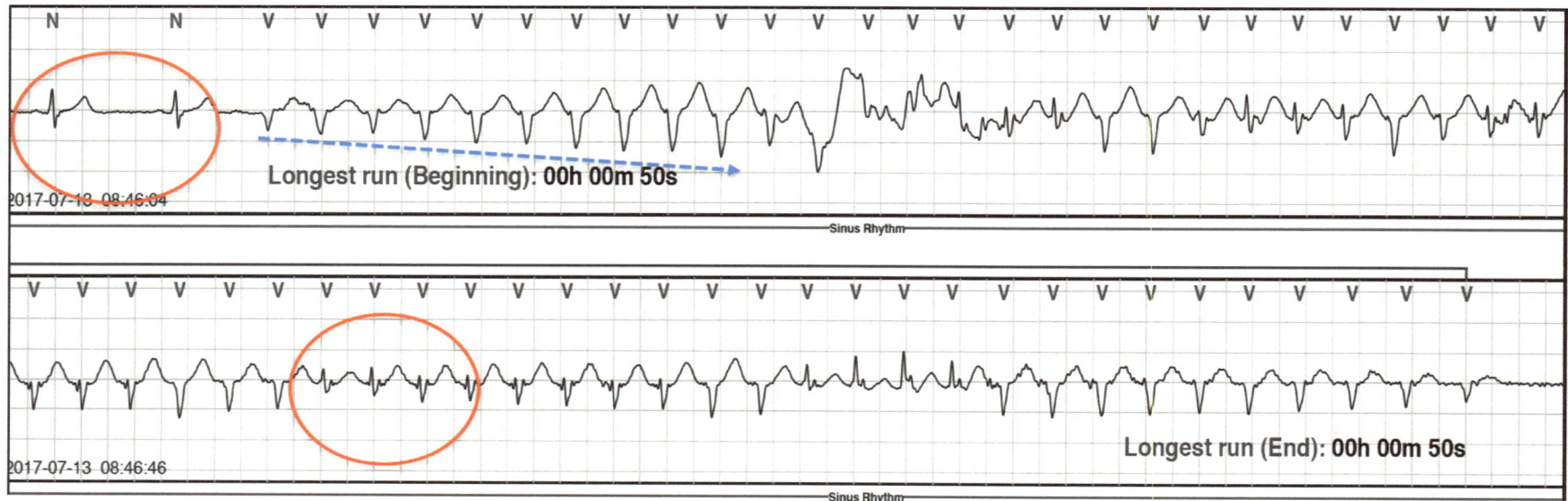

The patient was subsequently brought to the electrophysiology (EP) lab with a working diagnosis of probable AVNRT with WCT related to either bundle branch block or bystander preexcitation.

The catheters were placed and the arrhythmia shown in **Figure 1.1D** was induced during ventricular pacing. The first 2 cycles are the last 2 beats of ventricular pacing. In this and subsequent problems throughout the book, try making the interpretation before looking at the annotated versions. Ask yourself if you have a "strategy" to interpret the tracing or are just waiting to be inspired as you look at it.

Figure 1.1D

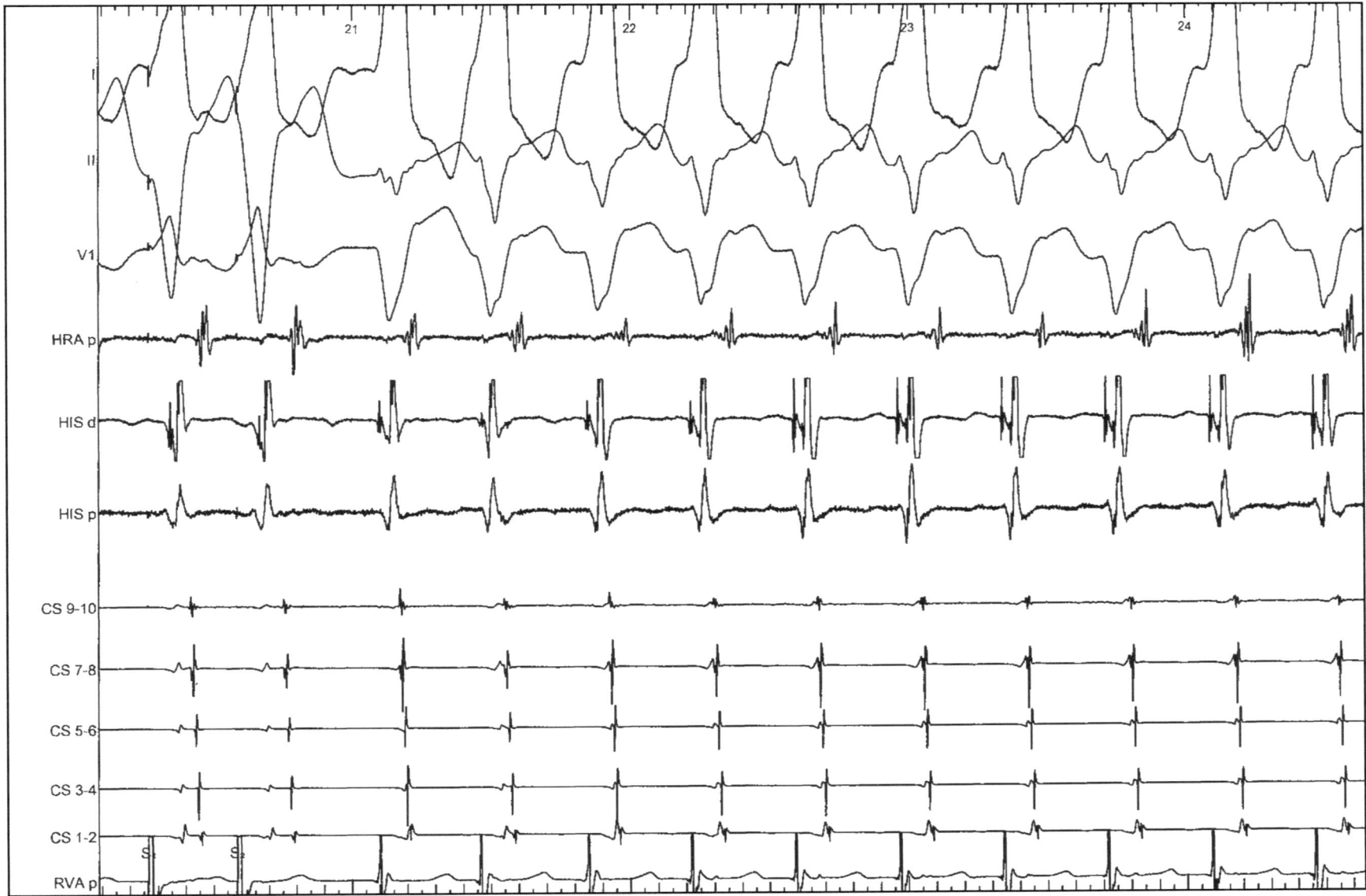

A broad look shows **2 zones**, namely a WCT and the transition zone with induction by the ventricular pacing (**Figure 1.1E**). I find it easier to focus first on a zone that looks more obvious and straightforward—and in this case, the WCT seems a good place to start. Walking through with calipers shows that the WCT is perfectly regular and the cycles are repetitive. The QRS has reasonably "typical" left bundle branch block (LBBB) and left axis deviation, suggestive of LBBB aberrancy, but is not diagnostically definitive. Applying a vertical cursor at onset of QRS (**blue line**) makes it obvious that the right ventricular (RV) apex is activated simultaneously with the onset of QRS (**time 0**). A rapid deflection at onset of QRS is identifiable as the His EGM and is also simultaneous with the onset of QRS.

With an HV of 0, we are considerably ahead since the WCT can ONLY be VT or a preexcited (Px) tachycardia. We now examine the atrial activation sequence (**dotted blue line**) and note that it is septal or central—that is, the coronary sinus (CS) orifice (CS$_{9-10}$) is earliest with HB atrial EGM not seen. This is not helpful in this instance and is compatible with any of the potential possibilities: atrial tachycardia (AT), AVNRT, or atrioventricular reentrant tachycardia (AVRT).

It is time to focus on the *transition zone*. The ventricular pacing beat starting tachycardia is followed by atrial activation with identical activation sequence to the tachycardia. *Such an induction can be thought of as analogous to ventricular overdrive pacing with entrainment.* The stimulus–atrial (St-A) interval is only 45 ms longer than the ventriculo-atrial (VA) during tachycardia (**red lines**) and the "post-pacing interval" after correction for prolongation of the AV interval is 80 ms. Furthermore, the HA interval with pacing is *identical* to the HA during tachycardia. The above informs us that the atrial activation during tachycardia is most likely retrograde and over the normal AV conduction system. The RV EGM is also most probably "in" the circuit.

If we put this together with the ECG data from prior to the study, we have anterograde conduction over an accessory pathway and retrograde conduction over the normal AV conduction system. The early RV activation at the RV apex is realistically only compatible with an atriofascicular pathway.

We now return to our initial ECG which was most compatible with AVNRT. Knowing that we have a functional atriofascicular pathway, we can now conclude that the slightly variable QRS morphology during AVNRT on the ECG was probably bystander AP conduction over the atriofascicular AP. Atrioventricular node (AVN) reentry coexists relatively frequently with AVRT in patients with atriofascicular pathways.

Figure 1.1E

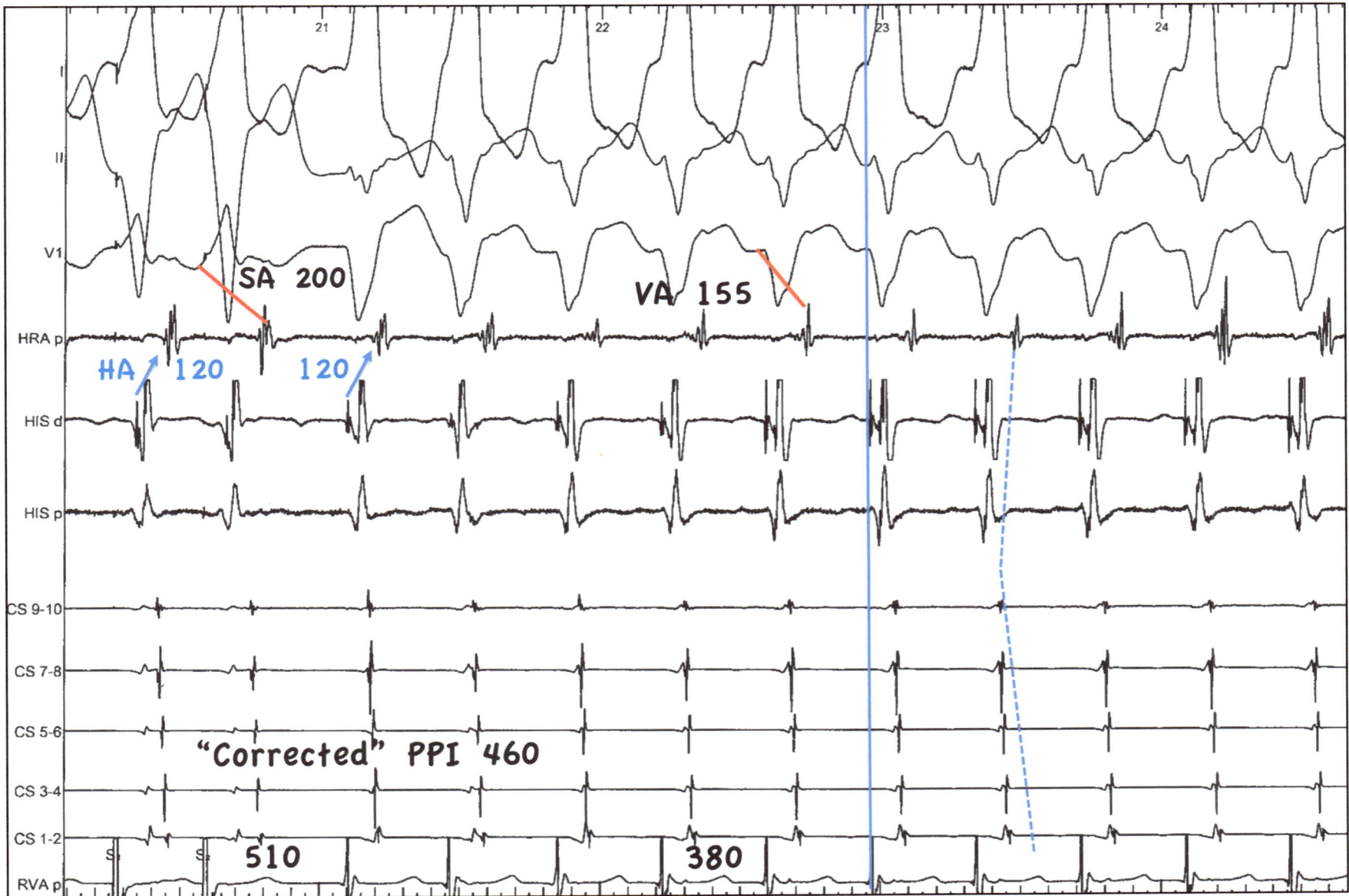

The "take-home" from this admittedly complicated case is the cognitive process: dividing a tracing into more manageable segments, focusing on parts of the tracing that are more understandable and building from there, having a checklist of questions to ask oneself, and being armed with a differential diagnosis when a problem is framed (for example, in this case, unequivocally knowing that a HV of 0 can ONLY be VT or preexcitation).

In going through the subsequent cases, the first tracing is always unannotated. It is optimal if the reader has a thorough go at this version before moving on to explanations. I have deliberately not provided multiple-choice questions since the idea is for the reader to frame their own problem and interpret more broadly. The chapters will highlight a specific tool or strategy but, of course, there will be considerable overlap as multiple "tools" are invariably used for most tracings.

Trusting you find this useful,

Chapter 2

Value of Diagnostic Tables, Framing the Problem, and Hypothesis Testing

Problem 2.1

Although the more experienced reader might recognize the "answer" to this tracing (**Figure 2.1A**) immediately, I always find it useful to verbalize the problem that I am trying to solve or "frame the problem." One can then begin to look at the universe of possibilities to explain what is observed and test each hypothesis according to the observations. In this example, we might initially frame our problem in this instance as "wide QRS tachycardia" (see "Wide QRS Tachycardia" section of Chapter 8) and note that the realistic list of possibilities includes VT, SVT with bundle branch block, or preexcited tachycardia. The other possibilities on the list—namely artifact, paced rhythm, and "pseudo" VT due to ST elevation—are readily excluded by inspection. P waves are not apparent, and the only clue would be the QRS morphology, which is relatively "typical" LBBB. This favors aberrancy, but doesn't exclude VT (such as bundle branch reentry) or preexcitation (specifically the atriofascicular type of AP).

Figure 2.1A

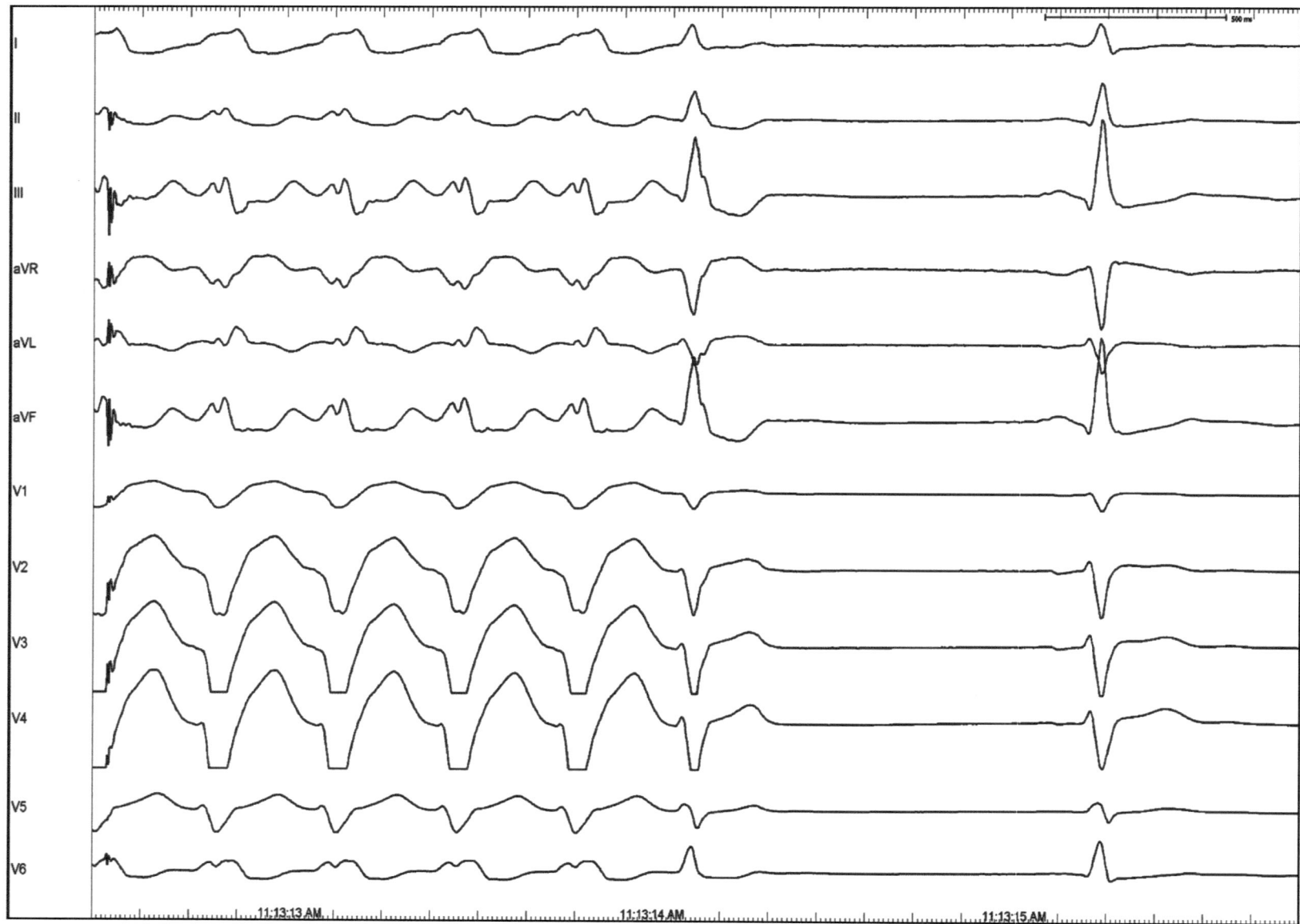

Then, we note that the last beat of tachycardia appears normal, and comparison to the sinus beat that follows shows it is a good match—that is, *the last cycle of the tachycardia has a normal QRS.* We then run our calipers along the tachycardia beats (**Figure 2.1B**) and note that the cycle length (CL) is regular and the coupling interval of the last cycle that normalizes—*does not change.*

Figure 2.1B

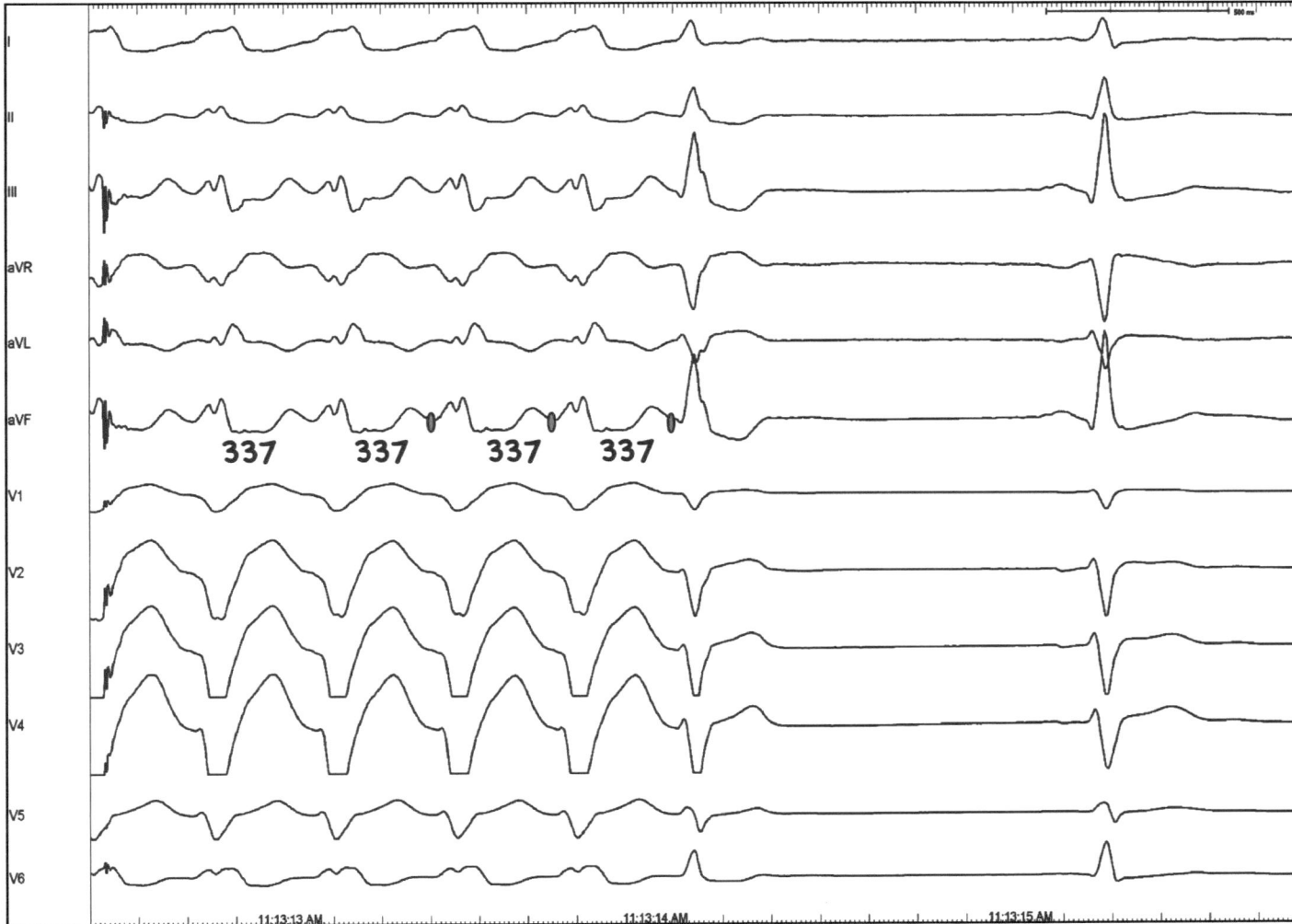

We now create a new and more specific "frame" and ask ourselves what the universal list of possibilities would be if a WCT ends with a normal beat (see "Wide QRS Tachycardia" in Chapter 8). There may well be others to add to our list that we have not considered or encountered. Nonetheless, the termination of the tachycardia with a normal beat without change in the coupling interval suggests that the tachycardia needs the wide complex to perpetuate itself. If we then go down our list and hypothesize that the WCT has LBBB aberration, termination with normalization suggests that the LBBB is important to the mechanism. A look at the intracardiac recordings in **Figure 2.1C** immediately shows the diagnosis, and the annotated version shows that the spontaneous normalization of the QRS results in a shorter VA interval with subsequent termination due to block in the AV node. Orthodromic AVRT with retrograde conduction over a left AP is evident from the atrial activation sequence. There is a larger circuit during LBBB (down the right bundle, across the septum and up the left pathway), which shortens with resolution of LBBB (now down LBBB and up the left AP), causing the VA interval to shorten. See **Figure 2.1D** for a pictorial version of this explanation. Ask yourself why the other hypotheses listed in "Wide QRS Tachycardia" section of Chapter 8 to explain this phenomenon don't work. For example, a capture beat could stop slower VT but it would have to be quite premature to get into a VT circuit.

Figure 2.1C

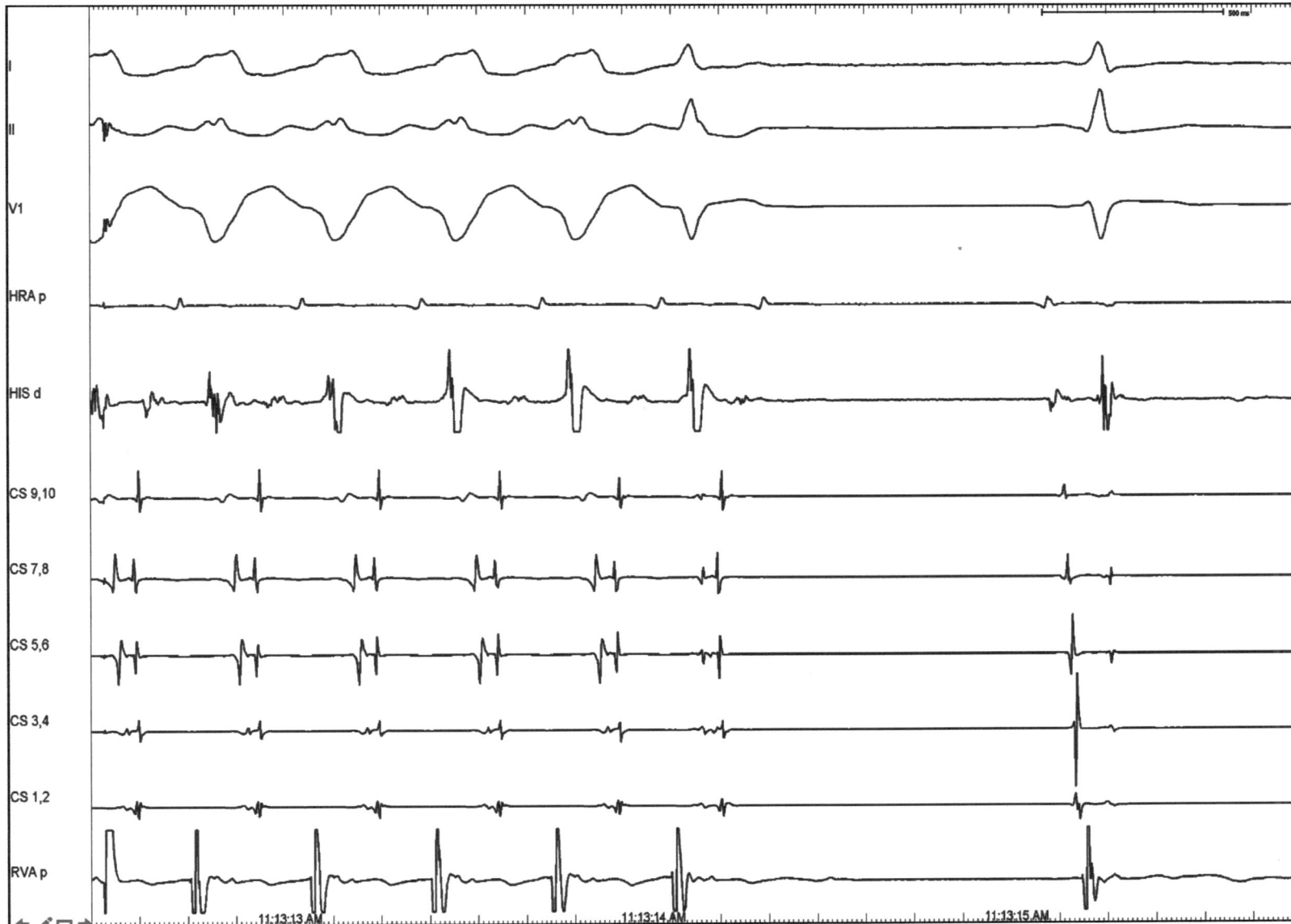

Figure 2.1D

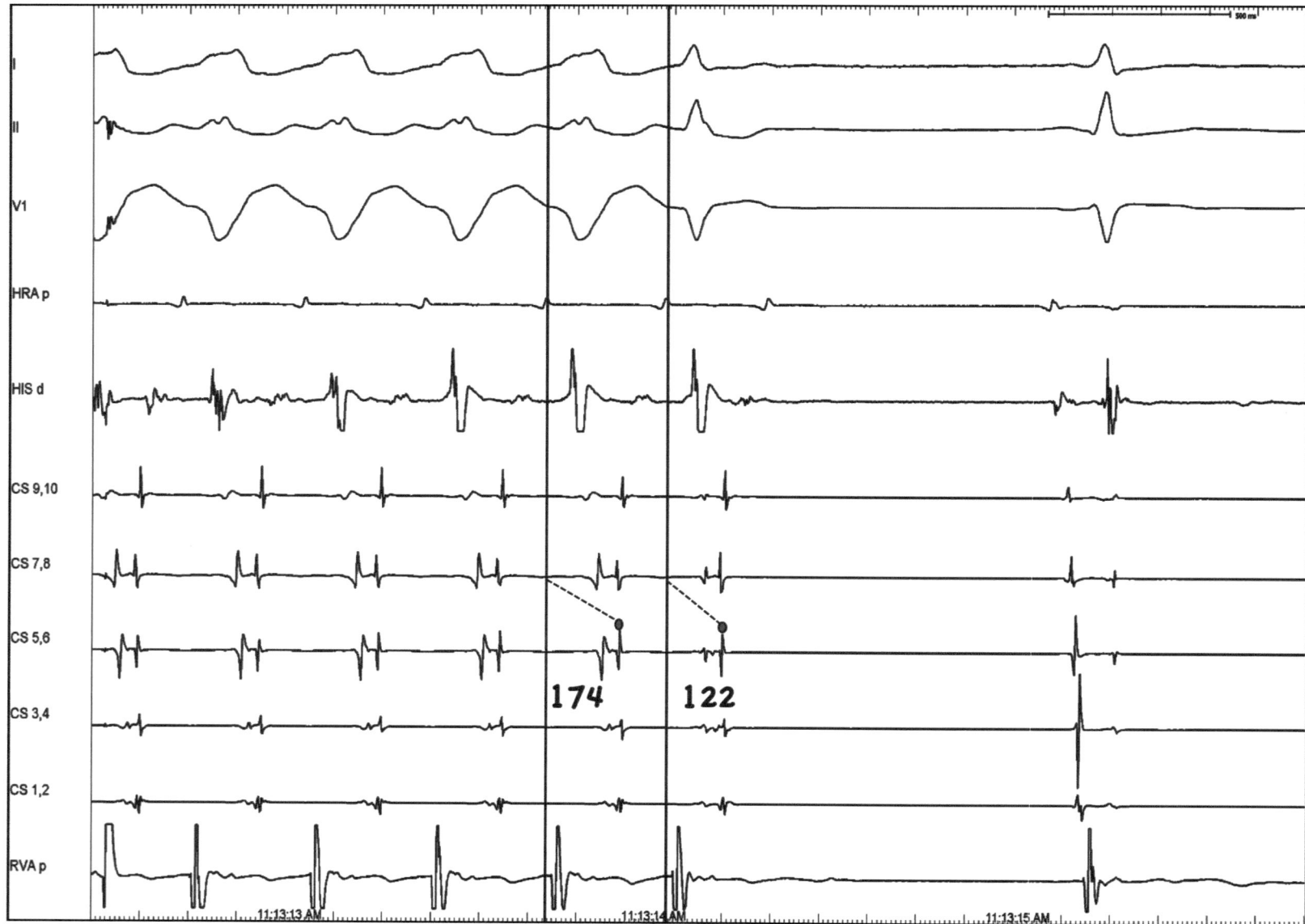

Problem 2.2

Problem 2.2 is obviously a WCT, and **Figure 2.2A** illustrates the result of overdriving ventricular pacing. The QRS morphology is compatible with a relatively typical LBBB pattern, but we don't see a His EGM, and the WCT has a 1-to-1 AV relationship. This leaves the differential diagnosis open at this point.

Figure 2.2A

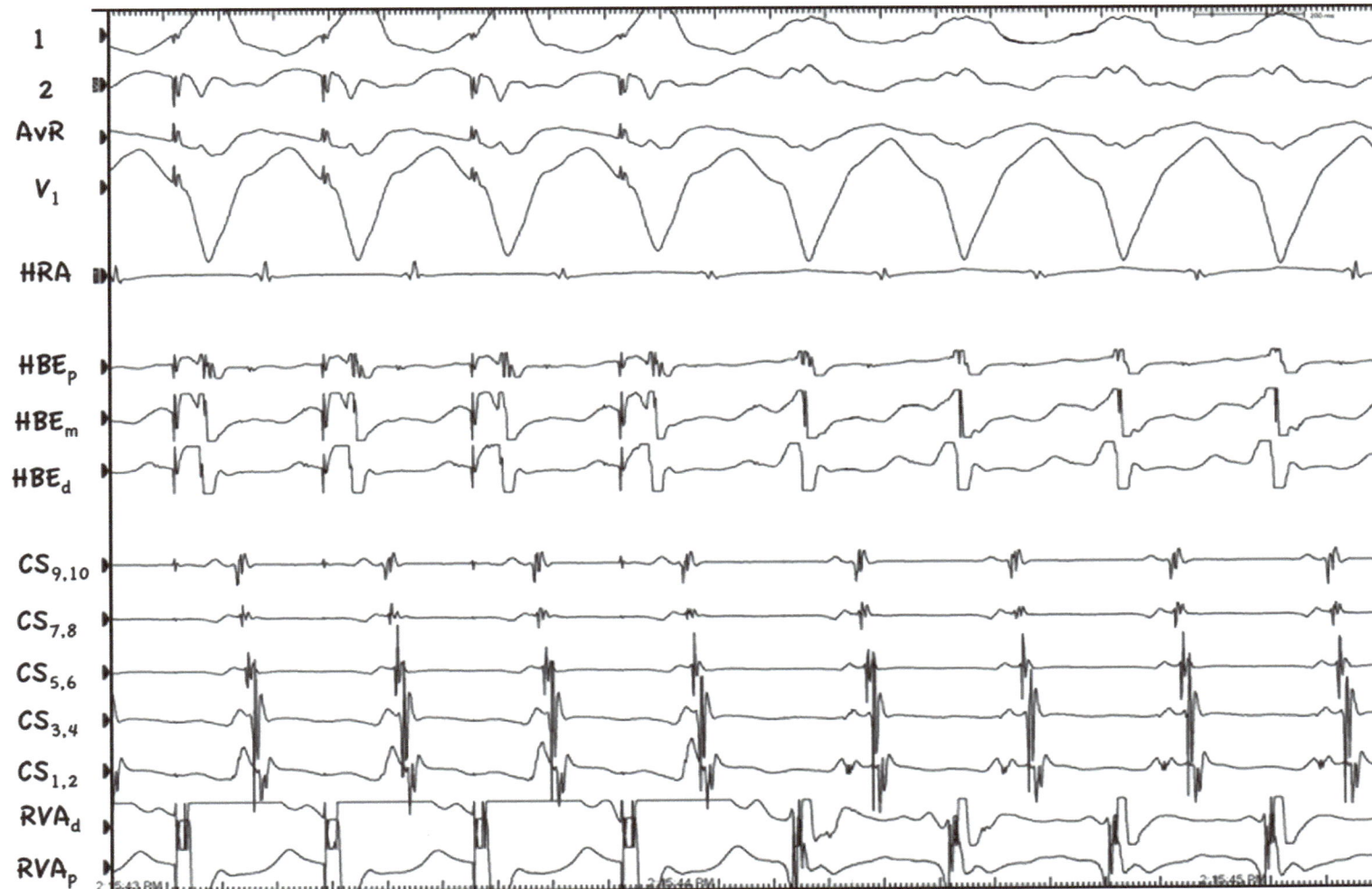

Overdrive pacing has resulted in stable entrainment, the QRS morphology during pacing being intermediate between pure pacing (**not shown**) and WCT. We identify the last atrial EGM at the paced CL and note that we have *a VAV response*, which excludes AT. The post-pacing interval (PPI) is 305 ms, and the PPI–tachycardia cycle length (TCL) is 20 ms, showing that *the RV is essentially "in" the circuit* (**Figure 2.2B**).

Figure 2.2B

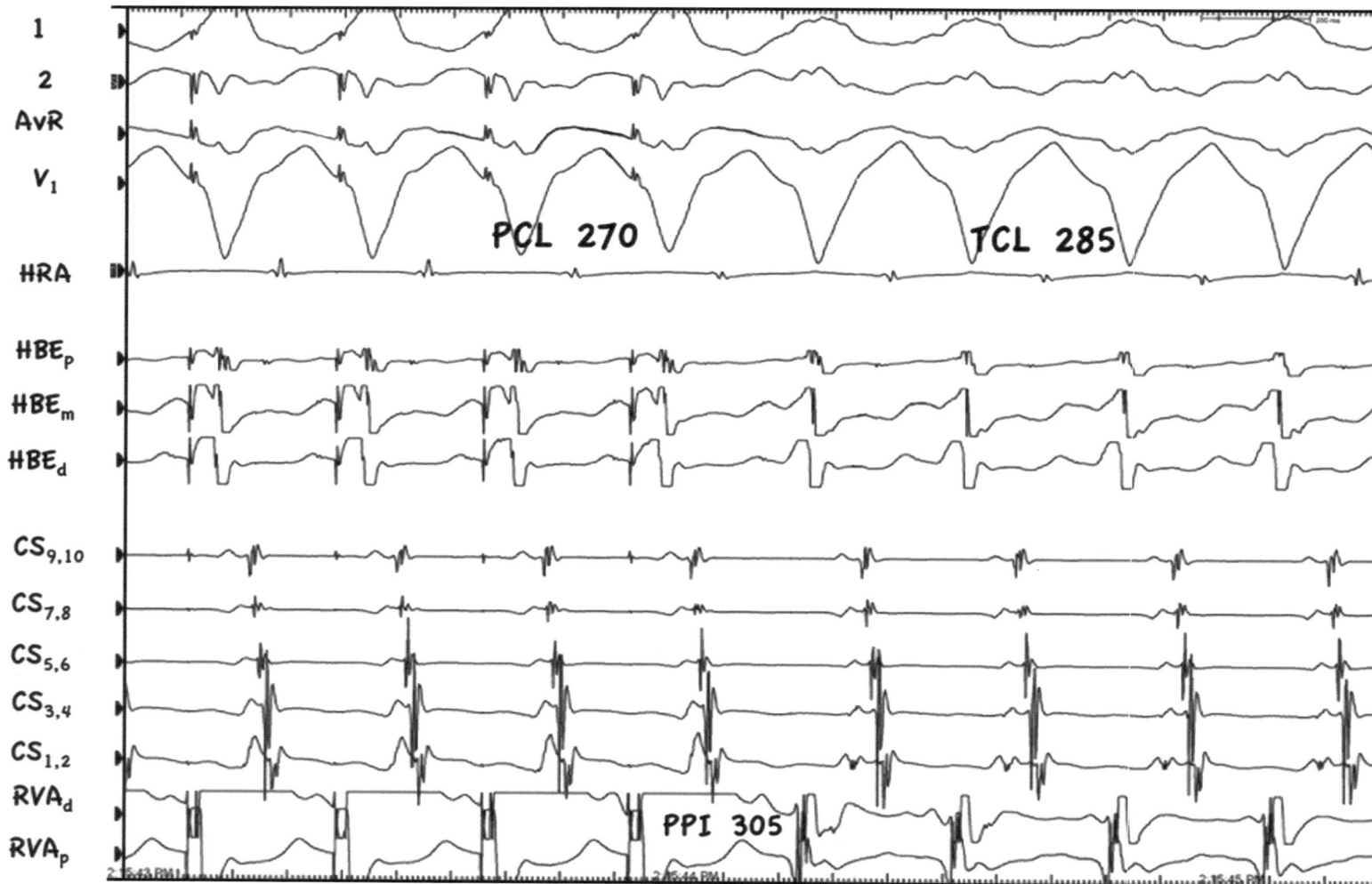

This, of course, excludes AVNRT as well as AT. More broadly speaking, we can say that we are now dealing with the universe of possibilities where *the RV is part of the circuit (AVRT, nodoventricular reentrant tachycardia [NVRT], or bundle branch reentry [BBR] VT)*. We now carry this thought into interpreting a fortuitous observation later in this study (**Figure 2.2C**).

Figure 2.2C

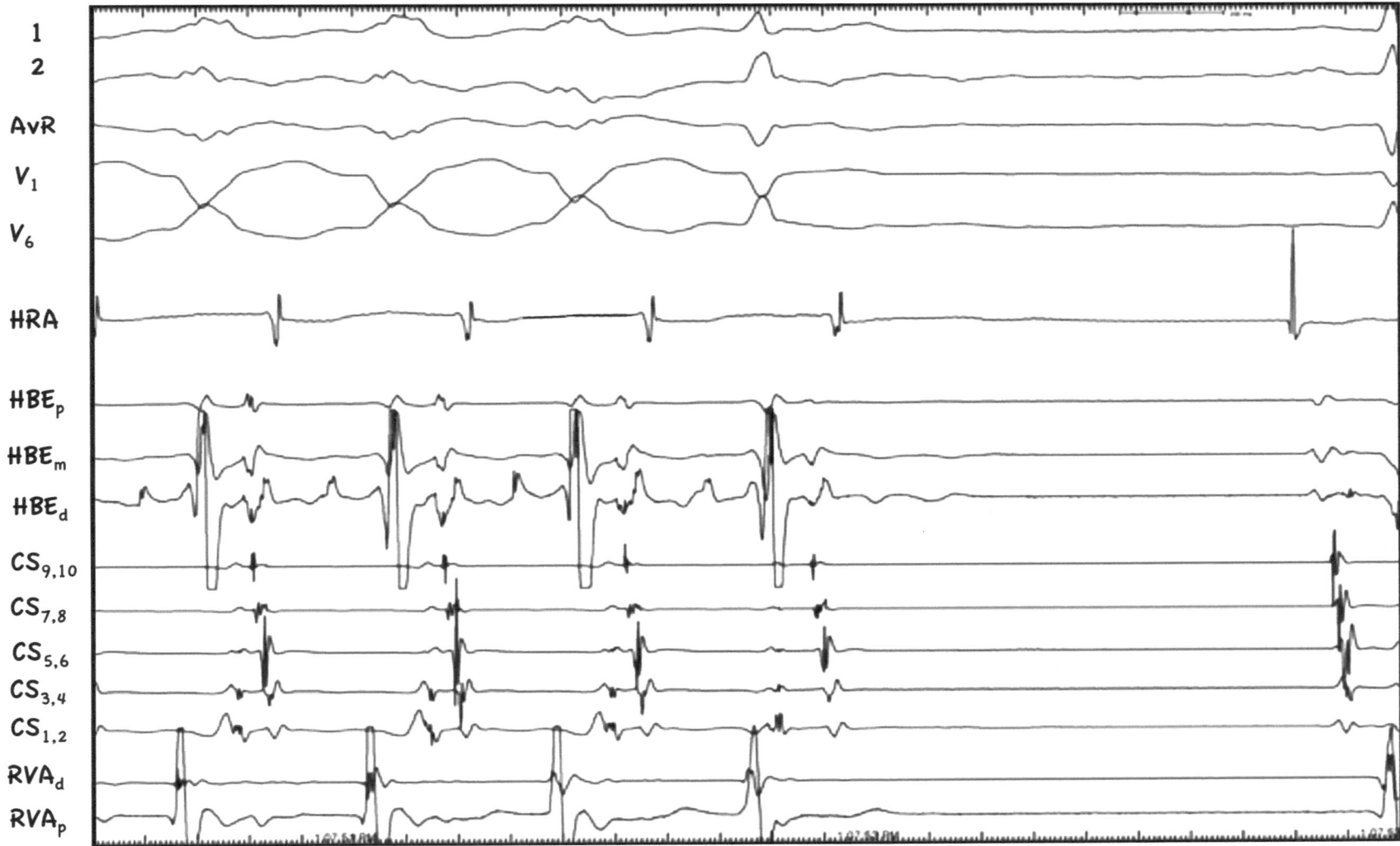

This tracing bears resemblance to Problem 2.1 and shows a spontaneous termination with a normal QRS being the last cycle. The His catheter has been moved, and we now see a deflection most compatible with the His (**Figure 2.2D**). The HV is 75 ms, comparable to the sinus cycle seen at the end of the tracing. The atrial activation sequence remains central after the normalized QRS.

We make our measurements, with the key observations being:

1. The atrial timing does **NOT** change, and the VA after the normal QRS is the same as the VA after the LBBB type QRS.
2. The ventricular timing at the RV EGM does **NOT** change (VV 365 to 370).
3. The far-field V EGMs at the coronary sinus (CS; **red ovals**) *advance* with normalization. This is most compatible with a normalization of LBBB. (Theoretically, it could be "pseudo" normalization by a left ventricular (LV) premature ventricular complex (PVC), although the latter would have to be perfectly timed relative to the tachycardia to provide such a perfect normalization.)

Figure 2.2D

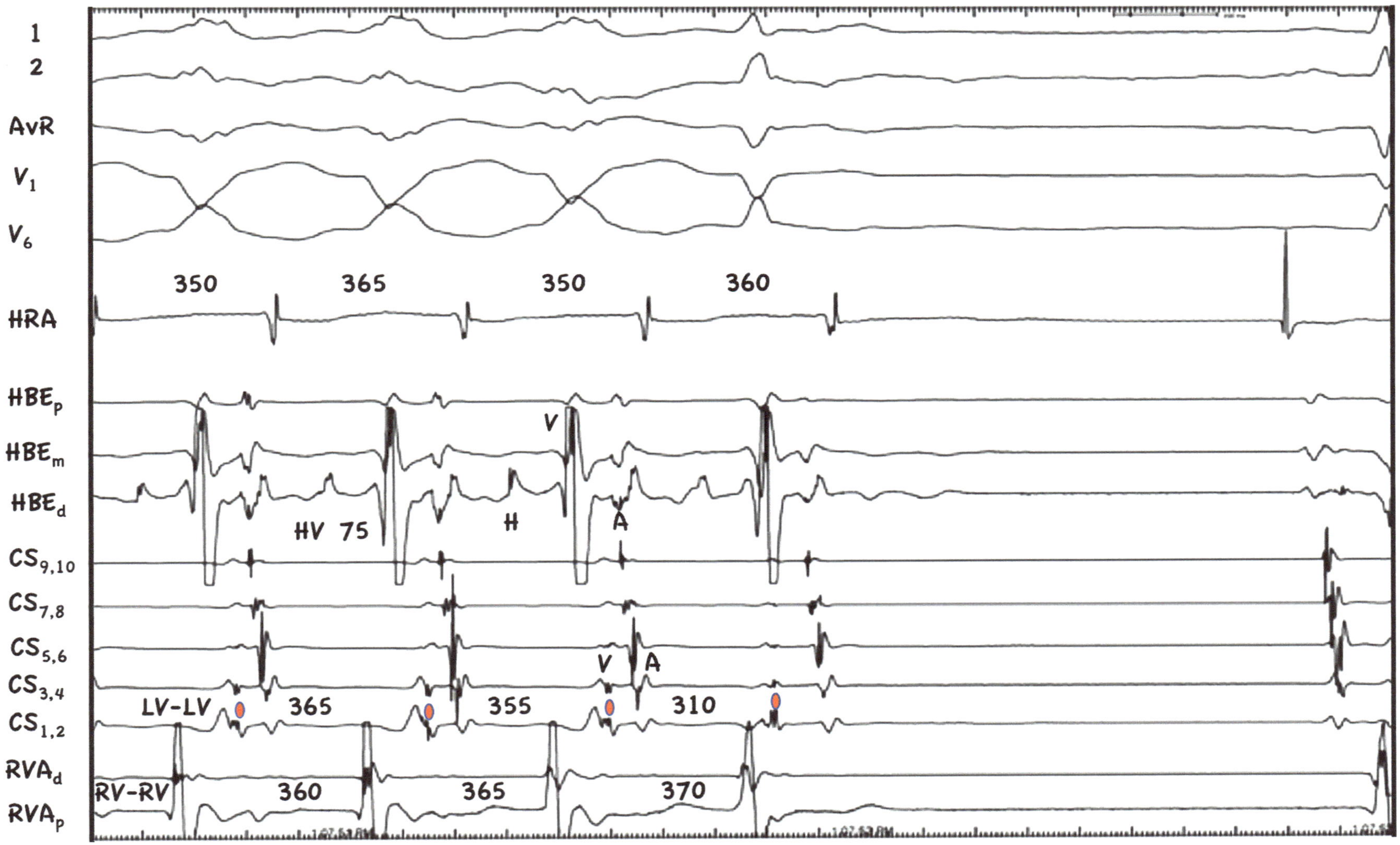
1
2
AvR
V1
V6
HRA
HBEp
HBEm
HBEd
CS9,10
CS7,8
CS5,6
CS3,4
CS1,2
RVAd
RVAp
350
365
350
360
V
HV 75
H
A
V
A
LV-LV
365
355
310
RV-RV
360
365
370

The preceding entrainment in **Figure 2.2** informed us that the RV was part of the circuit. The above tells us that the LBB (and the LV) is part of the circuit. ***Hence, we have a WCT where both the RV and LV form part of the circuit.***

We now ask, *how many tachycardia mechanisms involve both the RV and the LV?* It is a short list, as you see in **Figure 2.2E**, unless you can think of others. Each possibility on the list is now evaluated for feasibility.

When you examine the diagram in **Figure 2.2E**, it is difficult to envision a mechanism whereby BBR could terminate with a capture beat on time. Similarly, the HV interval is a little long but relatively normal and not compatible with anterograde preexcitation over an AV pathway, essentially eliminating option 4. Option 2 is more difficult to dismiss, but termination of LBBB AVRT by normalization as in Problem 2.1 is mediated by *shortening* of the VA interval, resulting in termination in the AV node by the prematurity of the A.

Thus, the only feasible explanation barring total coincidence remains option 3, nodoventricular (NV) tachycardia using a left NV pathway with concealed conduction into the node causing anterograde block (but not retrograde block) in the AV node.

Figure 2.2E

Tachycardia with both RV and LV "in" the circuit

1. **Bundle branch reentry**
2. **AV tachycardia with ipsilateral bundle branch block**
3. **NV tachycardia with ipsilateral bundle branch block**
4. **AP-to-AP reentry**

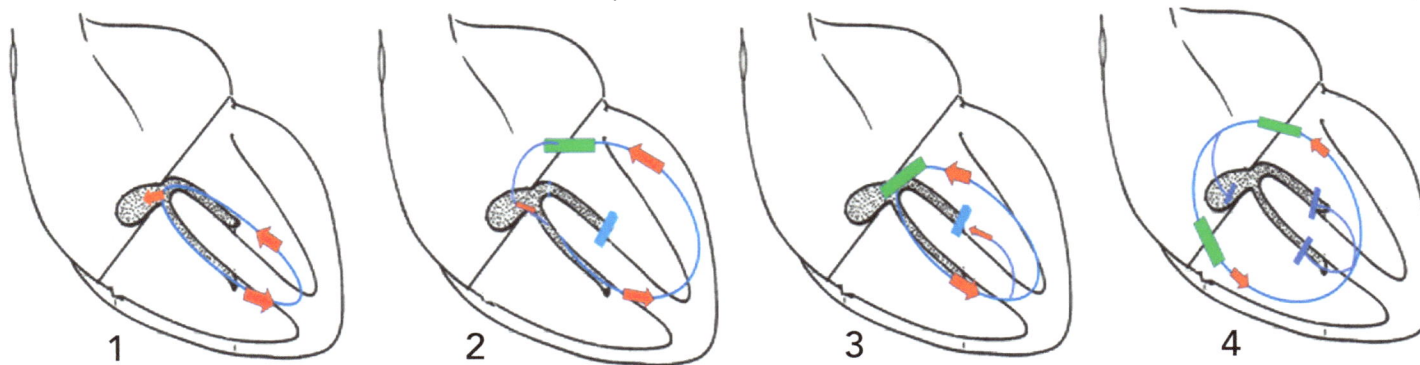

This is a potentially complicated case with a relatively rare mechanism, but its solution is identified simply by reviewing the mechanisms that could result in termination by normalization of the last cycle, showing that both the RV and LV are involved in the tachycardia, and running through the list of potential mechanisms that are compatible with these parameters.

EGM figures based on a case with the compliments of Dr. M. Scheinman.

Problem 2.3

An overview of **Figure 2.3A** shows a supraventricular tachycardia subject to a burst of ventricular pacing, which seemingly does not influence the SVT. We have a regular SVT with a 1-to-1 AV relationship of identical rate both before and after the burst. The differential diagnosis for this is wide open for all the SVT mechanisms, and we turn to our burst for enlightenment.

Figure 2.3A

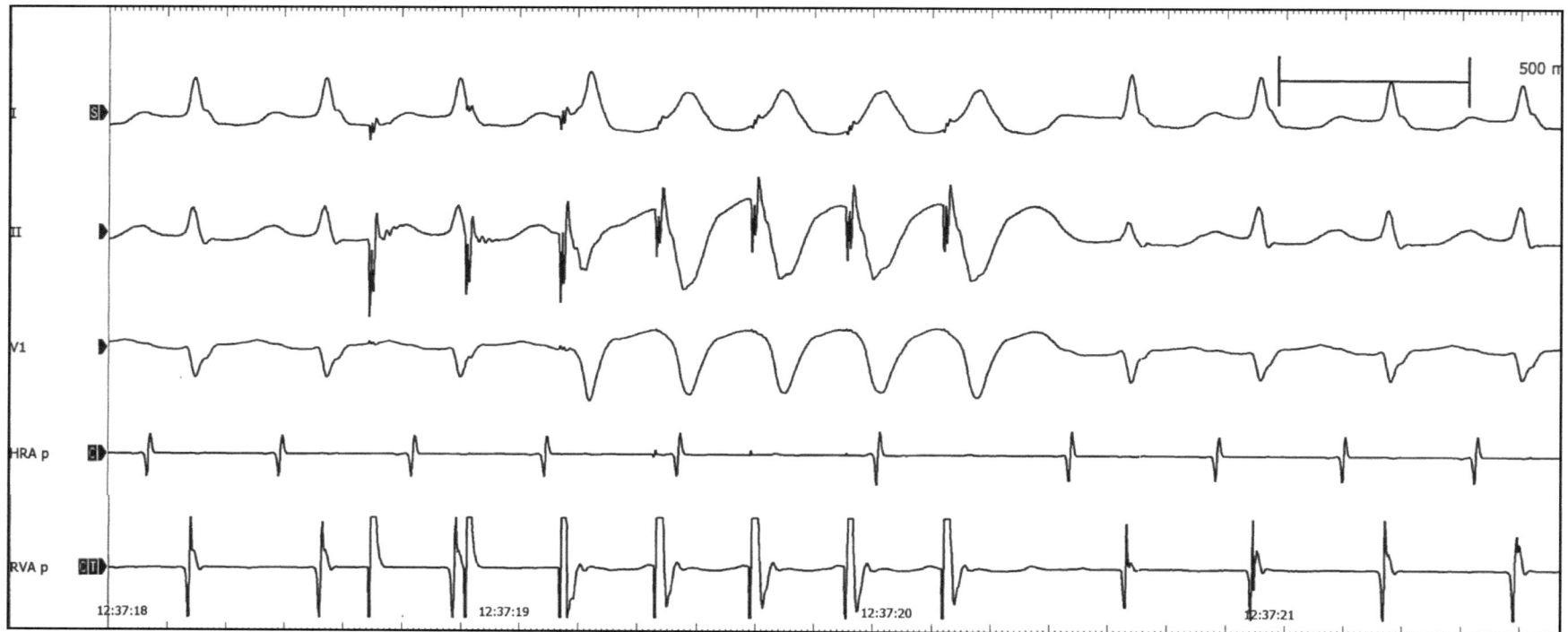

As we walk our calipers along the high right atrium (HRA) electrogram (**Figure 2.3B**), we note no change in the CL of 340 ms until after the 4th stimulus artifact, when it drops out to reappear after a longer interval. *This is a pivotal observation, as it is not physiologically possible to influence or terminate an AT by ventricular stimulation that doesn't make it to the atria.* Ventricular pacing or extra-stimuli can only influence AT mediated by prematurity of atrial activation resulting from VA conduction.

Figure 2.3B

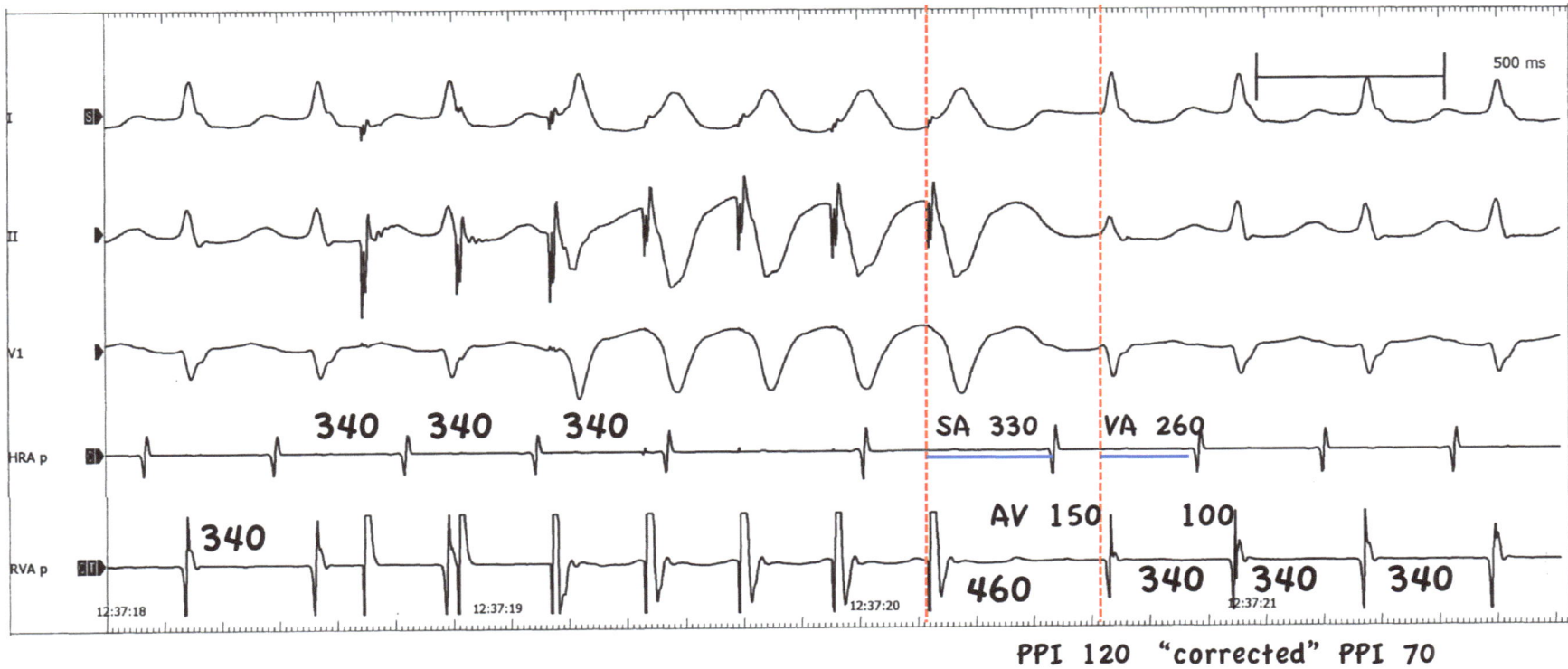

With AT ruled out, we ask ourselves whether the tachycardia has not been interrupted at all—or alternatively, whether the tachycardia was terminated and reinitiated. AVRT requires both the atria and ventricles as part of the circuit, so a diagnosis of AVRT would not be possible if we hypothesized that the tachycardia mechanism was not influenced by the burst. We can now measure the interval from the last spontaneous QRS prior to ventricular capture (3rd QRS) and the first one after the burst. This provides an interval of 1762 ms, which is NOT a multiple of the SVT CL (5 × 340 = 1700). Thus, the V burst has directly influenced the tachycardia, and it is more probable that we are dealing with a "terminate and restart" scenario with the last V restarting the arrhythmia with a relatively long St-A interval.

We can now use the fact that initiation of SVT from the V is analogous to entrainment in that both use the same VA routes to get to the atria. Looking at the "PPI," it is 460 and the PPI–TCL = 120 ms. When corrected for the AV delay of 50 ms, it is 70 ms, and this would rule out AVNRT by the Michaud criteria. Similarly, the St-A–VA is 70 ms, below the threshold for AVNRT by these criteria.

We come to a diagnosis of AVRT, but will proceed to **Figure 2.3C**, which includes the CS EGMs. At this point, the diagnosis is much easier but of course analysis without the CS EGMs forces a deeper understanding of the physiology, always a worthwhile exercise. We now use the atrial activation sequence and note that the distal CS EGM is earliest and we have an eccentric atrial activation sequence. Framing our problem as *SVT with eccentric atrial activation*, we have only 2 realistic possibilities (excluding the very rare AVNRT that has early atrial activation distally), namely AT and AVRT. Termination of SVT without getting to the A allowed us to exclude AT, making the diagnosis of AVRT without further discussion.

Figure 2.3C

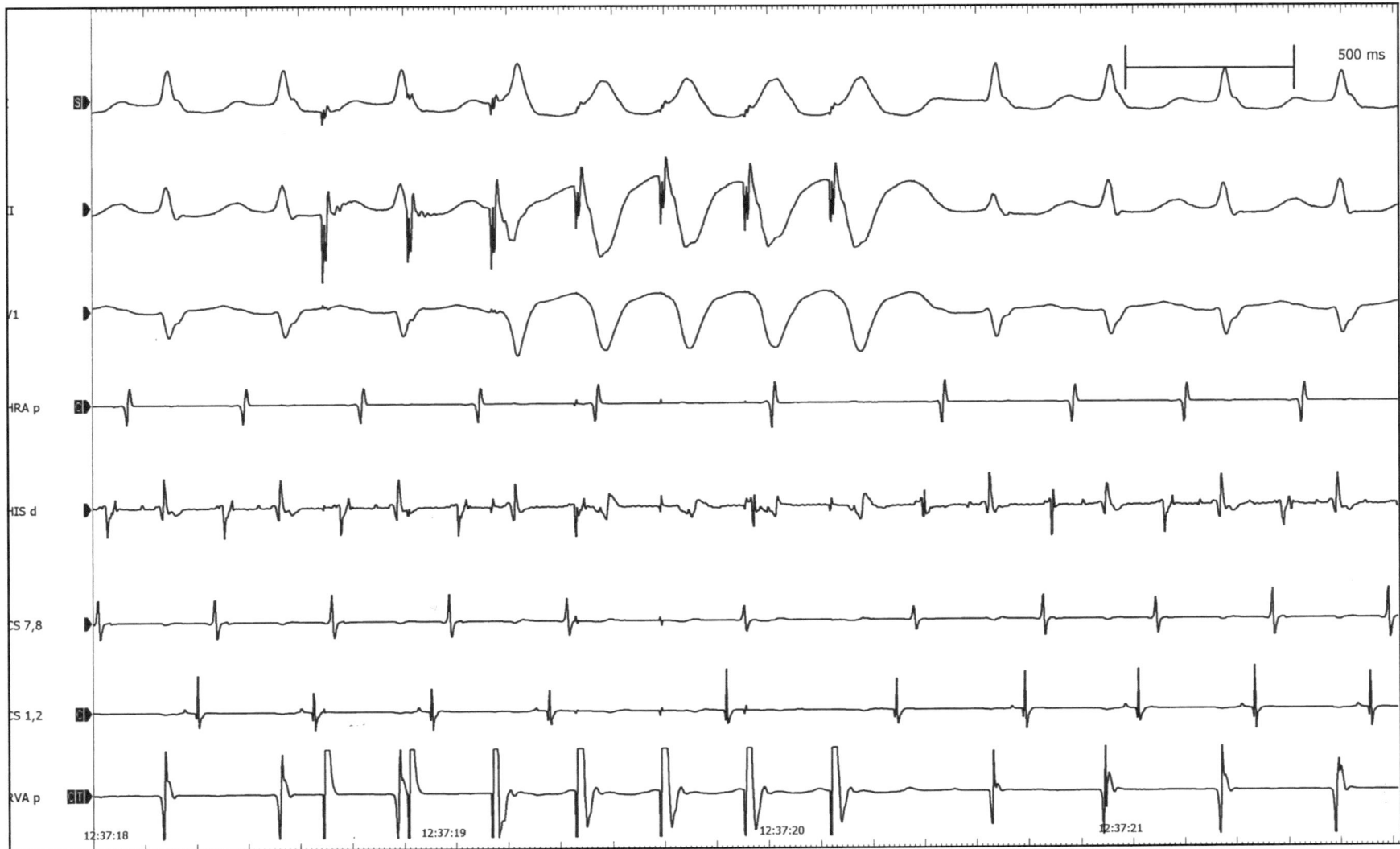

Some of you may ask whether we have excluded junctional tachycardia (JT) by our observations, and this is a fair question. Of course, this question does not come into play frequently, at least in the adult world, where JT as a cause of paroxysmal supraventricular tachycardia (PSVT) is uncommon. However, we can consider what the Michaud criteria tell us, namely that a PPI < 115 ms in this context is NOT seen with AVNRT.

This is because this measure is a reflection of the electrophysiological distance of the RV recording electrode from the circuit. A PPI–TCL < 115 ms is thus more or less "in" the circuit, or at least "close enough" for an AV reentrant tachycardia involving RV or septum. JT, although not formerly evaluated by a clinical study, would be expected to behave just like AVNRT in this context.

Problem 2.4

The patient from whom this tracing was recorded was originally referred for "atrial fibrillation" (**Figure 2.4A**). The QRS is normal, and atrial activity is not obvious. Running calipers through the tracing verifies the global visual impression of "group beating" or a repetitive pattern that, in this case, involves alternation between 2 or more beats at one CL and a few beats at another CL.

We can frame our dilemma as a "regularly irregular" tachycardia (**Figure 2.4B**). This involves a relatively short list of candidates (see "Supraventricular Tachycardia (AF Mimickers)" section in Chapter 8) and the absence of visible P waves makes the list even shorter, ruling out entities such as atrial flutter (AFl) or sinus tachycardia with "2-for-1" phenomenon.

Figure 2.4A

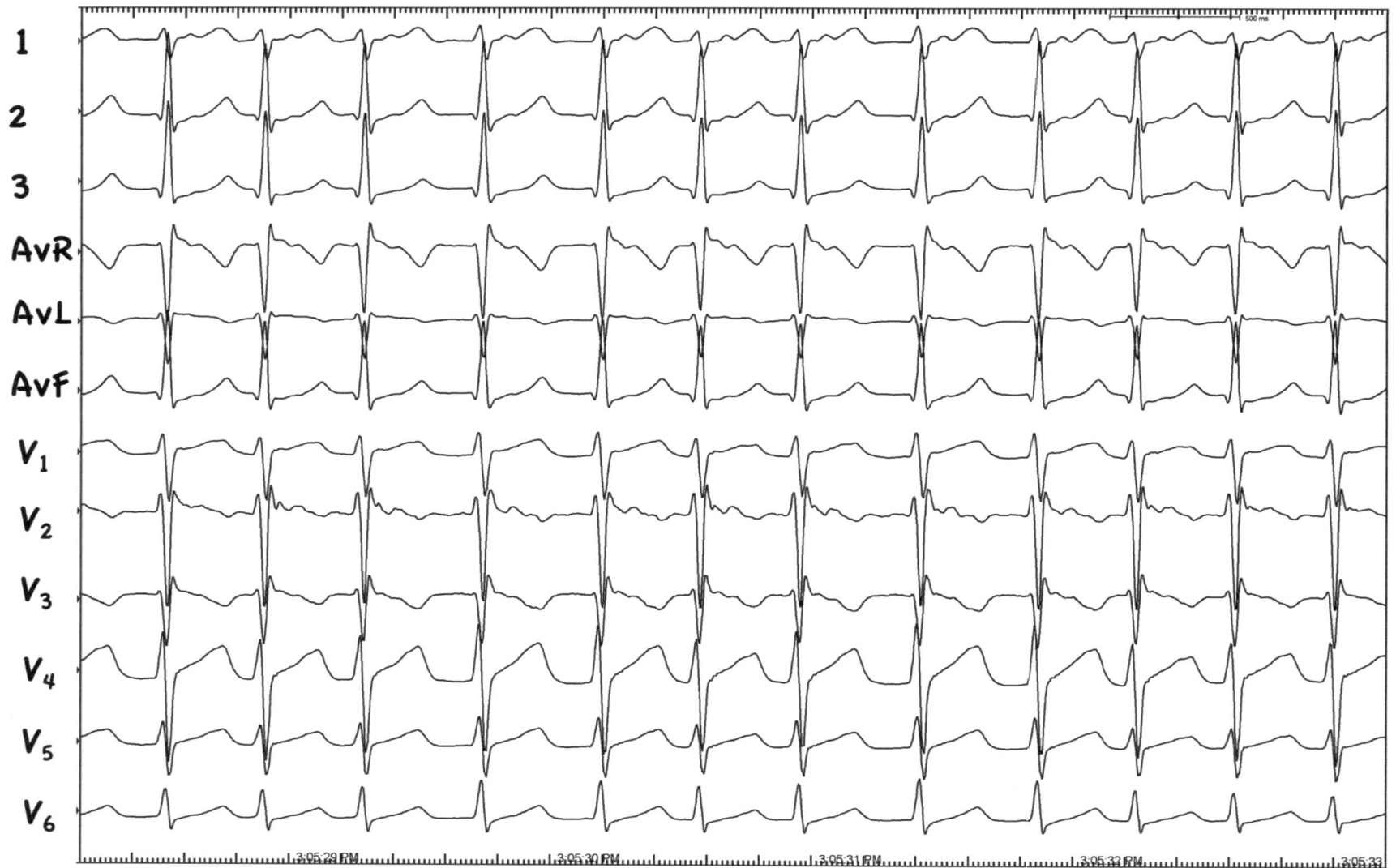

Figure 2.4B

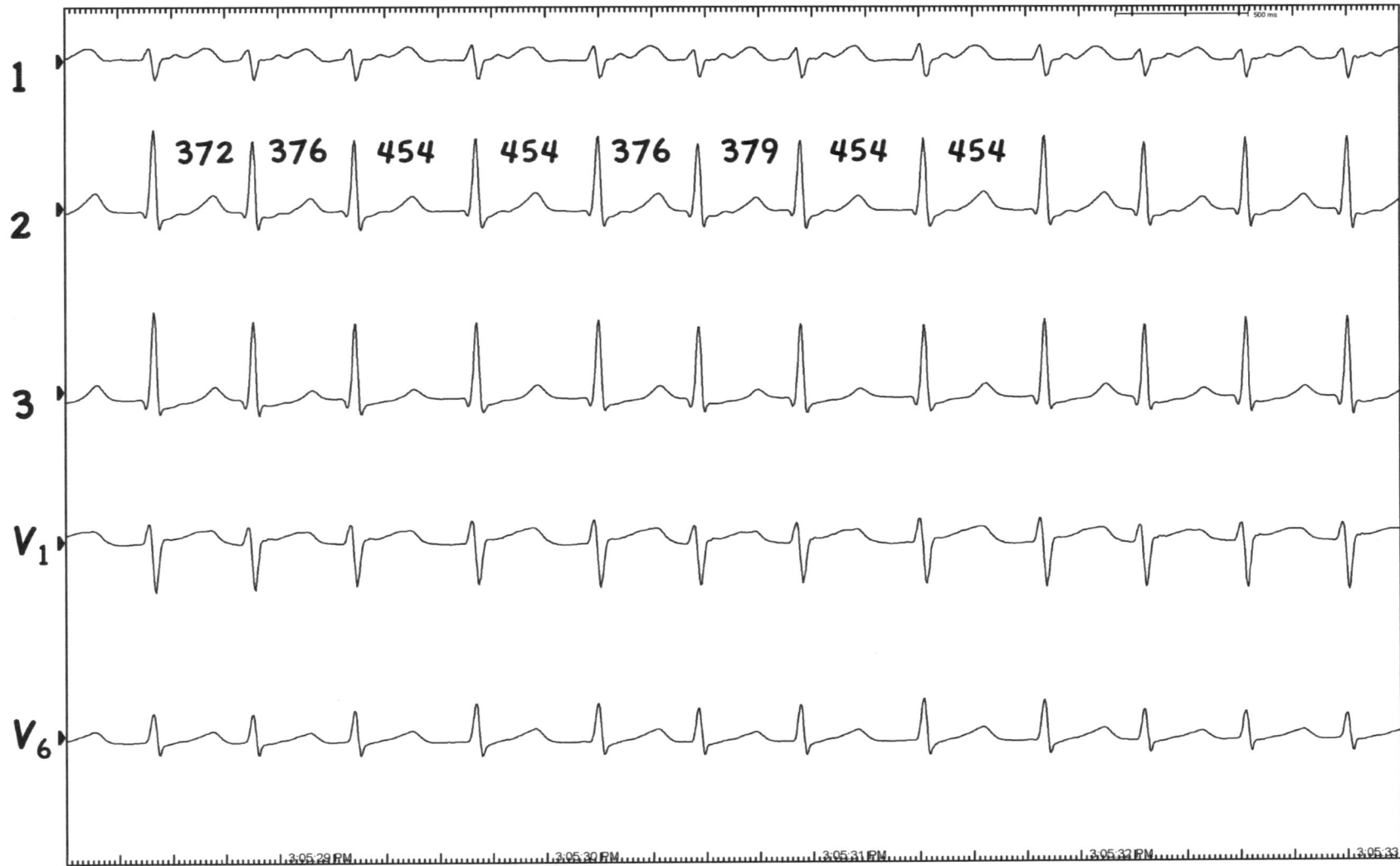

The best candidate on our list is thus AVNRT or AVRT with alternation between 2 slow pathways as the anterograde limb of the circuit.

We now look at the intracardiacs, which makes the issue much easier, showing atrial EGMs and atrial activation pattern. There is periodic AV block without affecting the tachycardia, and we can now refine our framing of the problem, namely referring to the list of SVTs that don't require the atrium ("Regular Supraventricular Tachycardia with VA Block" in Chapter 8). AVNRT would be the most common by far in this list and this was the final diagnosis.

You may have made another observation from **Figure 2.4C**. The switch from the shorter to longer anterograde slow pathway (for example, from the 3rd to 4th QRS) is *preceded by block of the retrograde fast pathway. This suggests that a single change in the actual circuit caused both phenomena*, and one can strain their imaginations to see how this could happen. The AVN is far from simple!

Figure 2.4C

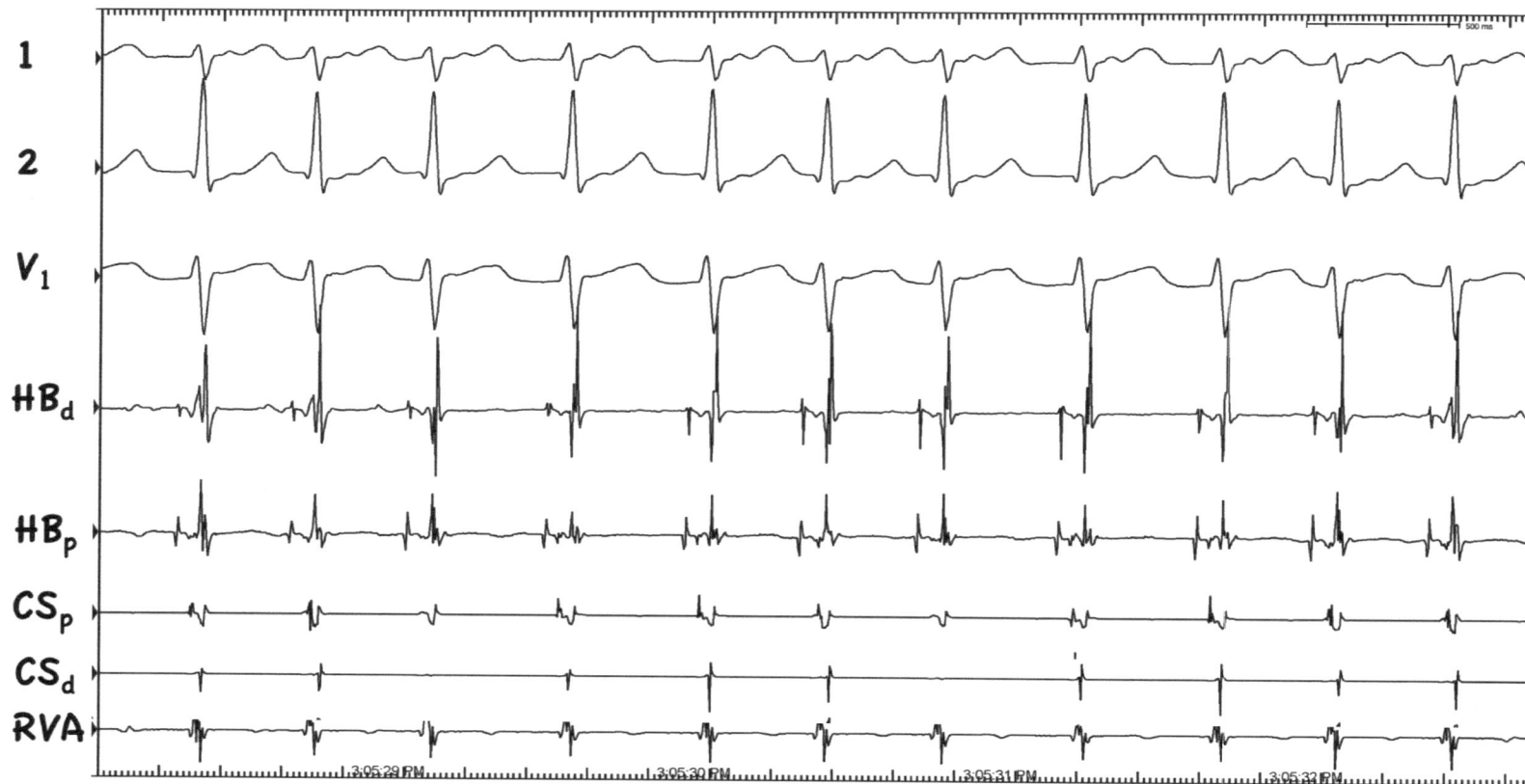

Problem 2.5

The patient whose ECG is shown was also referred for management of atrial fibrillation (AF) (**Figure 2.5A**). One can see why, as there are 3 or 4 distinct CL with the occasional wide complex beat thrown in. Nonetheless, readily identifiable P waves are evident in V_1.

Figure 2.5A

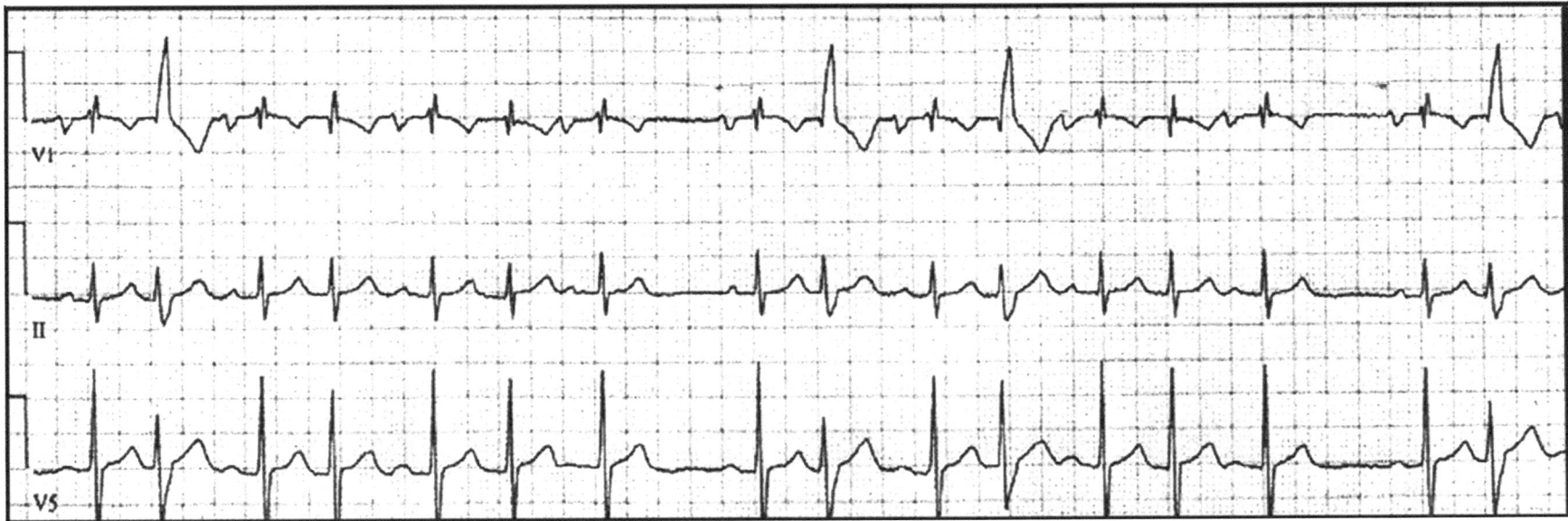

Identification of P waves is especially critical for this diagnosis. If one finds 2 consecutive P waves and marches the calipers through them (**Figure 2.5B, blue arrows**), it becomes readily apparent that:

1. The atrial rhythm is regular in spite of the ventricular response.
2. Many P waves are associated with 2 ventricular responses (**red dashed lines**) and some with only one.

This is quite typical of non–reentrant AVN tachycardia with anterograde conduction during sinus rhythm occurring potentially over a slow pathway (SP) or fast pathway (FP), both a SP and FP, or neither (i.e., blocked). This can readily mimic AF, especially when atrial activity is not as clear as it is in **Figure 2.5A**. In fact, all the "Irregular SVTs" may be "AF mimickers" (see "Supraventricular Tachycardia (AF Mimickers)" in Chapter 8).

Figure 2.5B

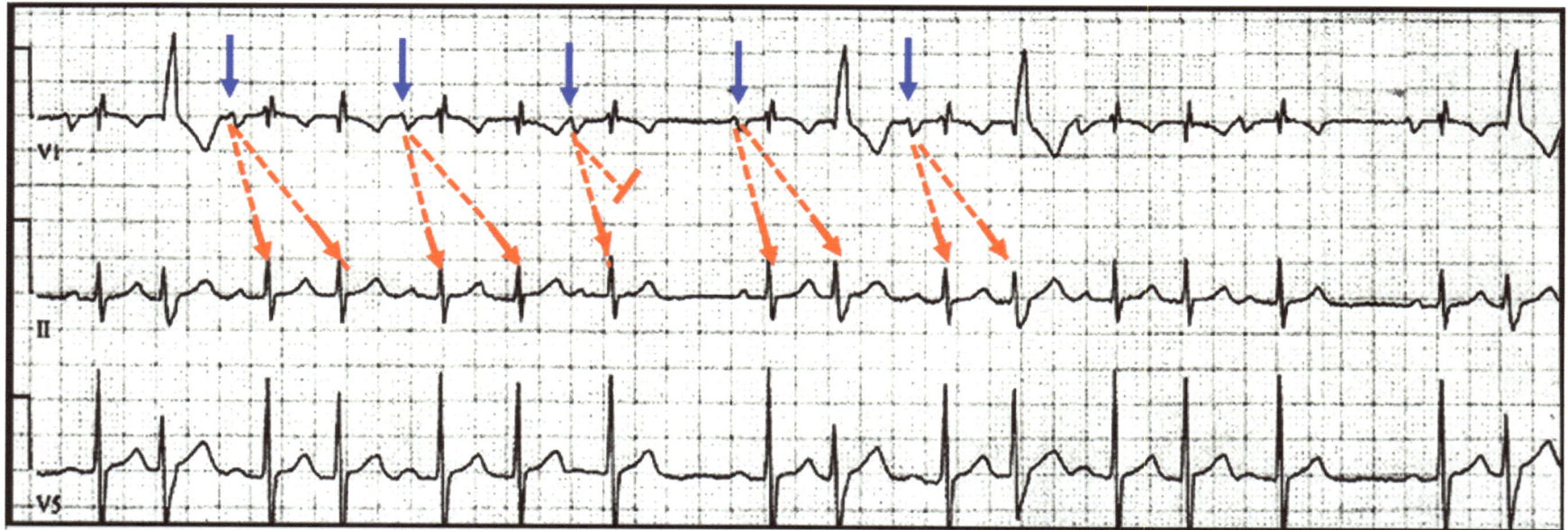

Figure 2.5C is from another individual but shows a slightly different twist on this where conduction occurs over the SP for several sinus beats after a brief atrial pacing burst initially and ends by several cycles with 2-for-1 conduction. All the while, regular sinus rhythm is present.

Of course, an alternate diagnosis of frequent junctional extrasystoles always comes in as when "2-for-1" rhythms are observed. The latter would likely be rare with a presentation like **Figure 2.5A**, but the only "definitive" exclusion of junctional extrasystoles is cure of tachycardia with SP ablation.

Figure 2.5C

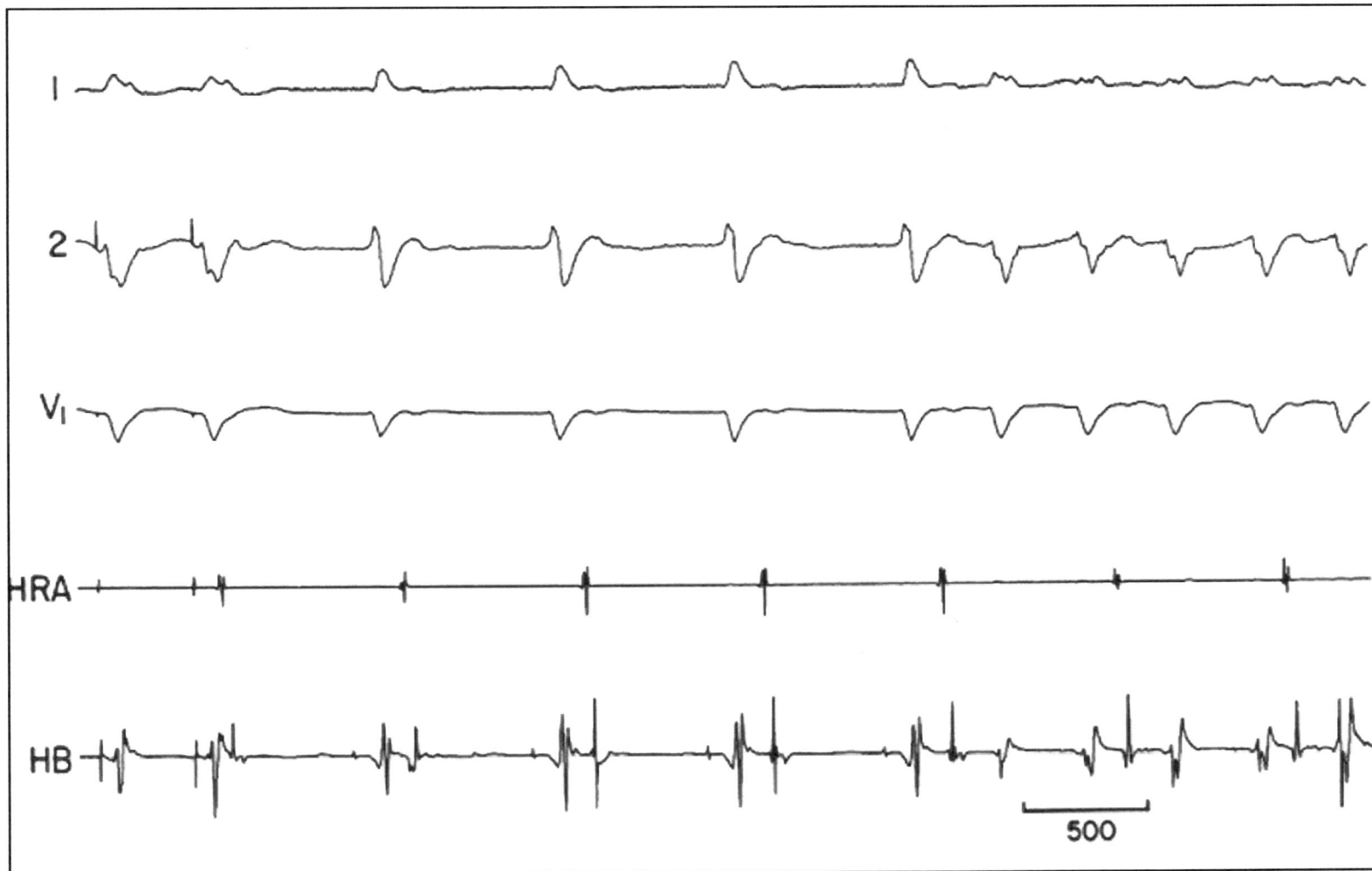

As a final note, one might ask why these patients do not have AVN reentry when dual anterograde AVN pathways are present and SP conduction occurs. Of course, one needs to complete the retrograde limb of the circuit for AVNRT to occur. Thus, one would expect that retrograde conduction does not permit AVNRT in most of these patients, or possibly the electrical connection between the anterograde slow and retrograde fast AVN pathway is deficient or absent.

Problem 2.6

The patient whose ECG is shown (**Figure 2.6A**) was also initially diagnosed with AF.

It is certainly a supraventricular rhythm without obvious atrial activity and seems irregular on overview.

Figure 2.6A

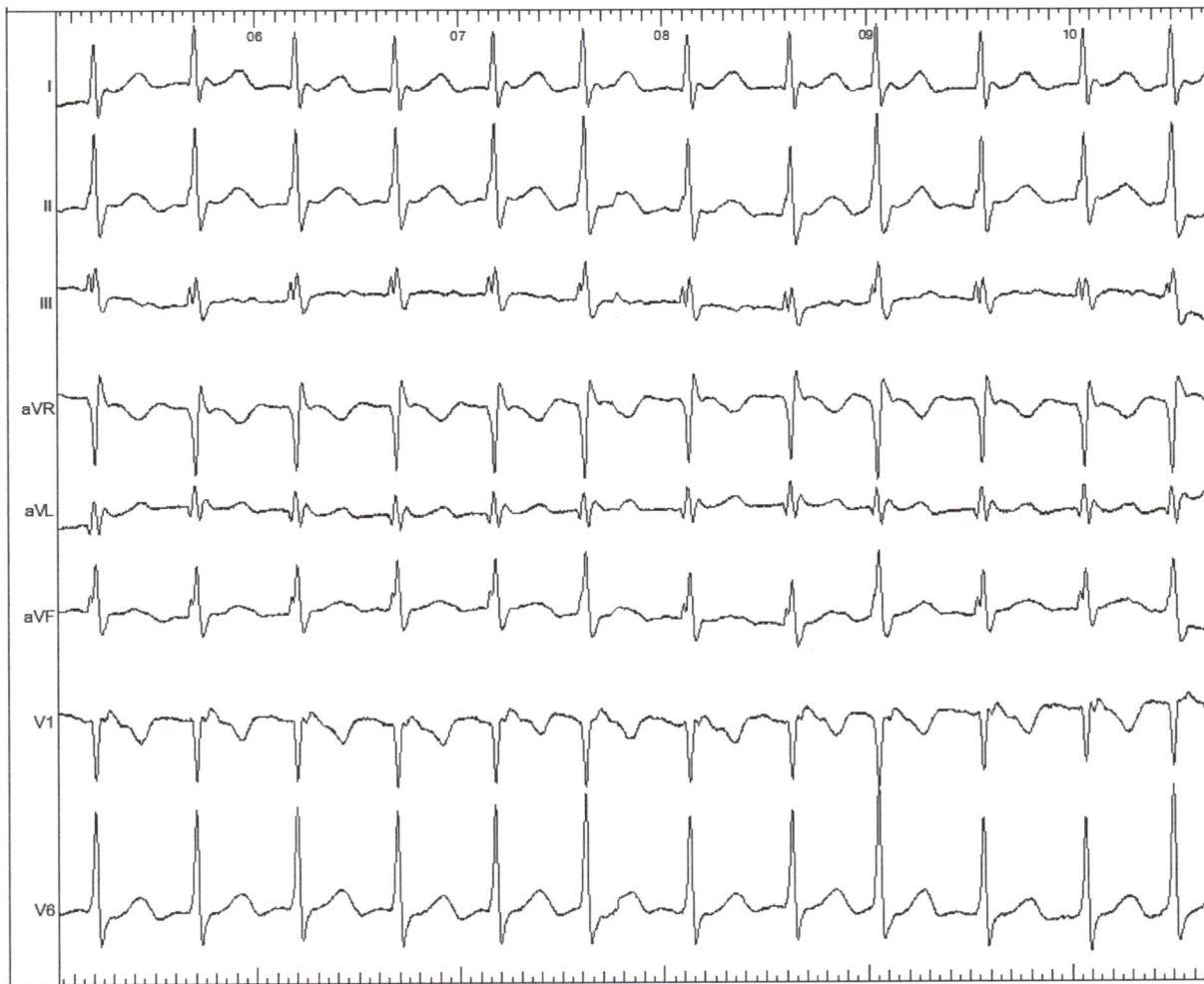

It is time to bring out the calipers and make some measurements (**Figure 2.6B**). When this is done, it is clear that it is *relatively irregular but with dominant cycle lengths* and obviously not AF. Rather, it also falls into the category of what can be called an "irregular SVT," whose differential diagnosis is found in "Irregular Supraventricular Tachycardia (AF Mimickers)" in Chapter 8 and also discussed in Problems 2.5 and 3.5.

Figure 2.6B

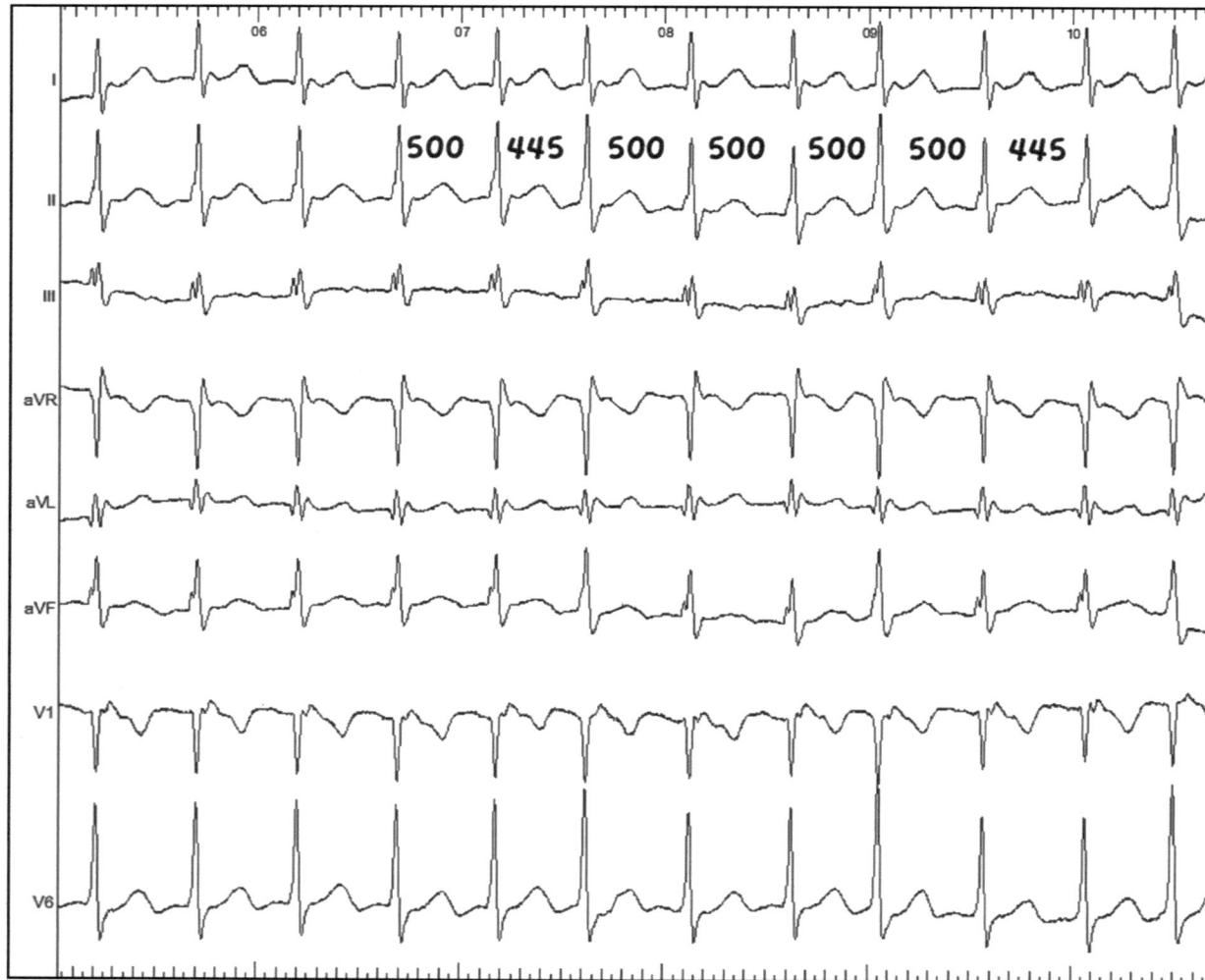

The definitive diagnosis awaits the intracardiac recordings, **Figure 2.6C**. This tracing readily reveals a very short RP ("P on QRS") interval that is fixed while the AH interval varies with 2 distinct AH times. Since a change in the AH interval predicts the arrival of the subsequent A (AA interval), *the AVN must be part of the circuit*, excluding AT. The very short VA interval (approximately 0) excludes AVRT. This leaves AVNRT (over 2 slow pathways anterogradely) as the most probable diagnosis. NVRT is not ruled out but much less likely statistically.

Figure 2.6C

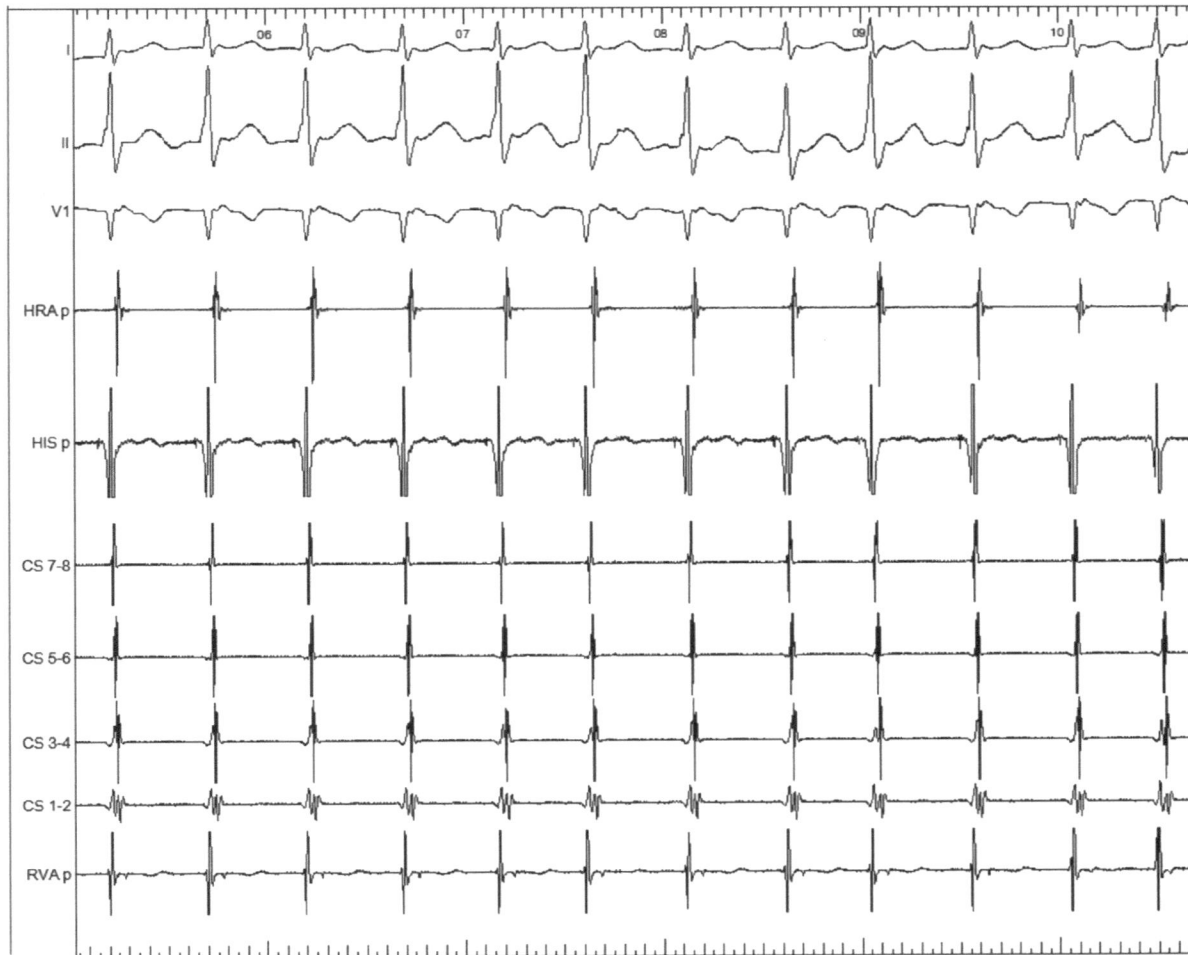

The interesting element in this scenario comes from the observation of reproducible spontaneous termination with PVCs as shown in **Figure 2.6D**.

I leave you to make the measurements yourself. You will observe that the PVC terminating the tachycardia is relatively late-coupled, perhaps premature by 70 ms if the last destined QRS pre-empted by the PVC is destined to come in at CL 445 ms (115 ms if the last destined QRS is to come in at 500 ms). This is arguably "His refractory" and does not advance the next A. If we accept this, the PVC must reach the AVN via a NV connection that has good access to the circuit, although it is not necessarily part of the circuit.

If there is a NV pathway, the SVT may be NVRT (rather than AVNRT with a bystander pathway), but the A is "on time" rather than being advanced with the PVC, which one might expect with NV reentry. It may not be advanced with AVNRT if the PVC gets there when the AVN circuit is underway and makes it to the retrograde limb first while the PVC is entering the anterograde limb.

All of the above may be a little speculative (and a little tangential to the main teaching point of this problem). What is relatively clear is that termination of SVT by a late-coupled PVC would be very unusual in AVNRT, and there is something very suspicious about such a PVC terminating garden-variety AVNRT.

Figure 2.6D

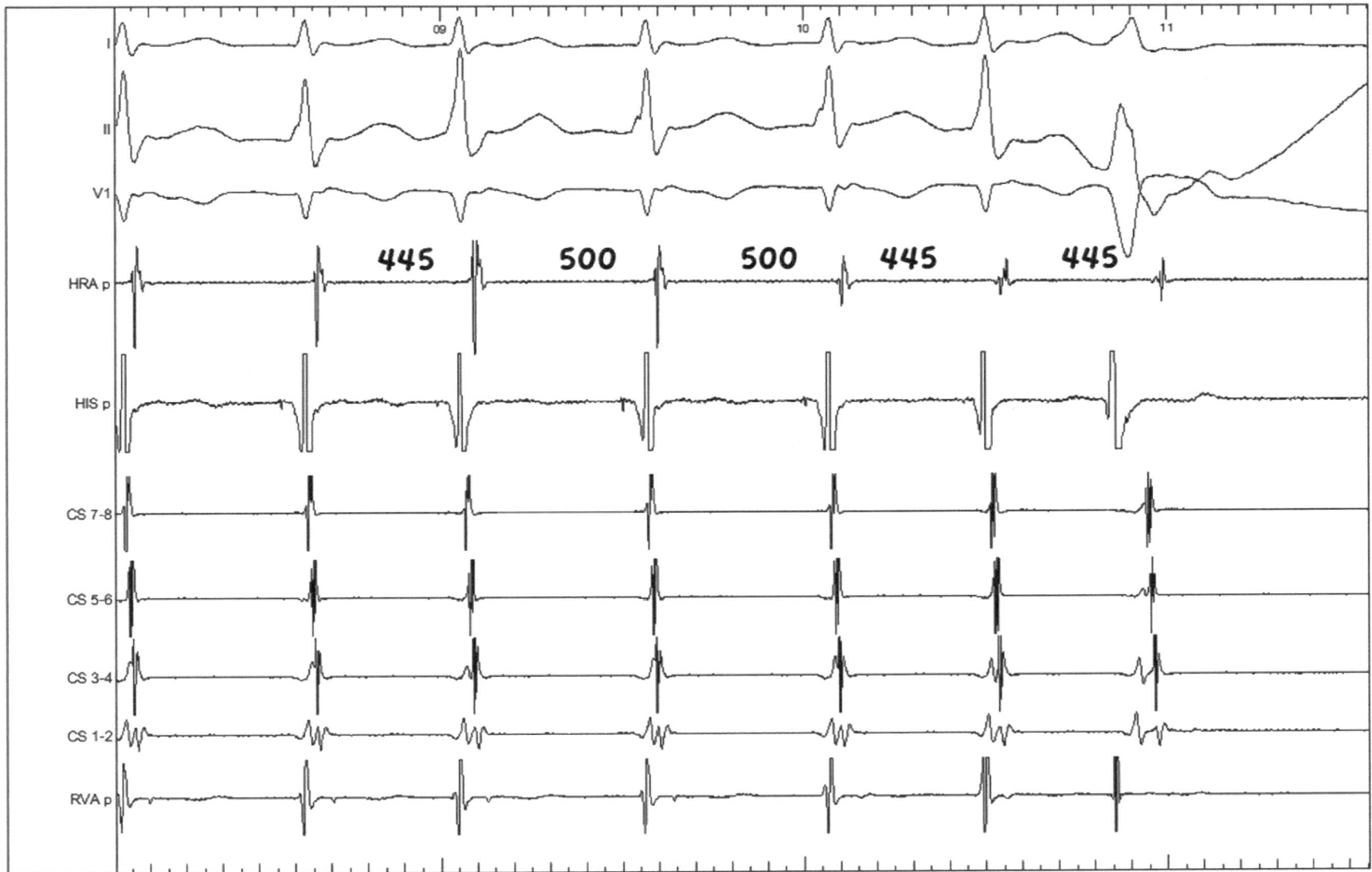

Problem 2.7

The overview of **Figure 2.7A** shows a regular WCT with a PVC introduced into the cardiac cycle. Focus initially on the zone *away* from the PVC initially before moving on to how the PVC affects WCT.

Figure 2.7A

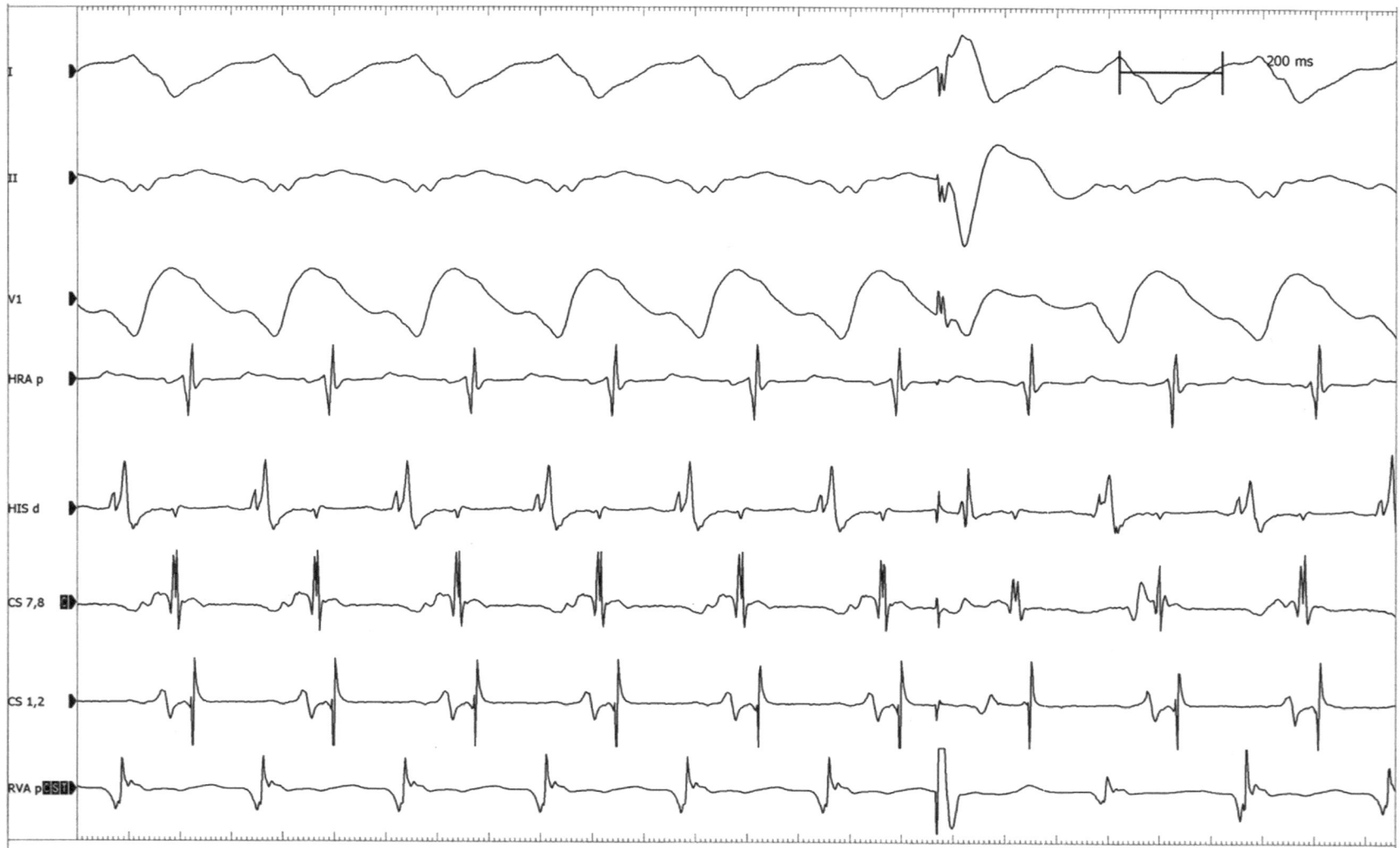

With the annotated **Figure 2.7B**, we start by focusing on the zone prior to the PVC. We run our calipers through the tracing and note that it is regular at approximately 272 ms. The QRS morphology is LBBB type (**QS in lead V₁**) and even with the limited leads available, it would be considered "atypical" for LBBB aberrancy and more likely to be VT or preexcited.

Figure 2.7B

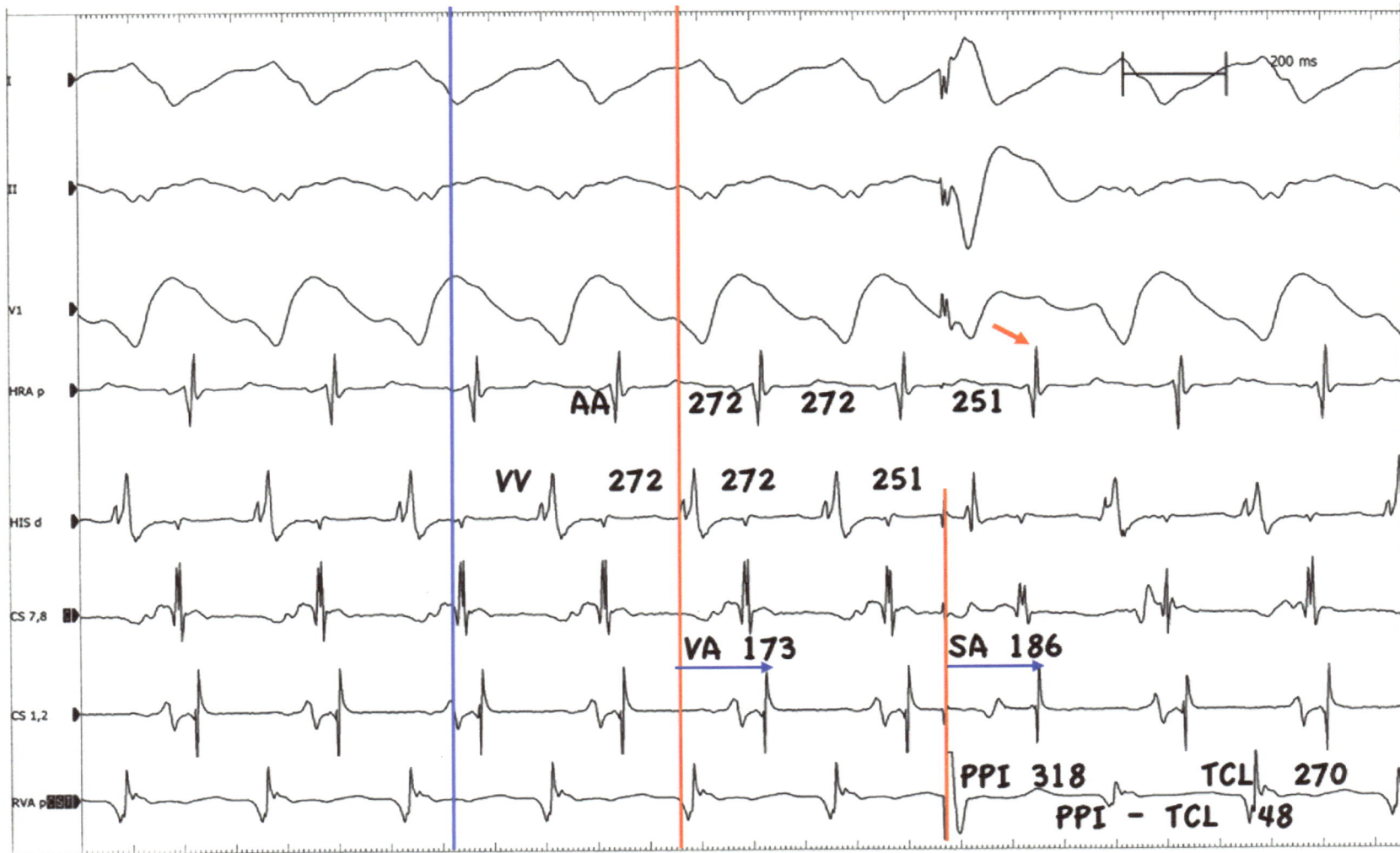

There is a 1-to-1 relationship between atrial and ventricular activation and, of course, we don't know at this point which is driving which. We note that atrial activation is "septal" (**earliest at orifice of CS and slightly later at HB site, blue line**).

We are able to obtain an approximation of ventricular activation from 4 sites, the RV apex, the HB region, and basal LV as indicated by the far-field V EGMs at the proximal and distal CS (**red line at earliest recordable ventricular activation**).

The His is not apparent, either because it is obscured within the QRS or because the catheter is out of position.

At this point, we can start "testing" our hypotheses with the information we have. I find it useful to consider one hypothesis at a time to temporarily reduce the traffic to my brain.

How well do our data fit with LBBB aberrancy? With LBBB, earliest ventricular activation would be expected at the RV apical EGM, since that is the nearest electrode to the exit from the RBBB. In this tracing, the earliest ventricular activation occurs at the HB EGM, which is at the base of the heart. *This is a key observation and rules out LBBB aberrancy, leaving only preexcited tachycardia or VT.* It also rules out BBR, which should have similar activation to LBBB aberrancy.

Thus, we have narrowed our list to two possibilities, namely VT (but not BBR) or preexcited tachycardia and can turn our attention to the PVC.

In broad terms, we have a RV PVC that is only 20 ms premature and so must be "fused" with the WC beat it advances. Yet, this late-coupled PVC advances the next A and also the next QRS associated with this advanced A—that is, it "resets" the WCT. This RV PVC must have extremely close access to the arrhythmia circuit and hence we must be dealing with an arrhythmia where the *RV is part of the circuit.* This is verified when we measure the PPI after the PVC (remember that advancing the cycle with a single, fused PVC is in essence entrainment for 1 beat). The PPI–TCL is only 48 ms. In addition, we note that the St-A–VA is only 13 ms, indicating that the pacing site is very close to the circuit, i.e., has the same distance to go to the A as the tachycardia beat.

The combination of "fusion" and "reset" is also the hallmark of macroreentry (see "Concept of Reset and Fusion" in Chapter 8). We are now dealing with a large, reentrant circuit where the RV is part of the circuit. This, of course, rules out AT and AVNRT. It leaves us with only 2 viable hypotheses, namely a macroreentrant RV VT (recall that we ruled out BBR) or AVRT. The AVRT would be preexcited, of course, and the most common preexcited AVRT with a 1-to-1 AV relationship is antidromic AVRT (anterogradely over the AP, return via the normal AVCS, the latter fitting with the septal atrial activation sequence in this tracing). The A follows the premature V and the next V follows with the same AV interval as the subsequent WCT, suggestive of a linking of the A to the next V. This is most plausible with antidromic tachycardia. In truth, one has not entirely ruled out macroreentrant RV VT with passive VA conduction following along in proportion to the V prematurity, with the next AV interval being fortuitously the same as the subsequent ones. However, this was in fact antidromic AVRT. The concept of "reset and fusion" is depicted graphically in **Figure 8.1A** in Chapter 8.

Chapter 3

The Power of Calipers, Measurement, and Magnification

Problem 3.1

This patient had recurrent PSVT and was referred to us with a preliminary diagnosis of "long RP" tachycardia (**Figure 3.1A**). It is not a complicated tracing, but I show it early in the book to highlight the utility of 2 useful "tools" I use after scanning any complicated tracing, especially an ECG where the search for the P wave is a critical part of the exercise.

Figure 3.1A

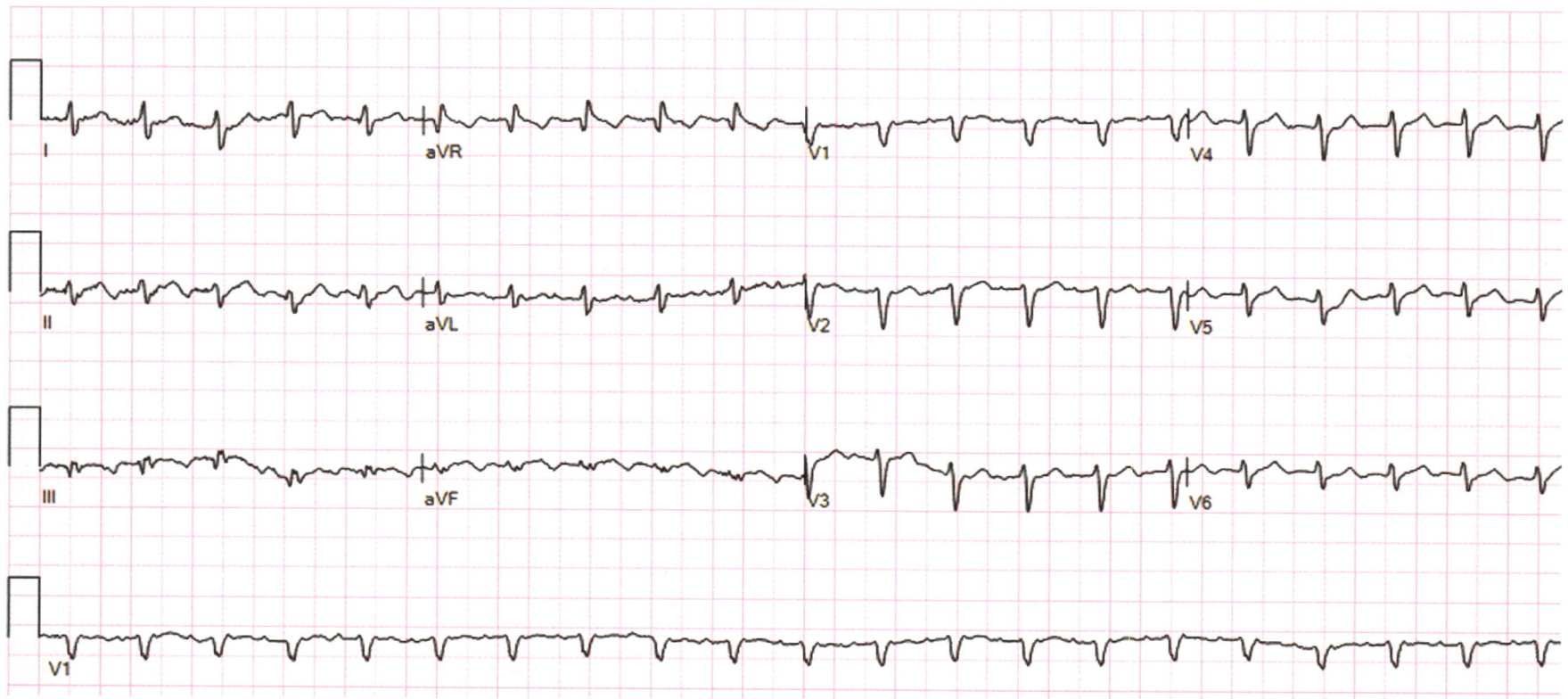

Our overview shows a narrow QRS with a 1-to-1 AV relationship. The P wave is in the latter half of diastole but almost mid-diastolic. It is negative in the inferior leads, clearly not "sinus" tachycardia.

At this point, we need to *enlarge* part of the tracing and have a closer look for detail (**Figure 3.1B**).

I have chosen V_1 since the P wave, although small, is clearly defined. I think of this as "moving to higher magnification" after I have had an overview. When you do this, you will more readily notice a slight notch at the end of the QRS (**blue arrows, Figure 3.1C**), raising the suspicion of a second P wave after the QRS.

Figure 3.1B

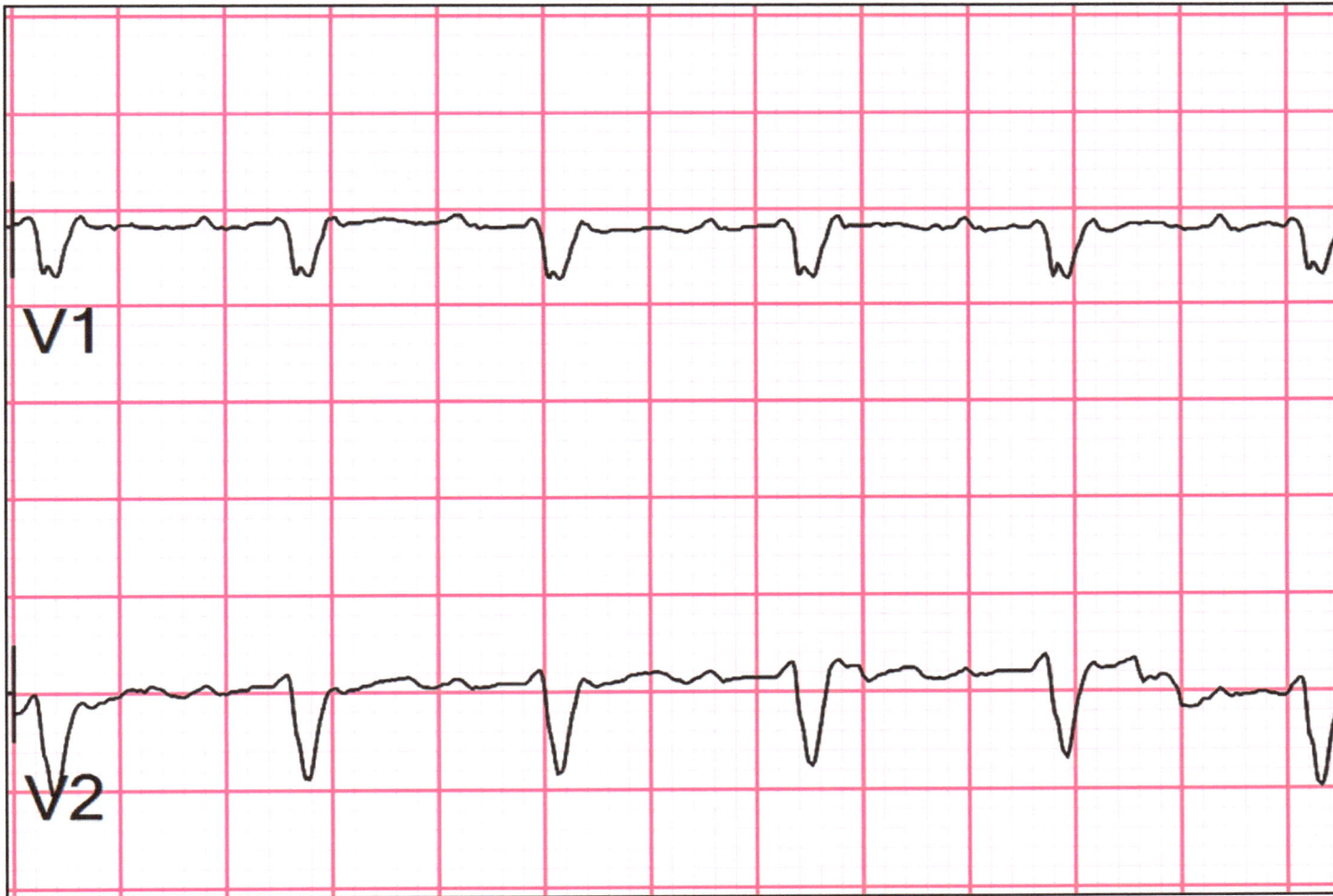

Figure 3.1C

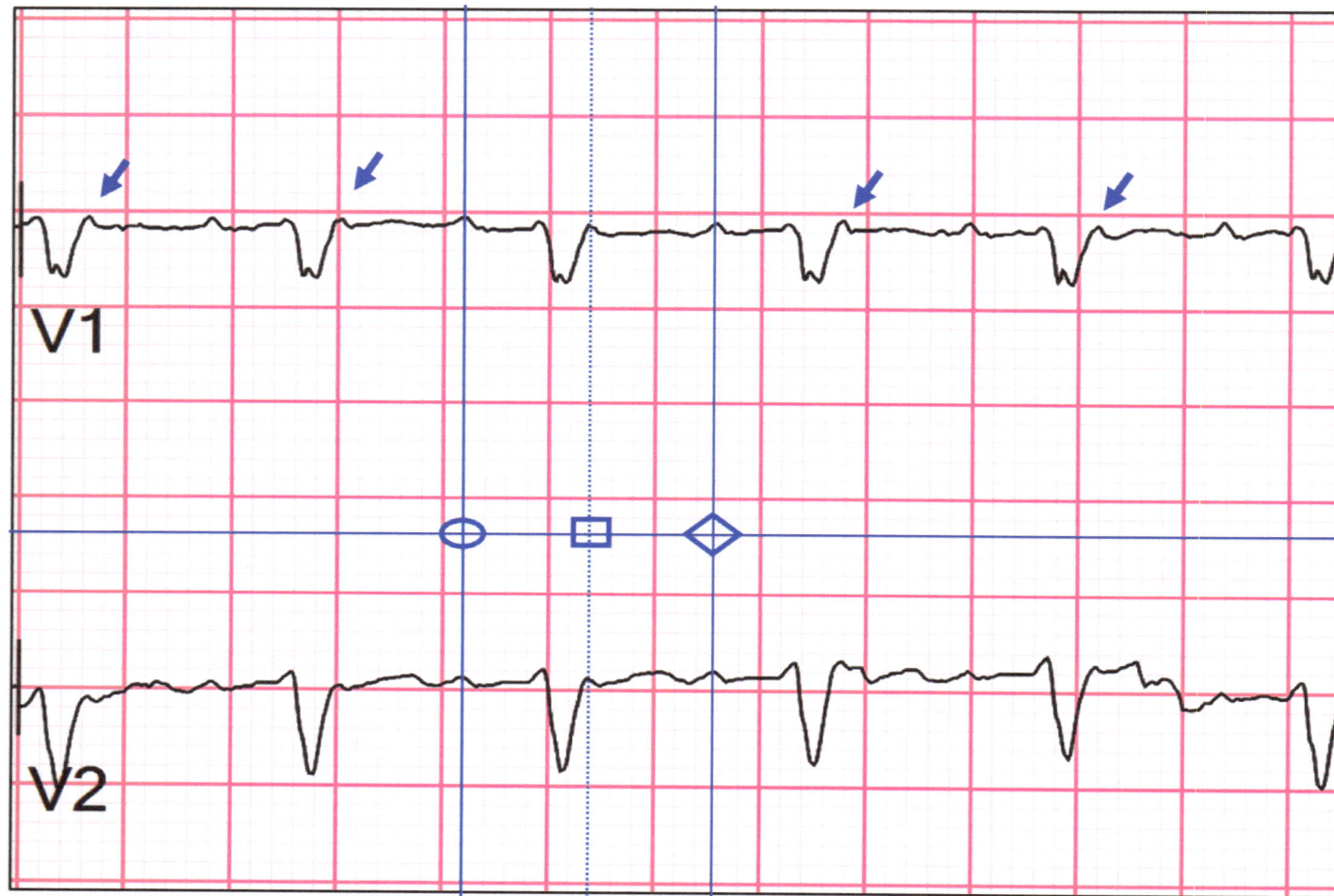

The second step is to start your caliper program and place the outer edges on 2 consecutive P waves. A very useful one is available on the Internet, known as PixelStick★ provides 3 lines, equally spaced (**blue lines** in **Figure 3.1C**).

Once you have positioned the outer lines on 2 consecutive P waves, the middle line shows the midpoint between the 2 P waves, effectively "pointing" to a hiding P wave between the 2 obvious ones. When you do this, the middle line shows the suspect P wave to be perfectly aligned and matching the outer,

★ PixelStick has no financial connection to me.

clearly seen P waves. It is now relatively obvious that there is a second P wave sitting at the end of the QRS segment at the mid-point of the 2 obvious P waves, allowing you to diagnose AFl with reasonable certainty. The diagnosis is verified on a later tracing where a brief period of AV block exposes the flutter waves (**Figure 3.1D**).

It is always wise to have a high index of suspicion for a second, cryptic P wave in any tracing and "check the midpoint."

Figure 3.1D

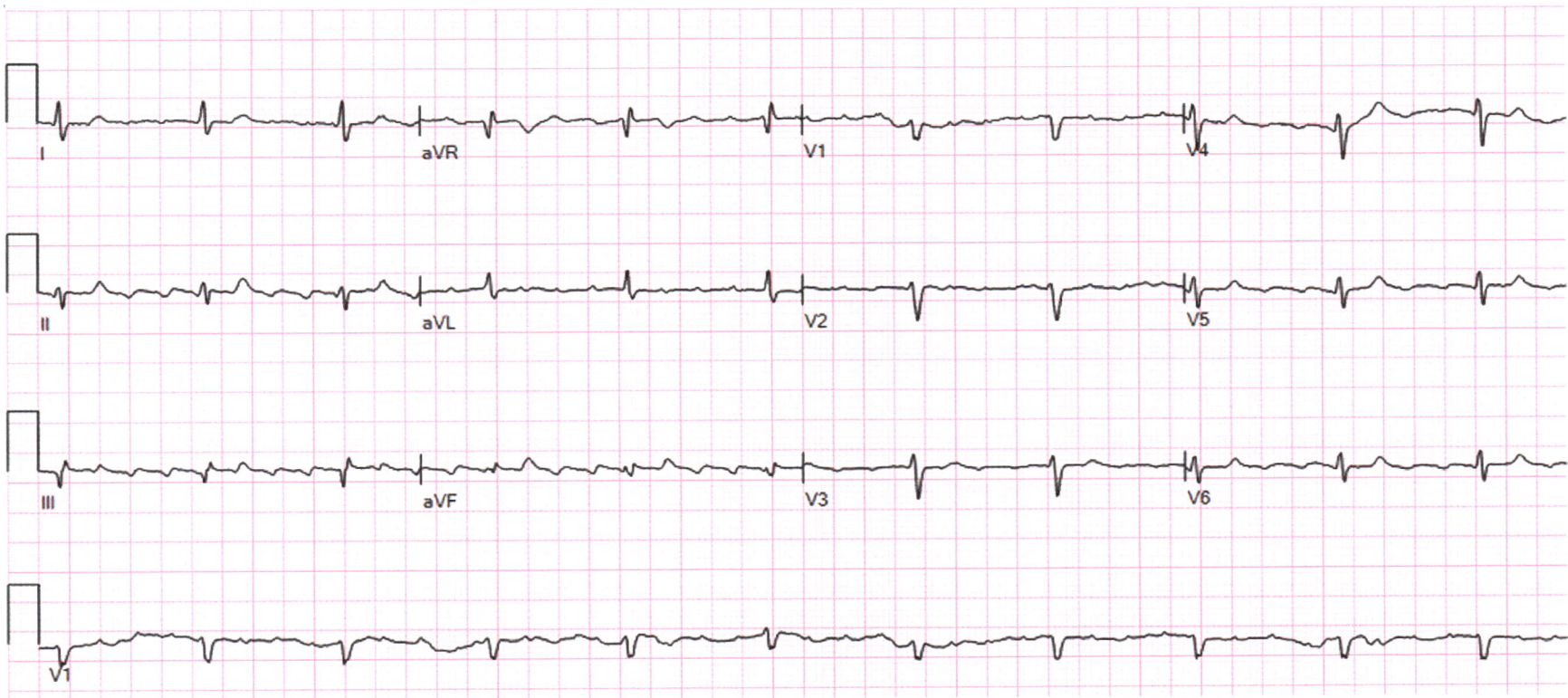

Problem 3.2

The tracing (**Figure 3.2A**) was recorded from a patient with recurrent SVT and a normal ECG during sinus rhythm.

An overview identifies 3 zones, namely before, during, and after the PVC.

Figure 3.2A

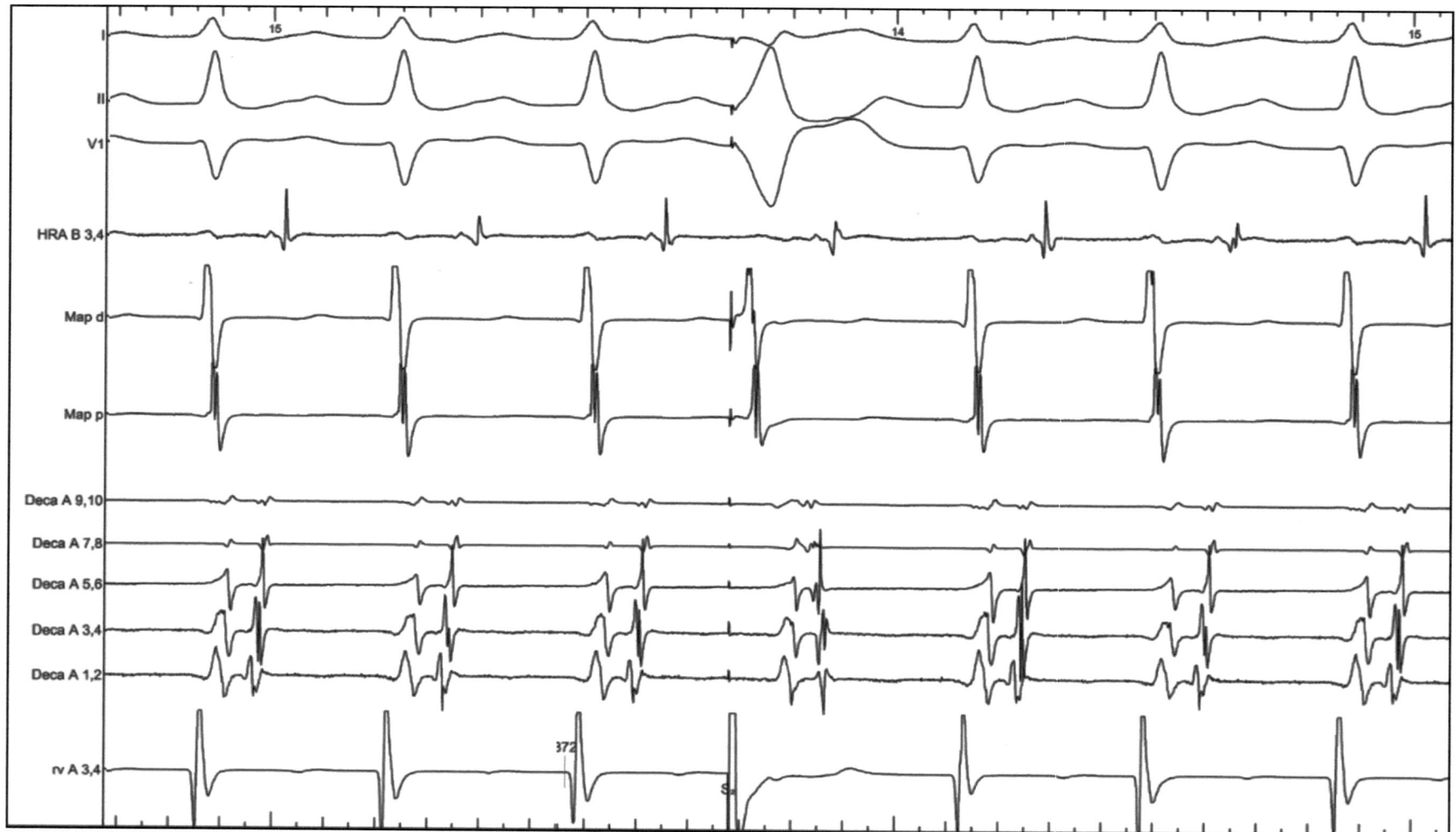

A scan through the recording with calipers (**Figure 3.2B**) shows that the SVT remains identical before and after the PVC with a CL of 350 ms. Focusing on the tachycardia, we note that the atrial activation is eccentric, i.e., distal CS (DecaA 12) atrial

EGM preceding the others. This can realistically only be AT or AVRT over a left pathway (discounting the rare eccentric atrial insertion site in AVNRT).

Figure 3.2B

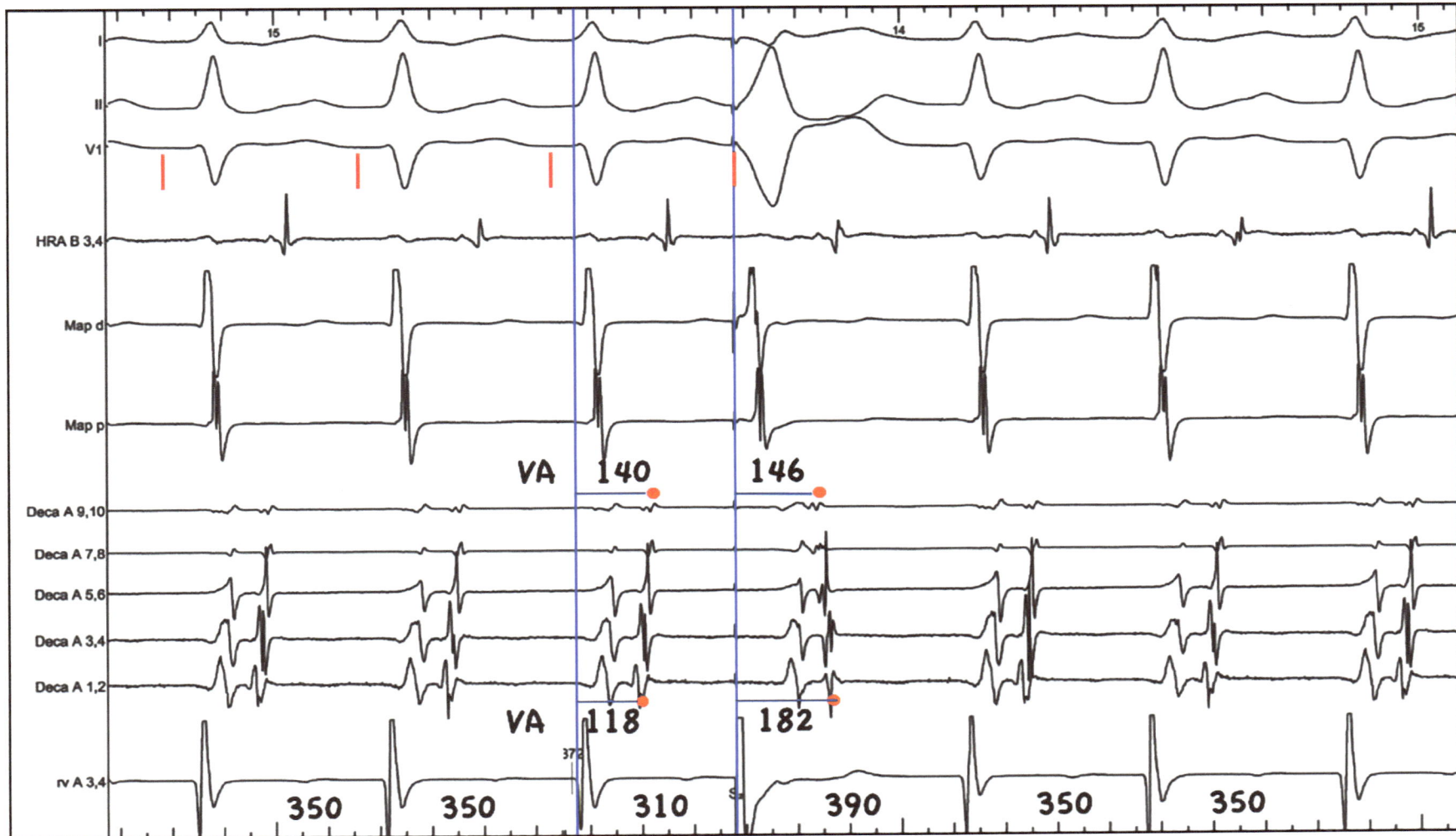

We move to the mid zone, the PVC, and note that the PVC did not reset or change the timing of the first QRS after the PVC. We note that there is no recorded His EGM but will estimate it to be approximately 50 ms prior to QRS onset (**red lines**). The PVC is rather late coupled (only 40 ms premature) and clearly "His refractory" (i.e., the QRS is a fusion of the PVC and the normal beat). This His refractory PVC clearly advanced the atrial activation, confirming the presence of an AP. The atrial activation sequence immediately after the fused beat has clearly changed. Running the calipers, one may note that the major shortening of the AA interval occurs at the proximal CS (Deca A 9-10), while the distal CS AA moves quite fractionally. That is, the atrium at the proximal CS is more preexcited by our RV PVC than at the distal CS.

How do we interpret this? Advancing the A during His refractoriness clearly confirms presence of an AP but not participation in SVT (although it almost universally is associated with participation of the AP as the retrograde limb of the circuit.) In this instance, the atrial activation indicates that it preexcited two AP, a left lateral and another more central, perhaps posteroseptal. The RV pacing catheter was closer to the atrial end of the posteroseptal circuit, resulting in more advancement at this site, with less advancement of the left lateral AP, which was more distant from the RV pacing site (requiring transseptal conduction).

We can thus reasonably hypothesize that atrial activation during SVT is a fusion of atrial conduction over a left and posteroseptal or right paraseptal AP. This is represented pictorially in **Figure 3.2C**, which shows a "double loop" reentrant

tachycardia with the normal AVCS being the common slow conduction zone.

This patient required ablation of 2 AP as hypothesized, a left and a right paraseptal.

Figure 3.2C

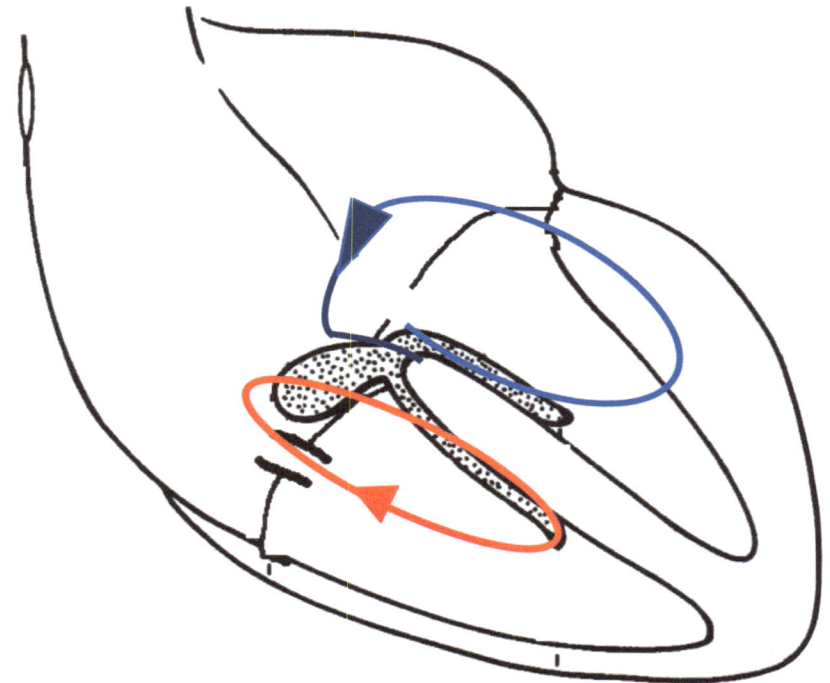

Problem 3.3

Figre 3.3A can be described as a WCT of relatively stable CL interrupted by a pause towards the end of the tracing with the emergence of arguably a supraventricular beat. One may reasonably assume a high probability that we are dealing with SVT.

Figure 3.3A

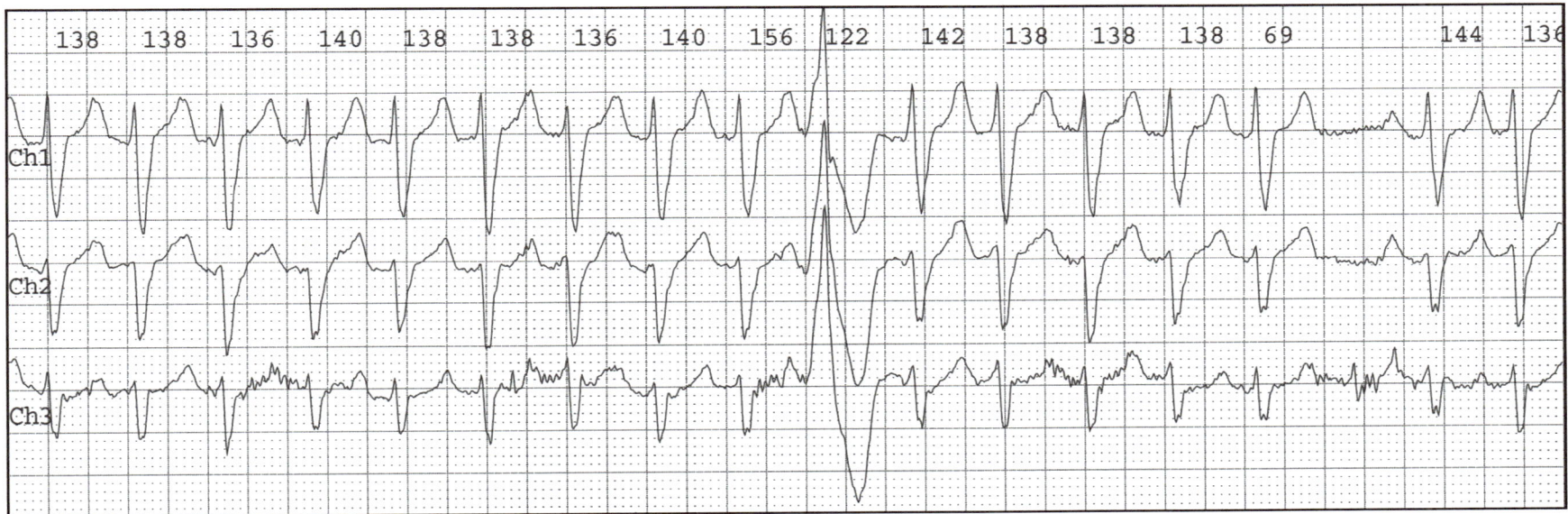

There are 2 obvious transition or zones where something is changing. The first is the PVC (**blue arrow** in **Figure 3.3B**). It is a PVC because there is no P wave preceding it. In addition, the basic supraventricular rhythm already has a bundle branch block morphology so that any beat *different* from that morphology is most likely ventricular.

Figure 3.3B

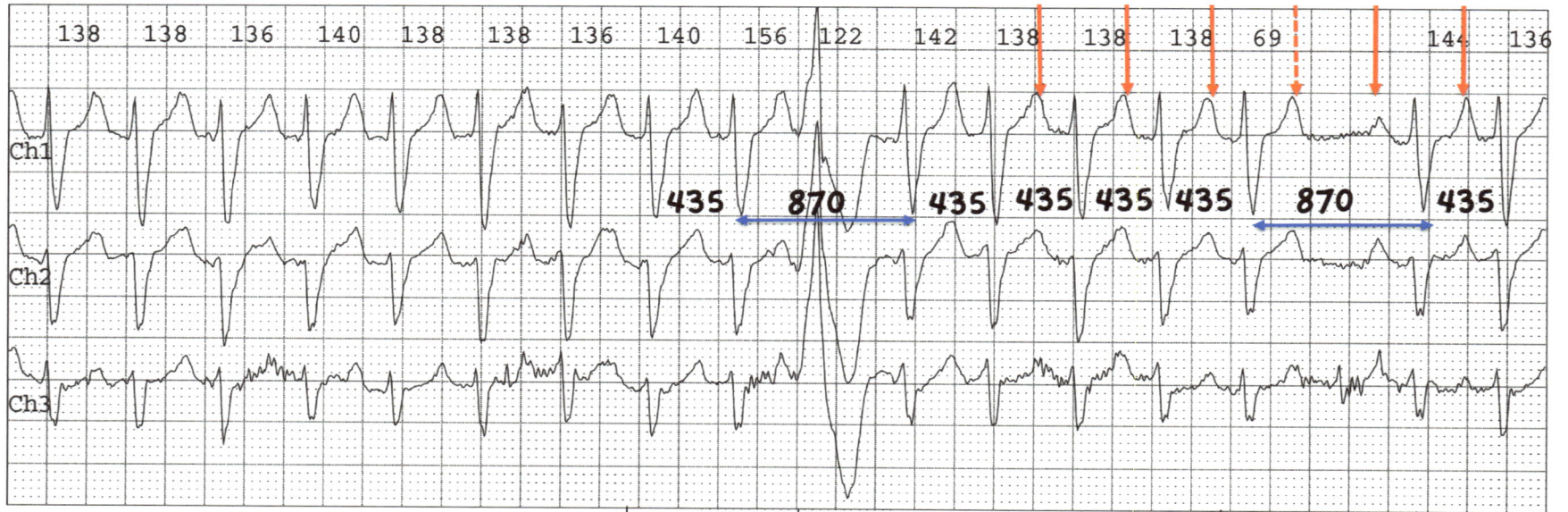

Measuring the intervals surrounding the PVC, we note that the PVC is straddled exactly by 2 CLs, i.e., there is no *reset* of the tachycardia. This is not terribly helpful in this instance. (The converse of course would be helpful, signifying that the PVC has good access to the mechanism or circuit, for example, a PVC from the LV would be more likely to reset a circuit using a left lateral pathway.)

Diverting to the pause at the end of the tracing, we set our calipers to one CL and place one point on the open P wave and "walk" the calipers before and after the pause (**red arrows**). The **dashed red arrow** is the presumed P wave that is blocked. This simple step "exposes" the P wave on top of the T wave (**the one after the first beat following the pause is more pointed**) and makes it clear that the P waves prior to the pause are also riding on the T waves. These are in effect slightly variable (**some more pointed**) with slight irregularity in the CL.

An AT has been reasonably exposed by merely setting up the calipers to one CL and "walking" through the tachycardia.

Problem 3.4

The ECG in **Figure 3.4A** was initially interpreted as AF, and it is not difficult to see why. I *routinely* "walk" my calipers through such a tracing from left to right, not trusting my ability to "eye-ball" the cadence of the rhythm. When I review the ECG using calipers (**Figure 3.4B**), it becomes immediately obvious that there is a recurrent pattern ("group beating") and recurring cycles. The rhythm is obviously not AF.

Figure 3.4A

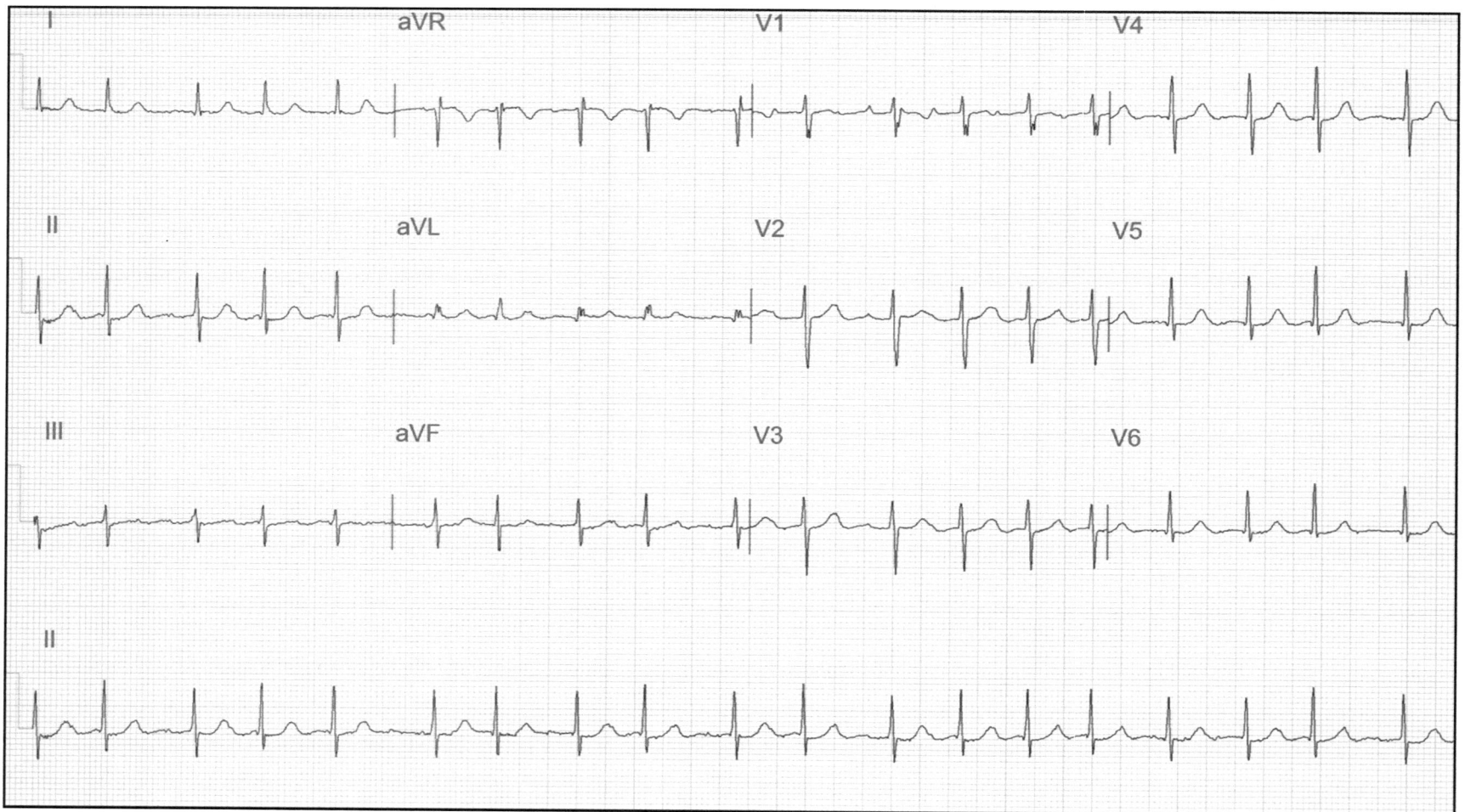

Figure 3.4B

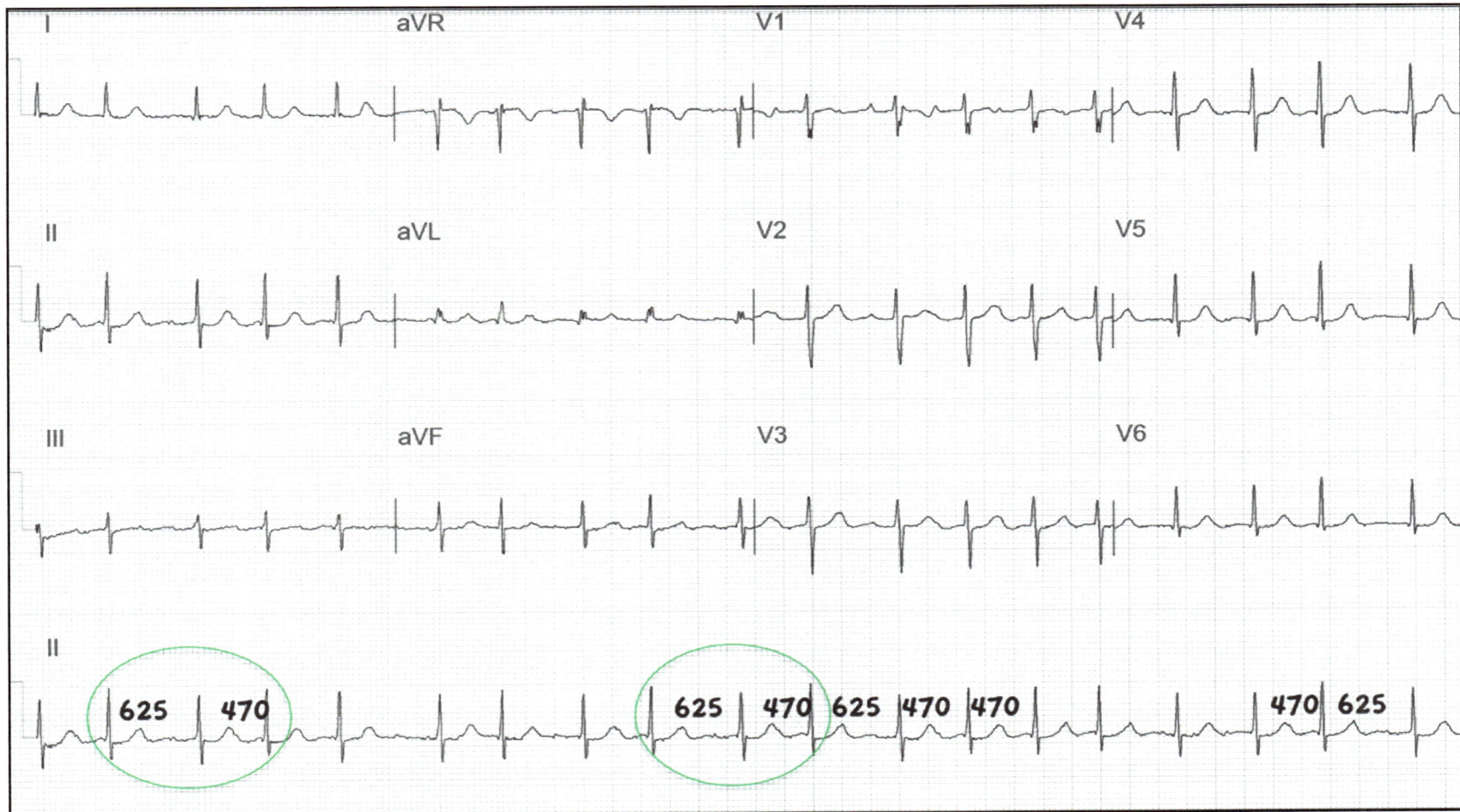

Our next task is to find P waves and V_1 in this tracing provides reasonable P-wave "candidates."

I will make life easier for myself by *enlarging* V_1 (**Figure 3.4C**).

Figue 3.4C

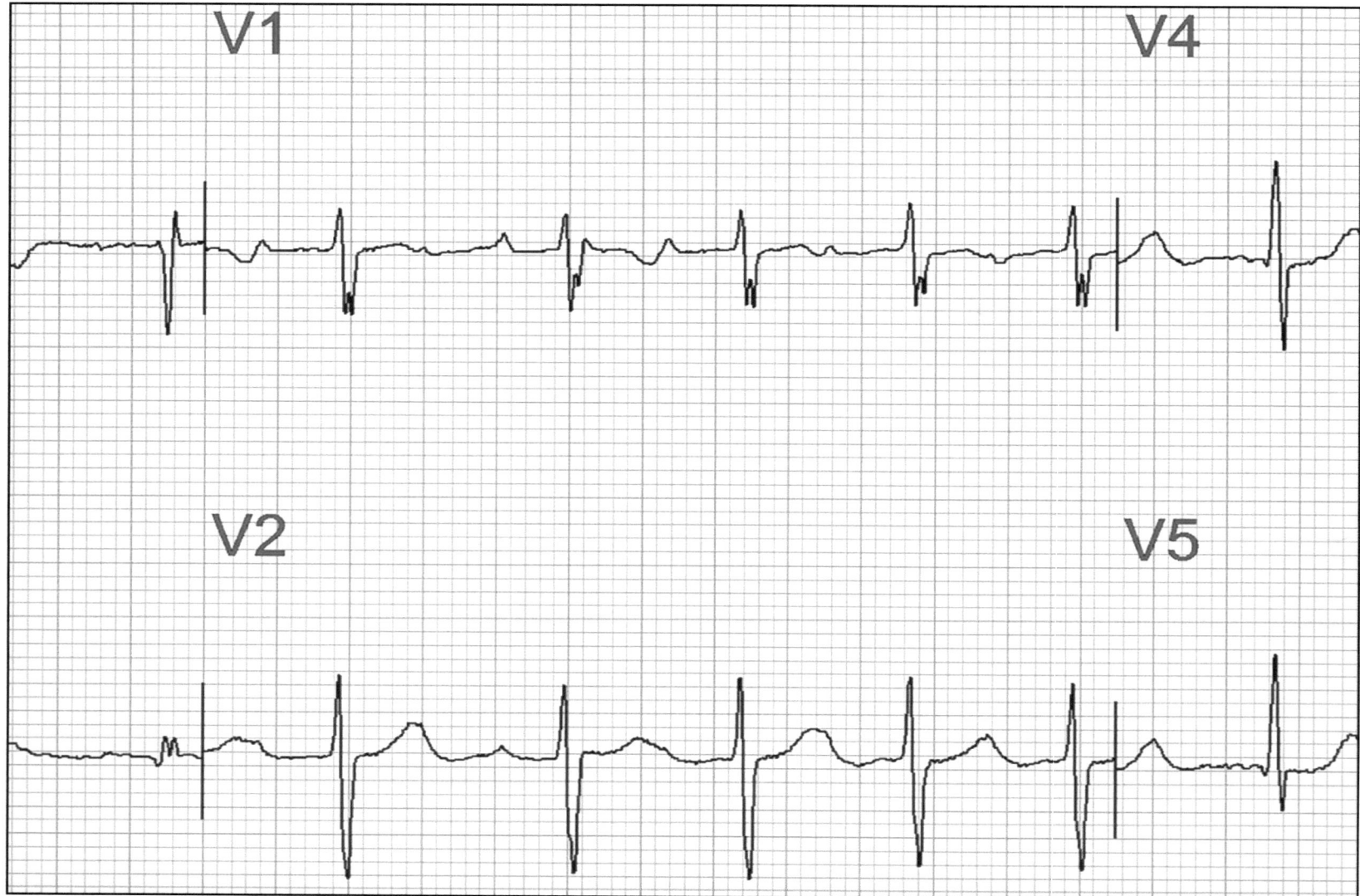

Again, I resist the impulse to just "eyeball" and bring out my electronic caliper with 3 lines (two at the ends and one in the middle: "PixelStick"). I place the ends of the calipers on the 2 closest P waves that I can reasonably identify. This is represented by **blue lines** in **Figure 3.4D**, **solid blue at the ends with the dashed blue in the middle**. This middle caliper now *"points"* to a deflection at the terminal part of the QRS that is undoubtedly a P wave. Note that this deflection is NOT there after the subsequent QRS. I now "walk" the calipers left and right and the AFl P waves now become obvious, even though fully or partially obscured by the QRS.

This is not a difficult tracing for an experienced electrocardiographer, but conscious use of a few simple "tools" should make it straightforward for everyone!

Figure 3.4D

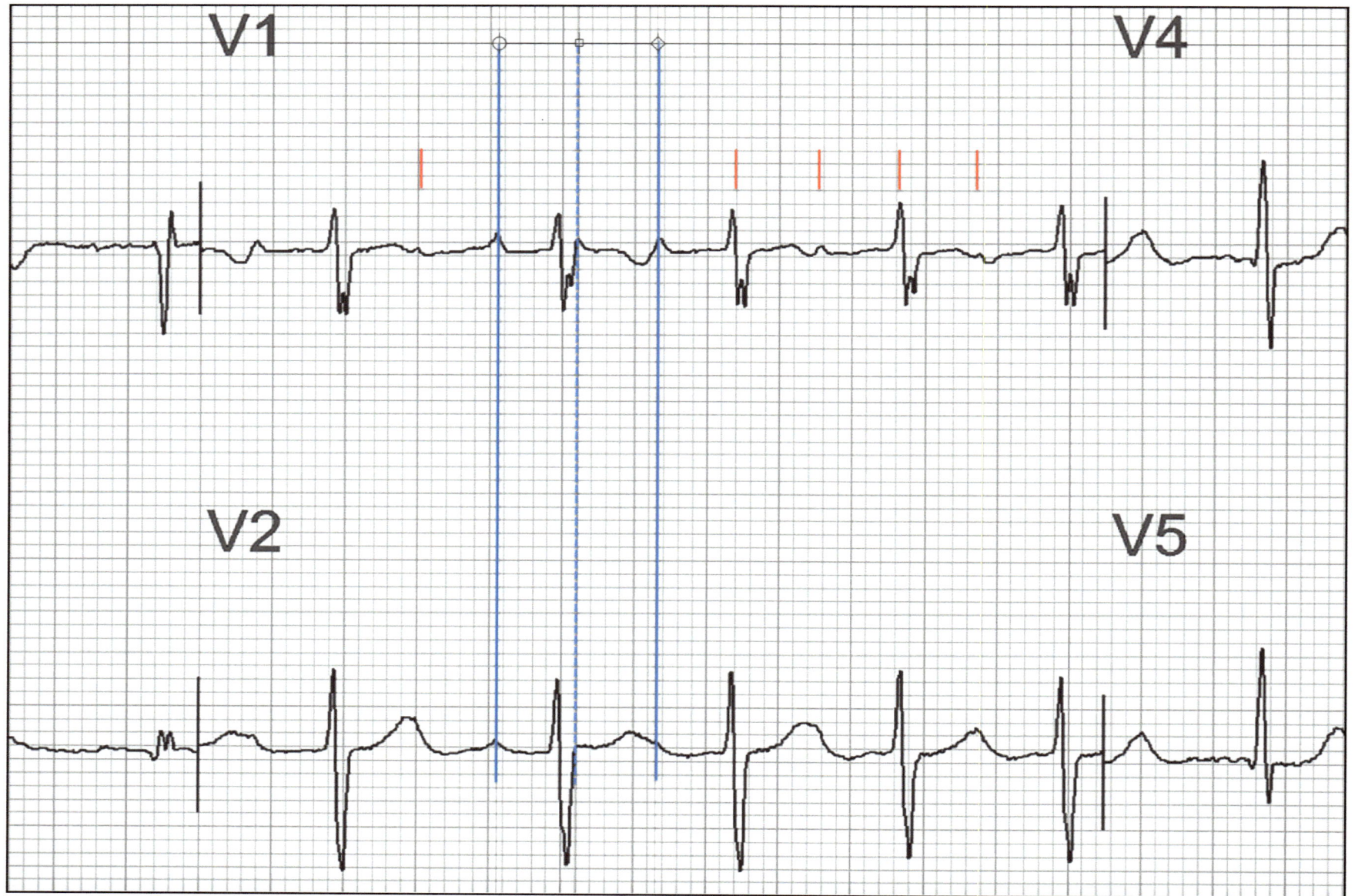

Problem 3.5

An overview of the tachycardia in **Figure 3.5A** suggests a narrow QRS tachycardia that is quite irregular. There are certain cycles that reappear periodically, so, allowing a bit of a stretch, it fits bet-ter within the category of "regularly irregular" (see "Irregular Supraventricular Tachycardia (AF Mimickers)" in Chapter 8). In addition, P waves are discernible with a low-to-high activation sequence and apparent variability of the PR interval.

Figure 3.5A

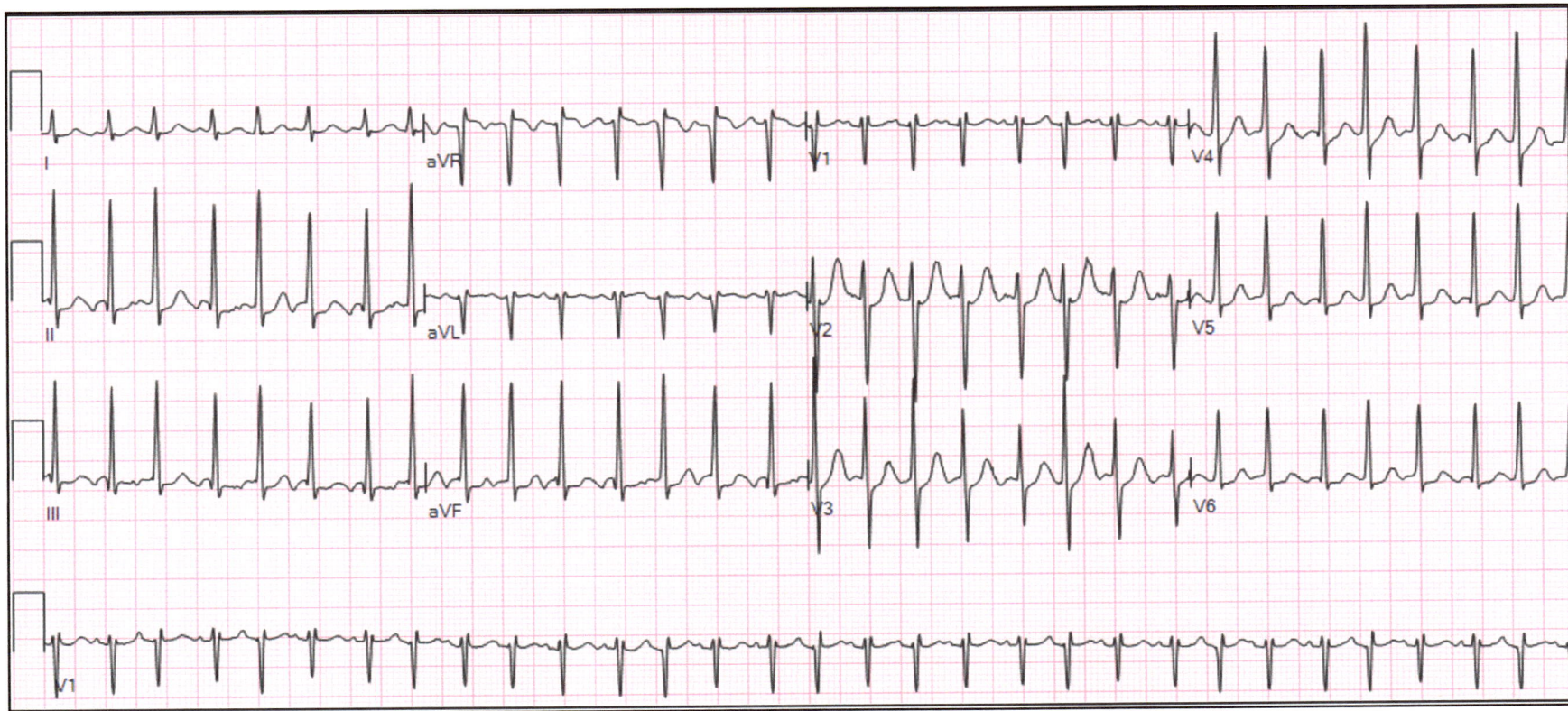

It is time to magnify a segment where the P wave is reasonably clearly identified (**Figure 3.5B**). This verifies the impression that there are 2 clusters of CL, one longer and one shorter. There is variability in both the PR and RP intervals. Going over our list of entities (see "Irregular Supraventricular Tachycardia (AF Mimickers)" in Chapter 8), the best fit is AVNRT.

Figure 3.5B

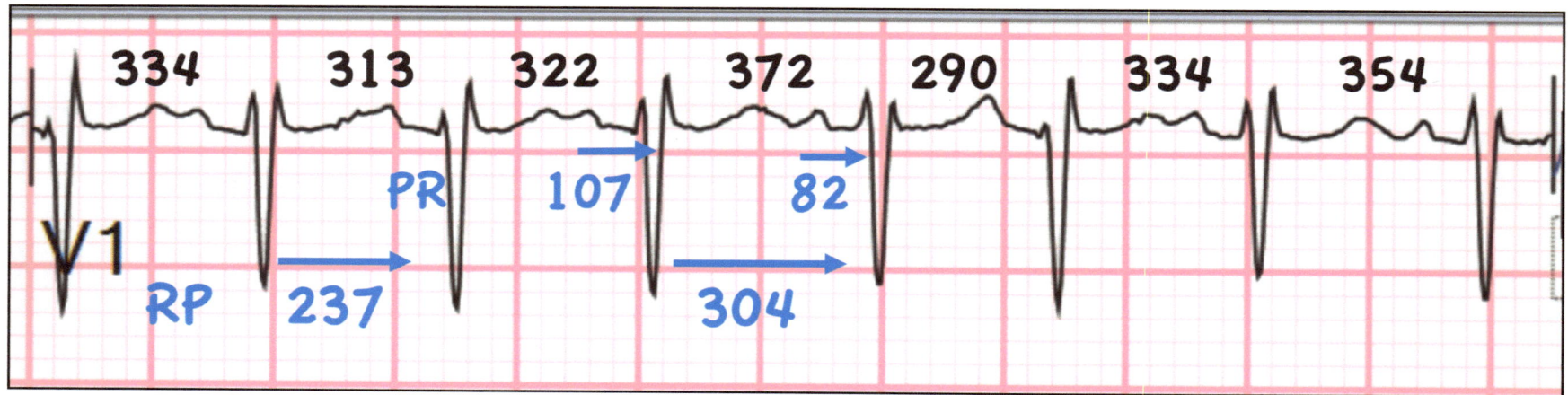

Moving to our intracardiac recording, we note that our key observations have already been made or strongly suspected from just the surface ECG. It is now easier to appreciate that the variability is related to irregularity in both the AV and VA intervals.

In my experience, variability if BOTH the PR and RP intervals has invariably led to a final diagnosis of AVNRT (atypical, of course), and slow pathway ablation in the "usual" area eliminated tachycardia in this instance.

Figure 3.5C

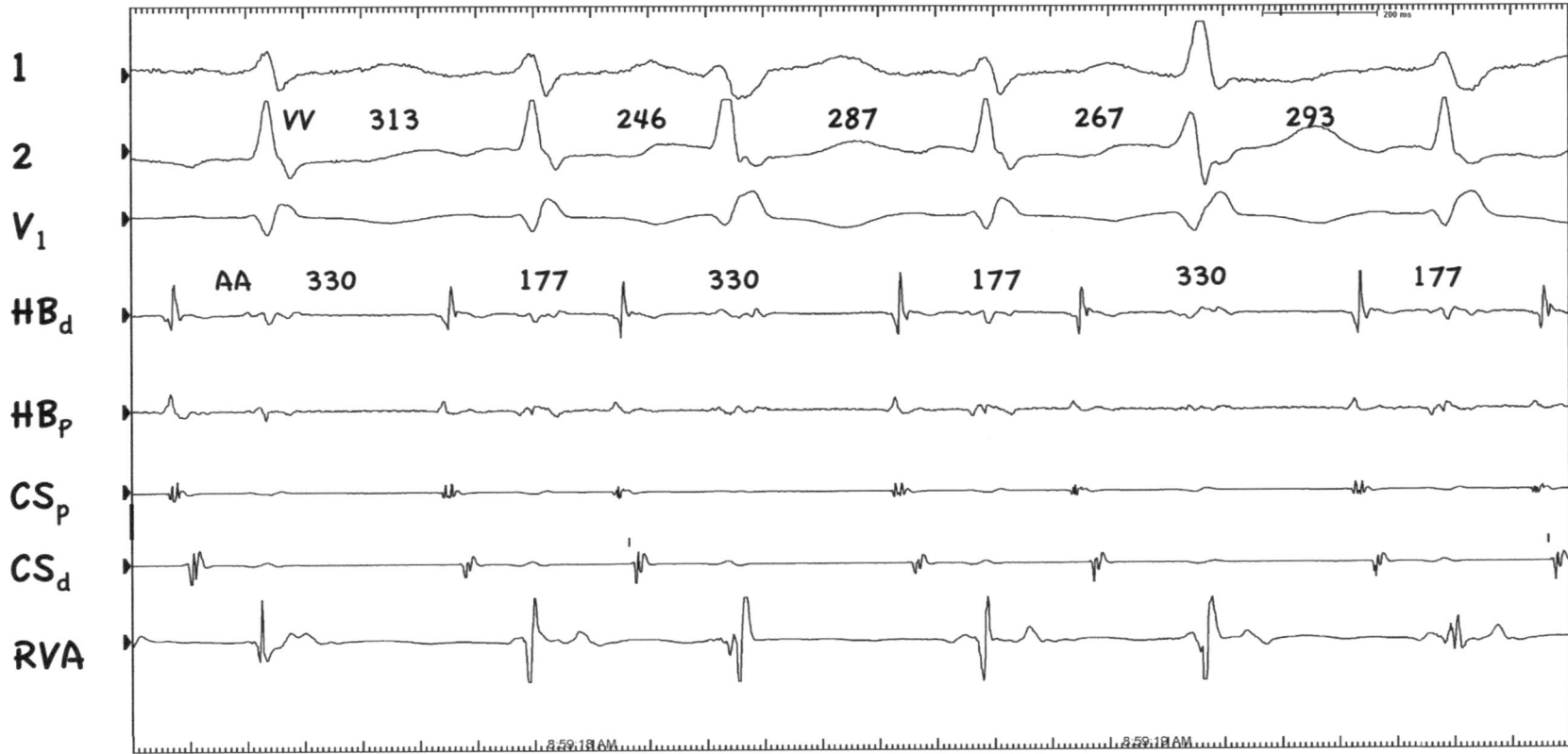

Problem 3.6

The "big picture" diagnosis of the tracing **Figure 3.6A** should not be difficult for most readers. We have a regular tachycardia, more WCT than narrow complex tachycardia (NCT), with intermittent interruption by normal QRS complexes with left axis deviation preceded by a plausible P wave. The tachycardia is thus AV dissociated with "capture" beats.

Figure 3.6A

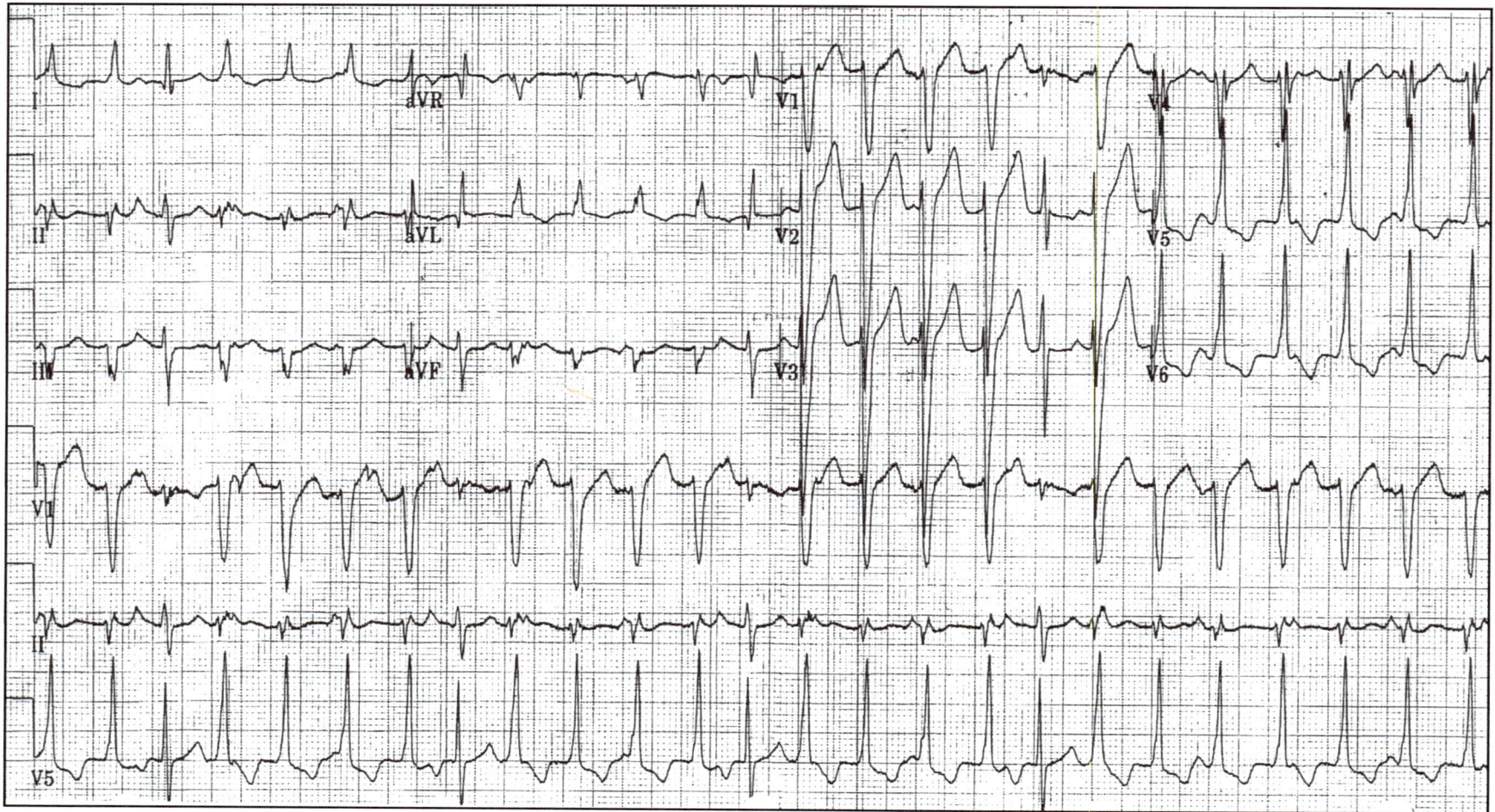

Our first "tool" is the differential diagnosis for a regular tachycardia not requiring atrial participation in the mechanism, a relatively short list that includes VT, AVNRT, and the relatively rare NV reentry. One would not expect the latter two to continue after an interpolated capture beat, leaving us with a diagnosis of VT. Can we do better than this?

Our next tool is enlargement and we magnify a strip of VT in lead 5 that shows the capture beat with reasonable clarity,

Figure 3.6B. I ask you now to simply use your calipers, either electronic or other, and simply "walk" along the top of the QRS complexes before looking at the annotated tracing that follows (**Figure 3.6C**). The capture beat is obviously early, but what happens to the next beat and the rest of the tachycardia? Now measure the CLs before and after the interpolated QRS.

Figure 3.6B

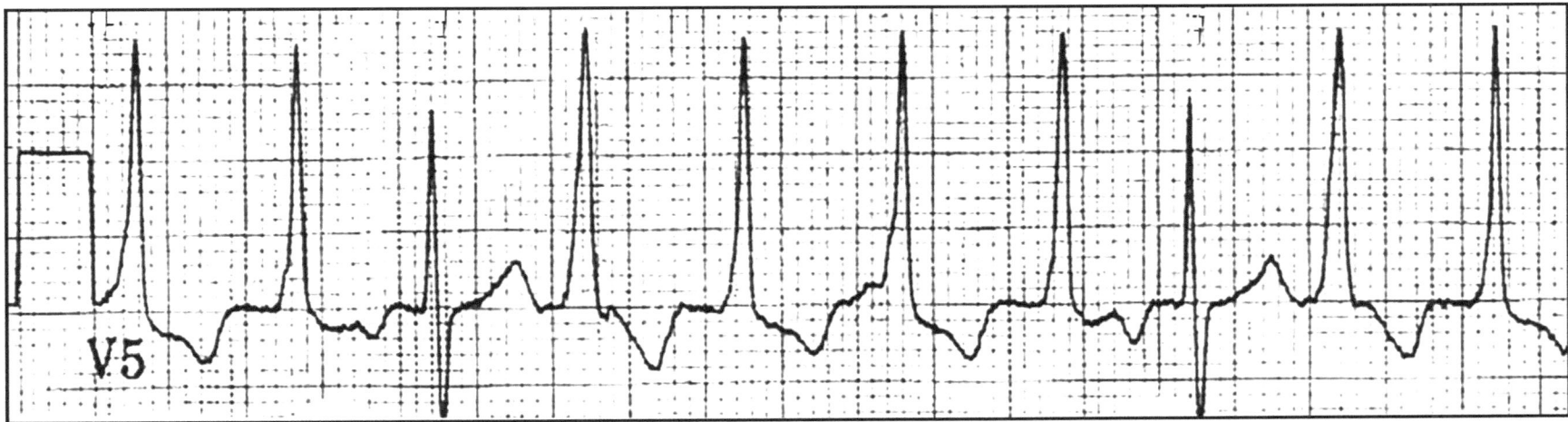

Figure 3.6C

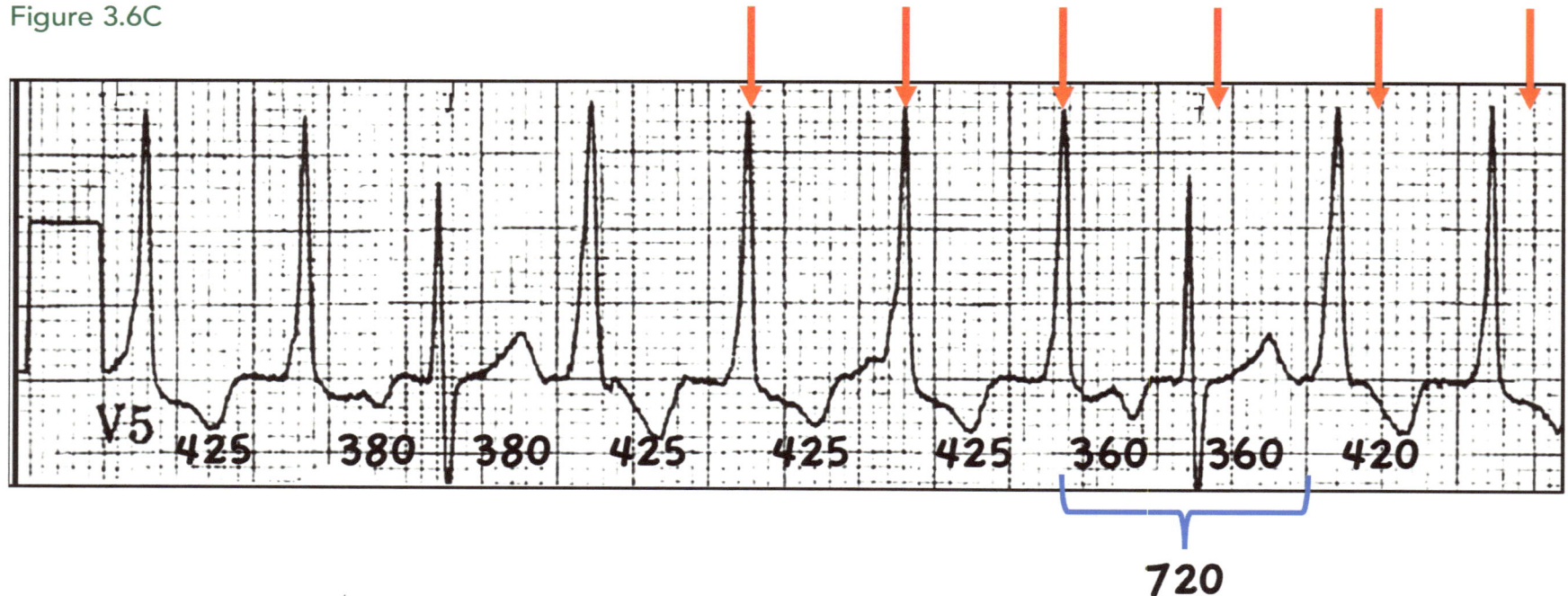

The **red arrows** in **Figure 3.6C** can be considered as calipers. When the measurements are made, it becomes obvious that a relatively late–coupled QRS *resets,* i.e., here advances, the next VT beat. This means that the normal AVCS has excellent access to the VT circuit, suggesting BBR or possibly reentry in the fascicular–Purkinje regions.

We now ask ourselves, if it's BBR, why doesn't the capture beat terminate the tachycardia? We note now that the capture beat has a left anterior fascicular block pattern. The postulated circuit for BBRT in this case is illustrated in **Figure 3.6D**. Because the capture beat has left anterior fascicular block (LAFB), we might reasonably assume that there is retrograde conduction up the left anterior fascicle (LAF) during BBRT.

Figure 3.6D

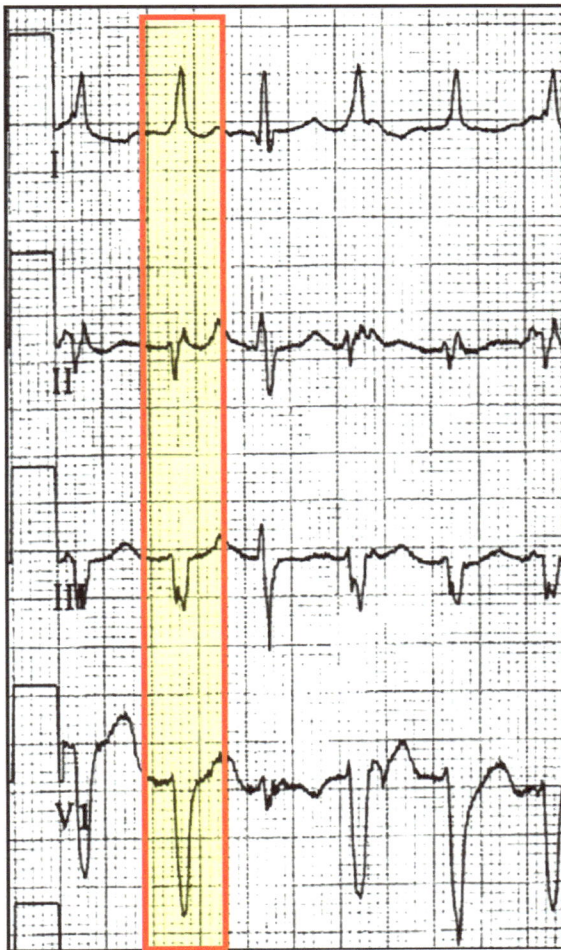

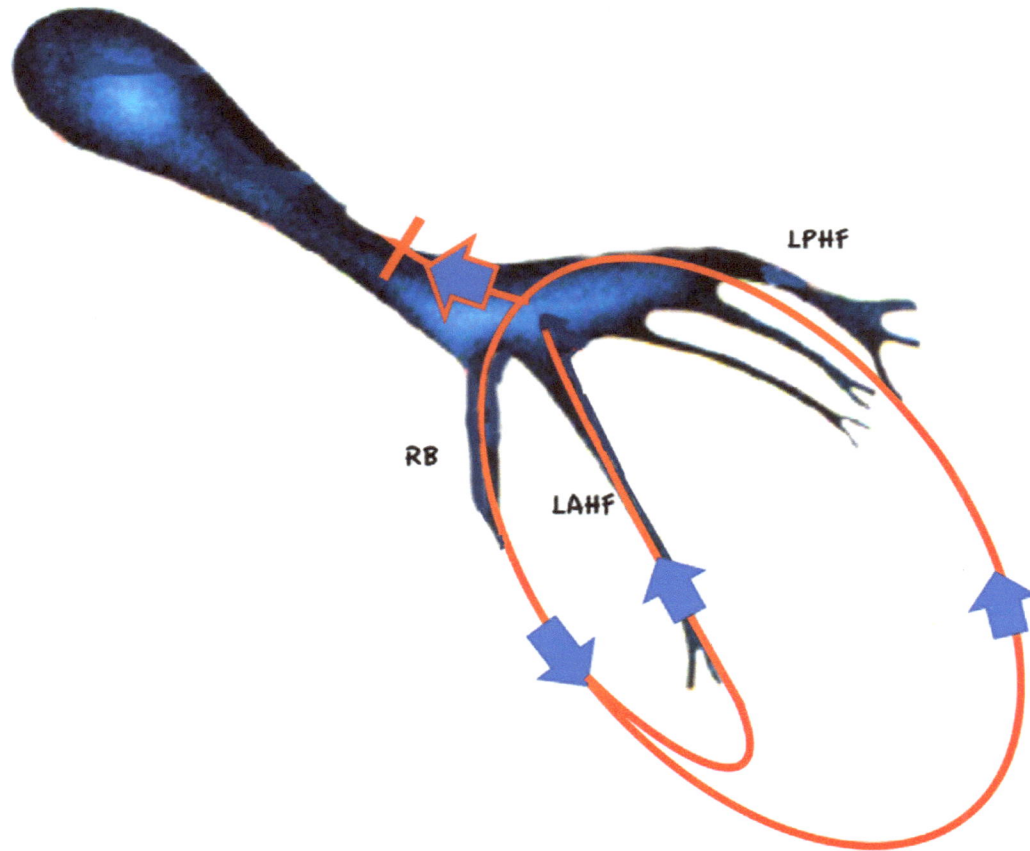

The circuit for the capture beat is depicted in **Figure 3.6E,** indicating why the capture beat doesn't extinguish VT. By this hypothesis, neither the capture beat nor the BBRT circuit conduct anterogradely over the LAF. This allows the LAF to conduct retrogradely after the capture beat and continue tachycardia. The capture beat has thus *reset* the tachycardia after entering the excitable gap of the circuit. Whether these are the exact circuits can't be certain without EP study, but reset of the circuit with a late-coupled capture beat indicates that the normal conduction system is almost certainly involved in the circuit, i.e., BBRT.

The point of this exercise is to approach the tracing systemati-cally within the limitations of ECG diagnosis using simple "tools" to aid the cognitive process.

Simply *measuring the intervals* surrounding the capture beat informs us about the underlying physiology!

Figure 3.6A was provided with the compliments of Dr. Nadia Sunni.

Figure 3.6E

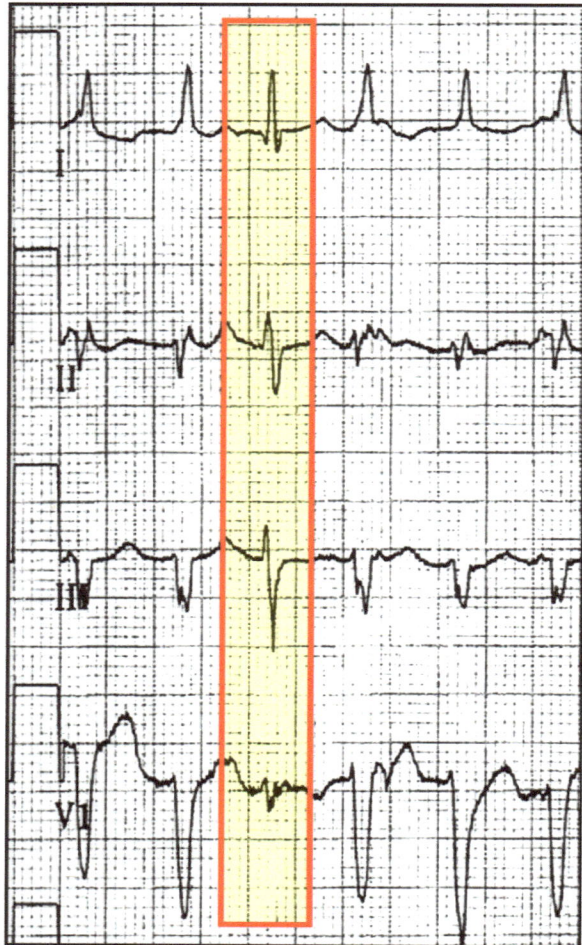

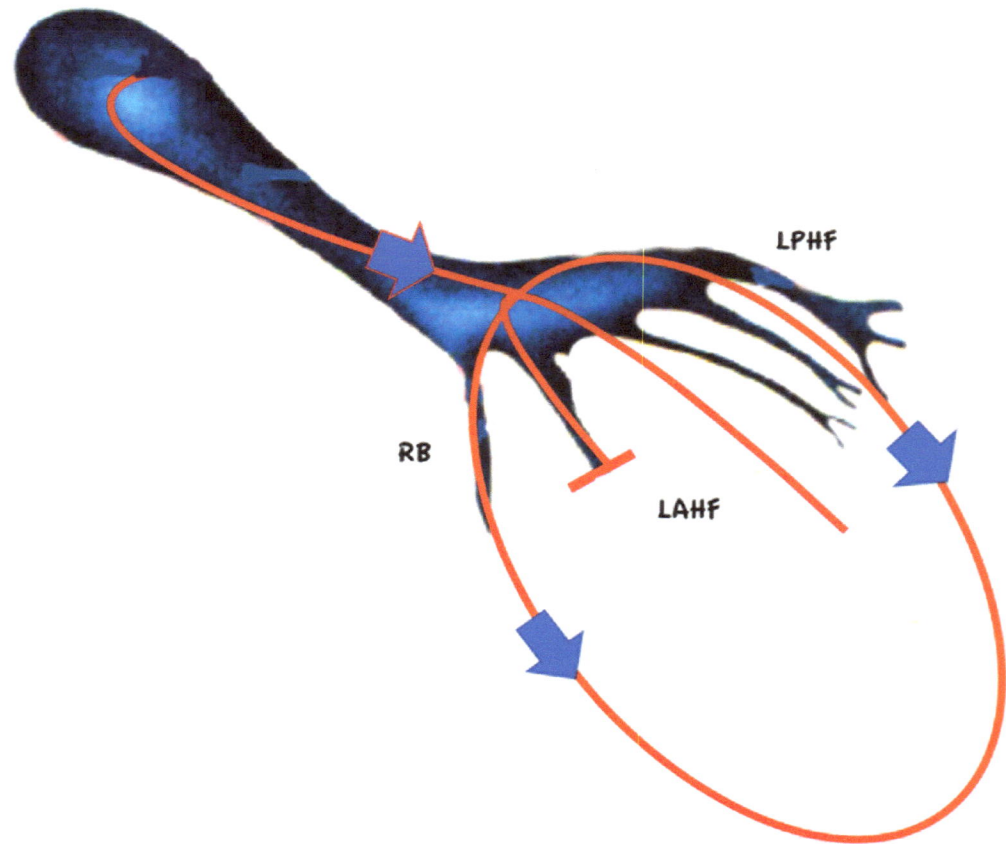

Problem 3.7

The tracing in **Figure 3.7A** may be thought of as a WCT with intermittent "normal" QRS (such as VT with capture beats) or conversely as an SVT with wide QRS cycles (such as AVNRT with intermittent aberrancy). Each of the 2 preceding broader headings or "frames" would have a list of possibilities in the differential diagnosis and it is useful for us to consider each separately as we look at our "evidence."

Figure 3.7A

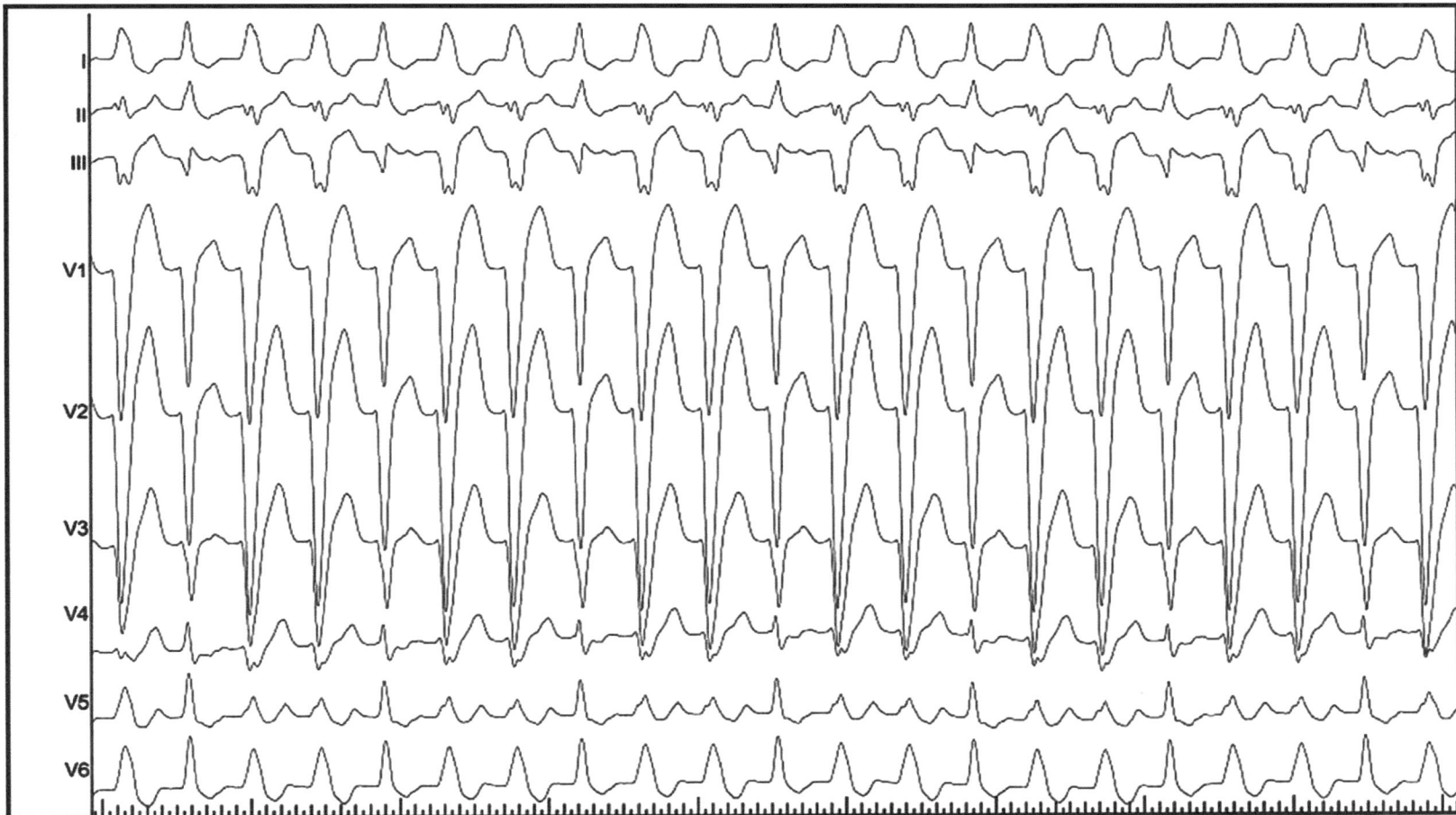

Our overview informs us that:

1. The tachycardia appears regular and two wide QRS complexes are followed by a narrow QRS in a repetitive fashion or "group beating."
2. P waves are not readily discernable.
3. The wide QRS is reasonably "typical" for LBBB (and hence less likely to be VT or preexcitation.)*

It is now time to enlarge a representative area of interest, run our calipers through, and make some measurements (**Figure 3.7B**). We observe that the tachycardia is not entirely regular with the dominant CL of 450 ms shortening **after** each normal QRS to a CL of 400 ms before reverting to 450 ms after the subsequent wide QRS. This consistency makes VT with intermittent capture beats now highly improbable. Intermittent bystander AP conduction is not in the cards, as this would have a constant CL. The same holds for AT or AVNRT.

---

* Preexcitation due to the less common atriofascicular pathway may have a relatively typical LBBB morphology.

Figure 3.7B

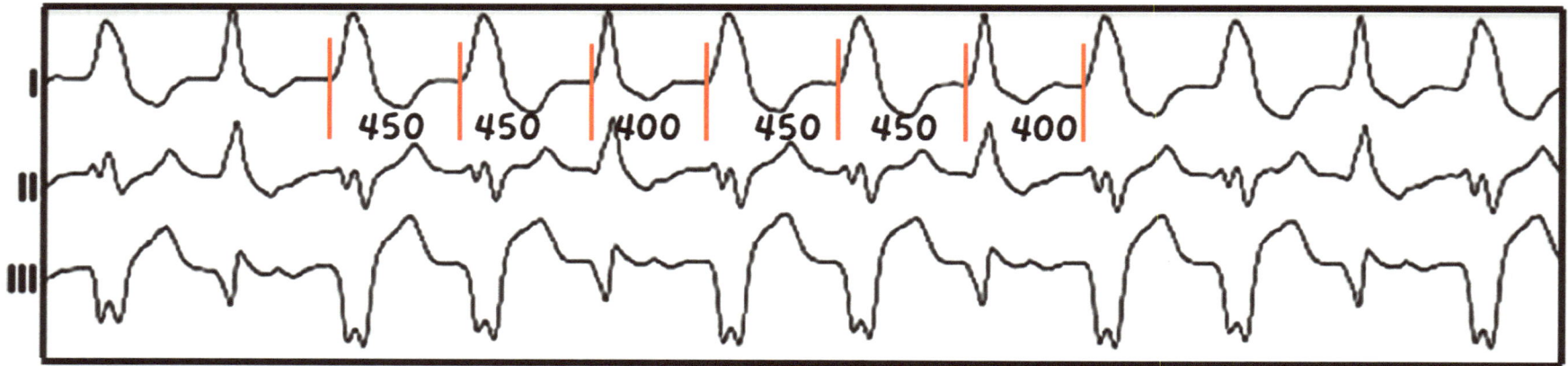

The SVTs that would involve such regular alternations of CL between wide and narrow QRS are limited. Conceivably, we could be dealing with interplay of 2 simultaneous tachycardias such as antidromic tachycardia and AVNRT but "Occam's razor" would suggest that a single tachycardia is a more probable explanation. There are only 2 possibilities where the presence of LBBB in a circuit makes a difference in CL, i.e., where the *LBB is part of the circuit*. These are orthodromic AVRT or NV tachycardia with a left nodoventricular pathway as the retrograde limb of the circuit. By virtue of its overwhelming relative frequency, our preferred presumptive diagnosis must be orthodromic AVRT over a left lateral AP.

This is readily evident when we examine our intracardiac recordings, **Figure 3.7C**. The atrial activation sequence is eccentric with earliest activation in the distal coronary sinus. Intermittent normalization of LBBB shortens the VA interval, shortening the CL of the next beat and reintroducing LBBB aberration (presumably CL dependent). The sequence is then repeated.

Consider the "tools" used in our analysis of the ECG after our overview has "framed" our problem, namely enlarging the area of interest, running our calipers through the tracing and making measurements, and finally testing each tenable hypothesis against the observations. This is the overriding theme of this book.

Tracings adapted from those provided by Dr. Mark O'Neill.

Figure 3.7C

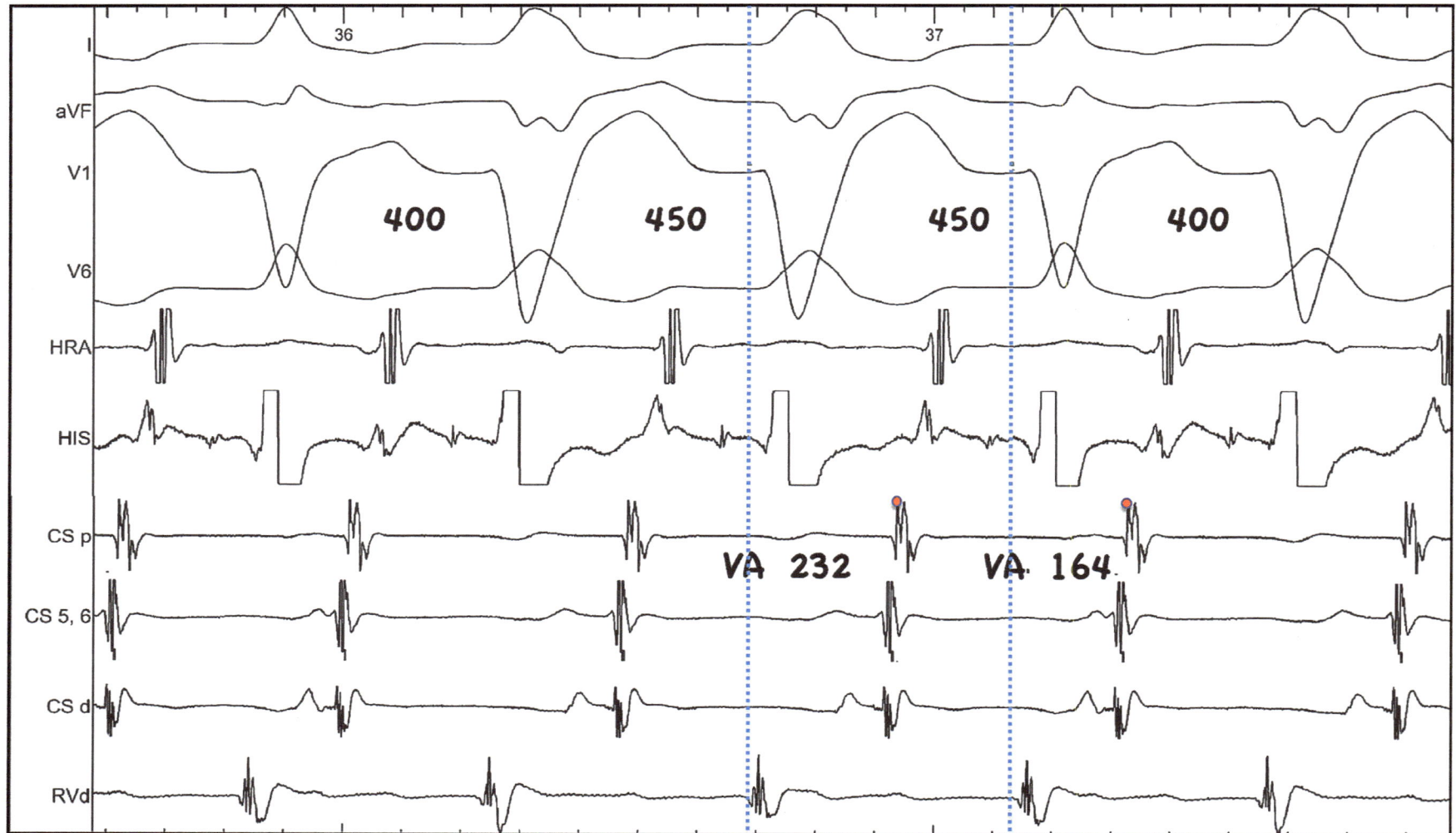

Chapter 4

The Complex Tracing: The Zone Strategy

Problem 4.1

The interpretation of the tracing with more than one apparent tachycardia exemplified in **Figure 4.1A** appears to be complicated but is facilitated by what I term a "zone" strategy. As the name suggests, it is essentially breaking up the tracing into zones to be focused on individually. In this case we see a WCT, a NCT, and a "transitional" zone, which we can refer to as zones 1 to 3, respectively. I find it easiest to do a broad overview and then starting, *not necessarily* at the beginning, but with the zone that I find easiest to understand. This provides a differential for each tachycardia that facilitates interpreting the transition. I also prefer to measure relevant intervals within each zone, moving on after I finish one.

Figure 4.1A

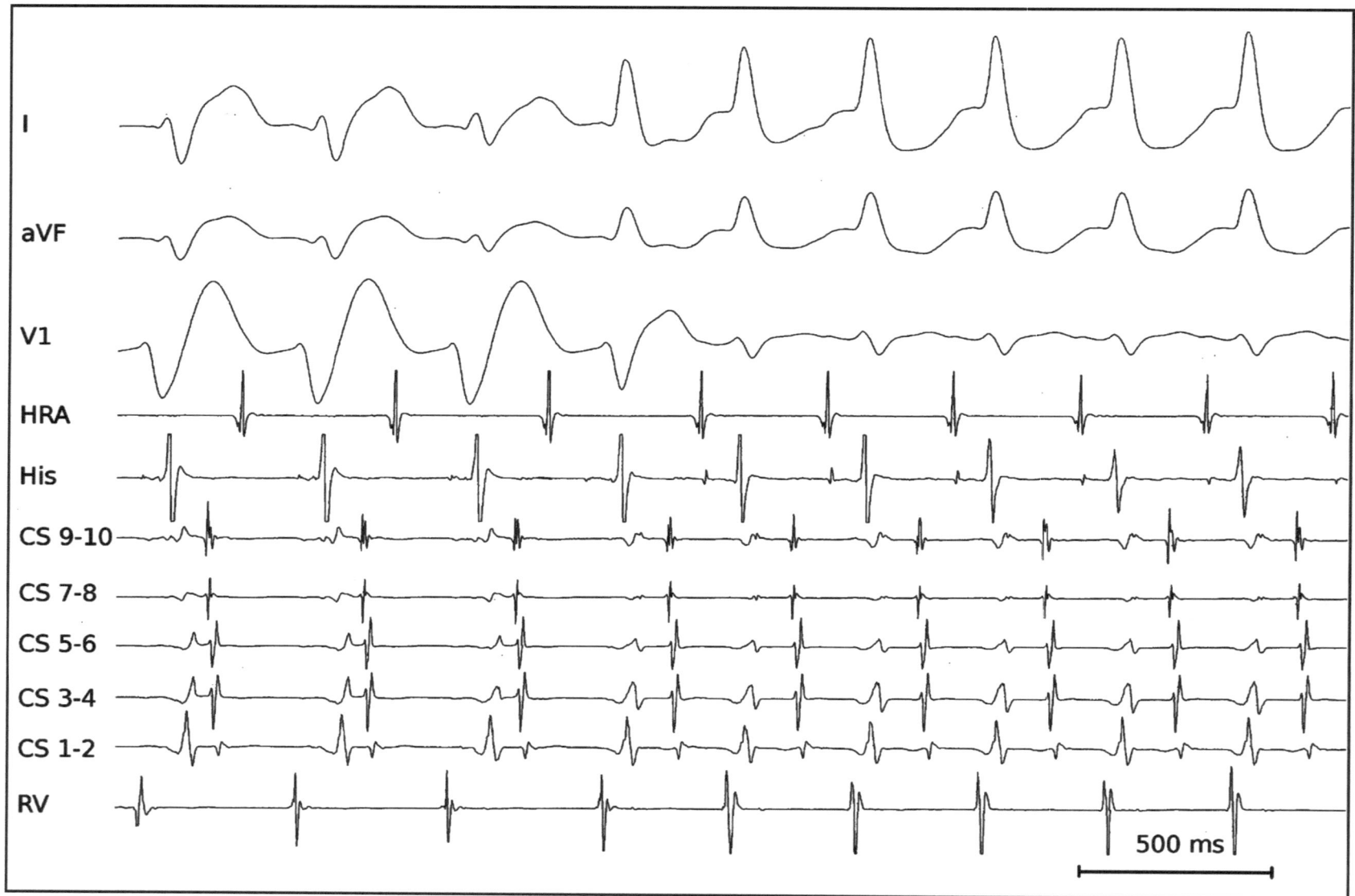

Starting with the NCT zone, I move calipers over the tachycardia and note that the tachycardia is regular, with a CL of 330 ms (**Figure 4.1B**). A light line (**blue**) is drawn marking the earliest recorded ventricular activation, in this case coincident with the onset of the EGM at the RV. Drawing these lines routinely facilitates interval measurement and makes activation sequence more obvious. The H is clear but small and the atrial EGM at the His site is relatively flat, suggesting the recording is more distal, towards the RBBB. The HV is 70 ms and the VA interval at the RA is 260 ms. We note that the VA is only an interval and does not in itself prove that conduction is actually moving from the V to the A.

Figure 4.1B

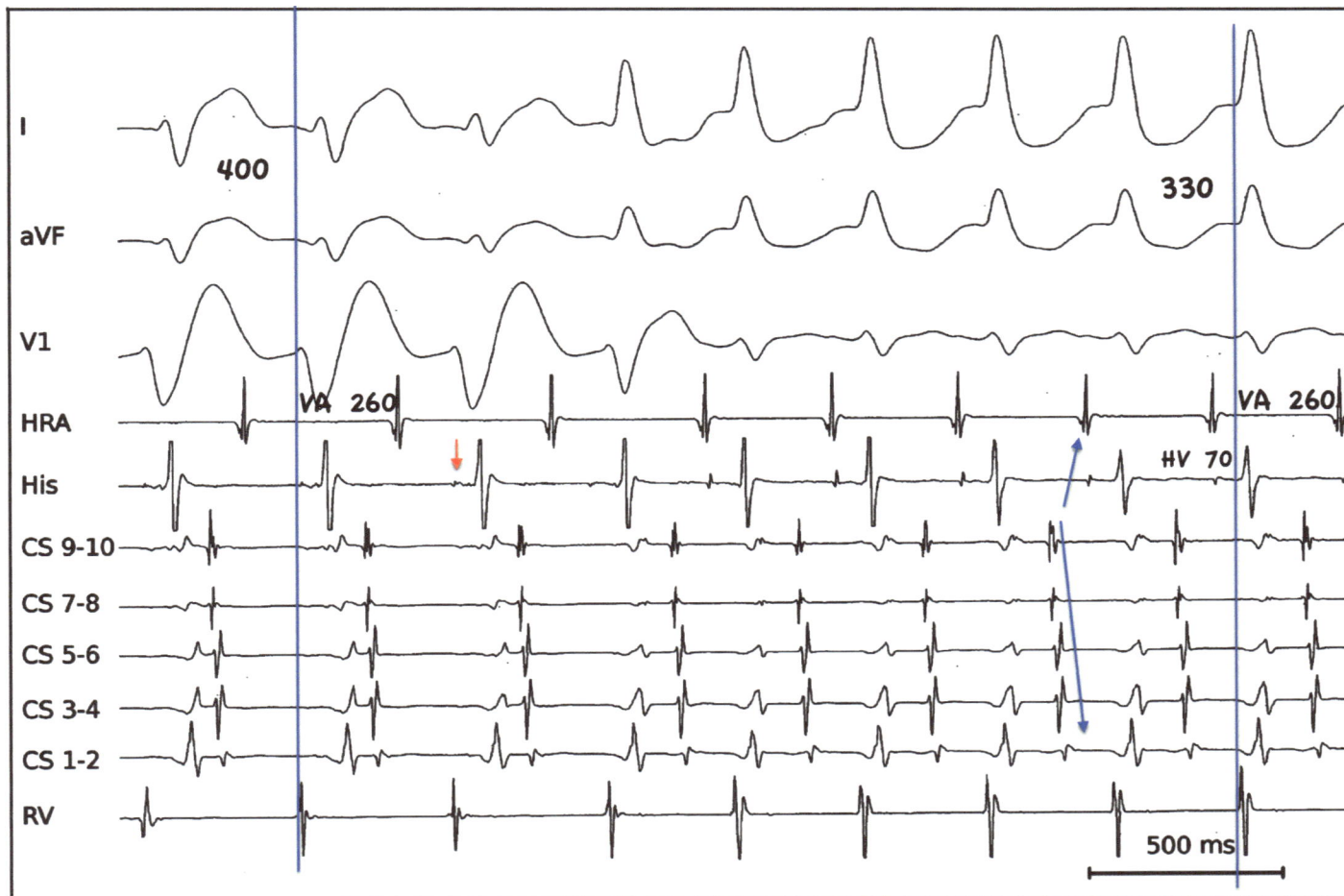

The earliest atrial activation is at the proximal CS, CS9–10 (His A not seen clearly) and this is more or less "central" activation.

Zone 3 thus shows a regular NCT with central atrial activation sequence. At this stage, the whole range of SVT mechanisms remains on the table, i.e., AT, AVNRT, AVRT, or JT.

Moving to the WCT zone at the beginning, we will similarly draw a line at the onset of ventricular activation and measure our key intervals. Several facts become obvious when this is done.

1. The CL of the WCT is *longer* than the NCT. This means that the 2 tachycardias have an entirely different mechanism or at least a change in the circuit if the fundamental mechanism is the same. We can rule out, for example, a single tachycardia mechanism such as SVT with and without a bystander AP or AVRT with and without contralateral BBB.

2. Earliest ventricular activation remains at the RV apex.

3. The atrial activation sequence and the VA interval *remain the same* as the NCT. This most probably means that the WCT and NCT share a retrograde limb of a circuit.

4. The HB (**red arrow**) is now simultaneous with the onset of ventricular activation (HV = 0). *Thus, we can conclude that the WCT can ONLY result from preexcitation or VT.* We can further observe that the apparent HA interval lengthens with the NCT but the VA remains the same. Thus, if atrial activation is indeed retrograde, conduction is *independent of the His bundle and can only be due to an AP for each of the WCT and the NCT.*

We now have considerable information but really need to o to the transition zone (**Figure 4.1C**) for a diagnosis. We observe that there are 2 transition cycles on the ECG, suggesting variable QRS fusion.

Figure 4.1C

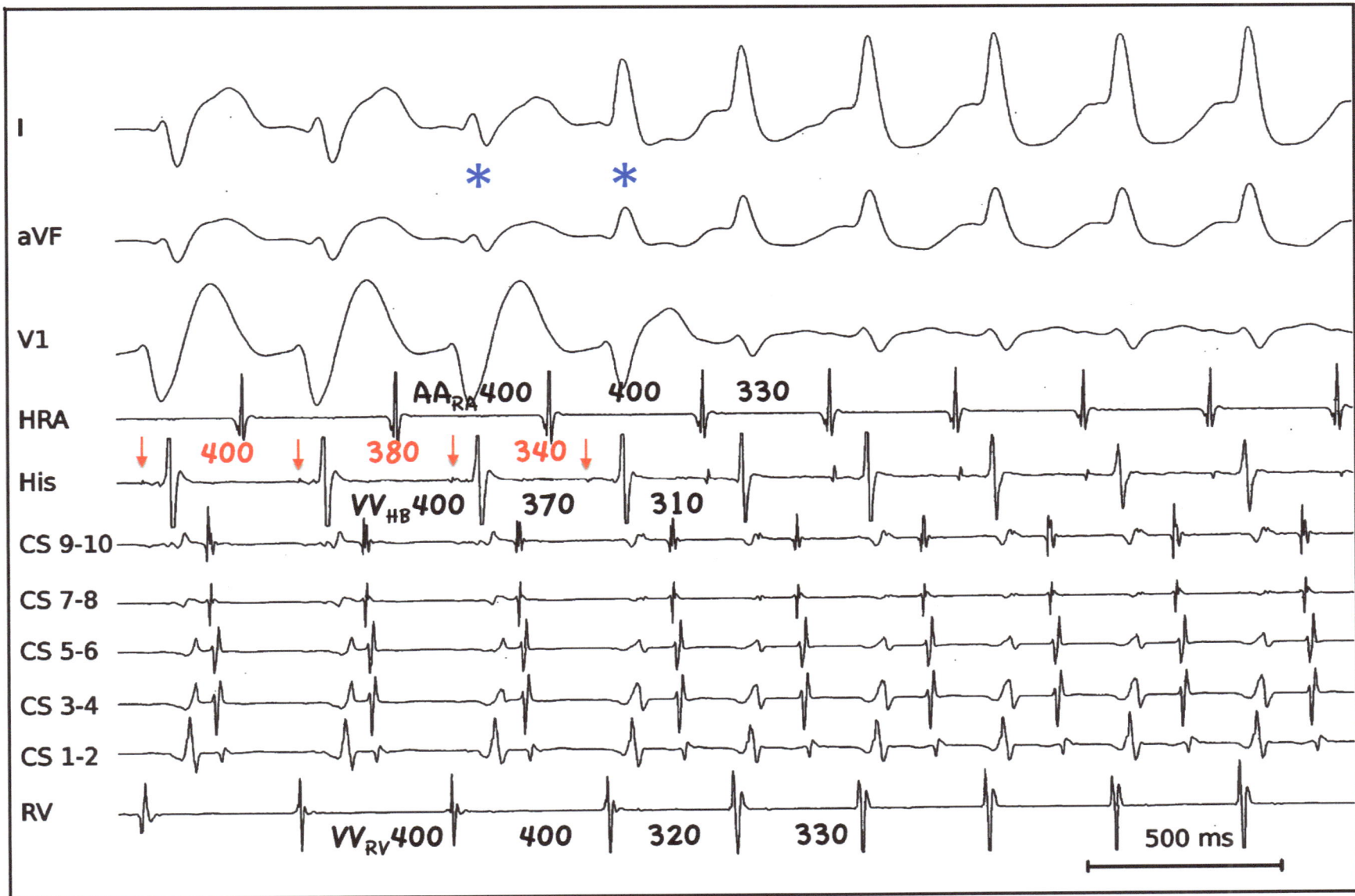

A key step now clarifies, that is simply measuring the intervals at all the EGM sites and determining which initiates the change, *i.e., which moves first?* It is then obvious that the first EGM to move (**red arrows**) is the HB! The V EGM moves next followed by the A EGM. This rules out AT completely, recalling that *the cause of change cannot be downstream from the result of change*. VT is also ruled out since only BB re-entry is possible with the H changing occurring first and our WCT is not really compatible with BB re-entry (HV of 0 would be very unusual for BB re-entry).

If we have ruled out VT, the wide QRS is preexcited, and the only preexcitation that results in the V at the RV_{apex} so early (i.e., HV essentially 0) is the atriofascicular AP, which this was. If we have ruled out AT, the atrial activation must be retrograde and the same for each tachycardia. In this case, it was a septal AP.

Retrograde conduction over the AVN was ruled out since the VA interval did not change simultaneously with the lengthening of the HA.

The change was initiated by a shortening of the AH interval which resulted in anterograde conduction shifting to the normal AVCS. The reason for AH shortening during the WCT is conjectural but probably related to increased sympathetic tone.

This might be summarized in **Figure 4.1D**, where the left panel depicts the WCT mechanism, the circuit anterogradely over an atriofascicular AP (**red arrowhead**) and retrogradely over a septal AP (**blue arrowhead**). The right panel depicts the NCT with anterograde conduction over the AVN (**red arrowhead**) and retrograde conduction over the septal AP (**blue arrowhead**).

Figure 4.1D

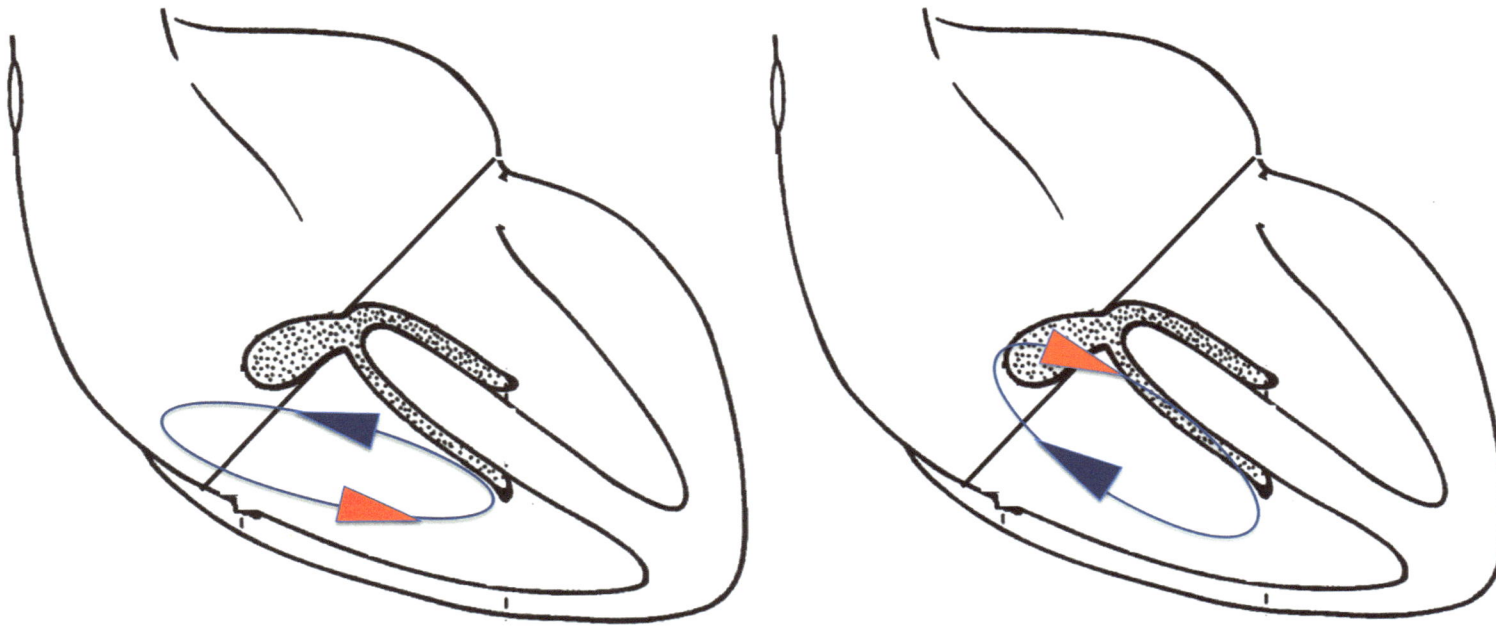

This is admittedly a complex tracing, but the message lies in the strategy for interpretation and the "tool" box. Breaking the tracing into more digestible parts or zones facilitates a difficult exercise.

Figure 4.1 was provided with the compliments of Dr. Raja Selvaraj and based on a publication with colleagues Rohit, M. and Krishnappa, D. (*Journal of Cardiovascular Electrophysiology*, 2018).

Problem 4.2

Continuing our theme of transition of a tachycardia, we start with the ECG (**Figure 4.2A**). An overview shows a WCT transitioning to a NCT after a PVC.

The fundamental question, is this a single tachycardia or more than one? The first step is to run our calipers through the tracing (**Figure 4.2B**).

Figure 4.2A

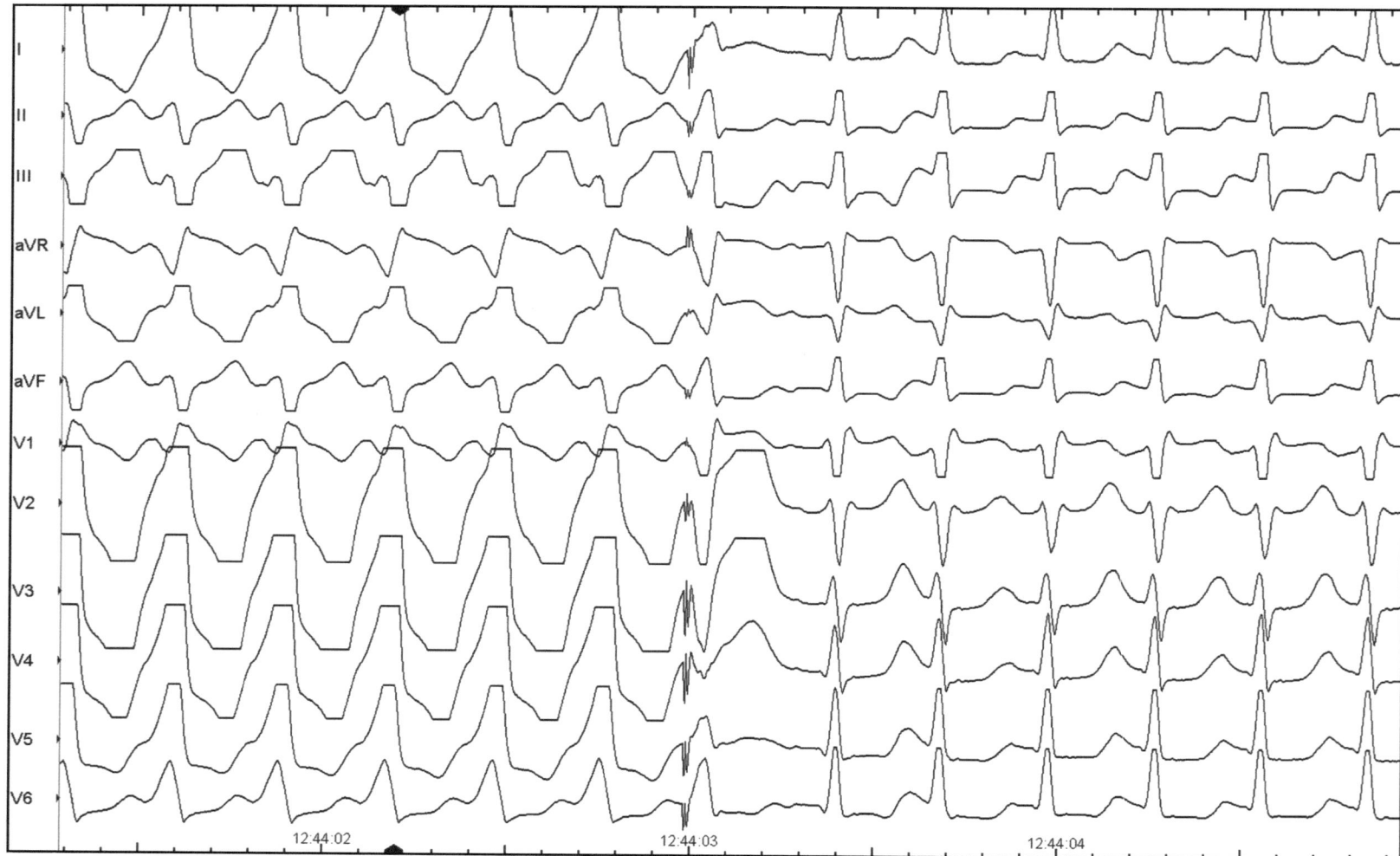

Figure 4.2B

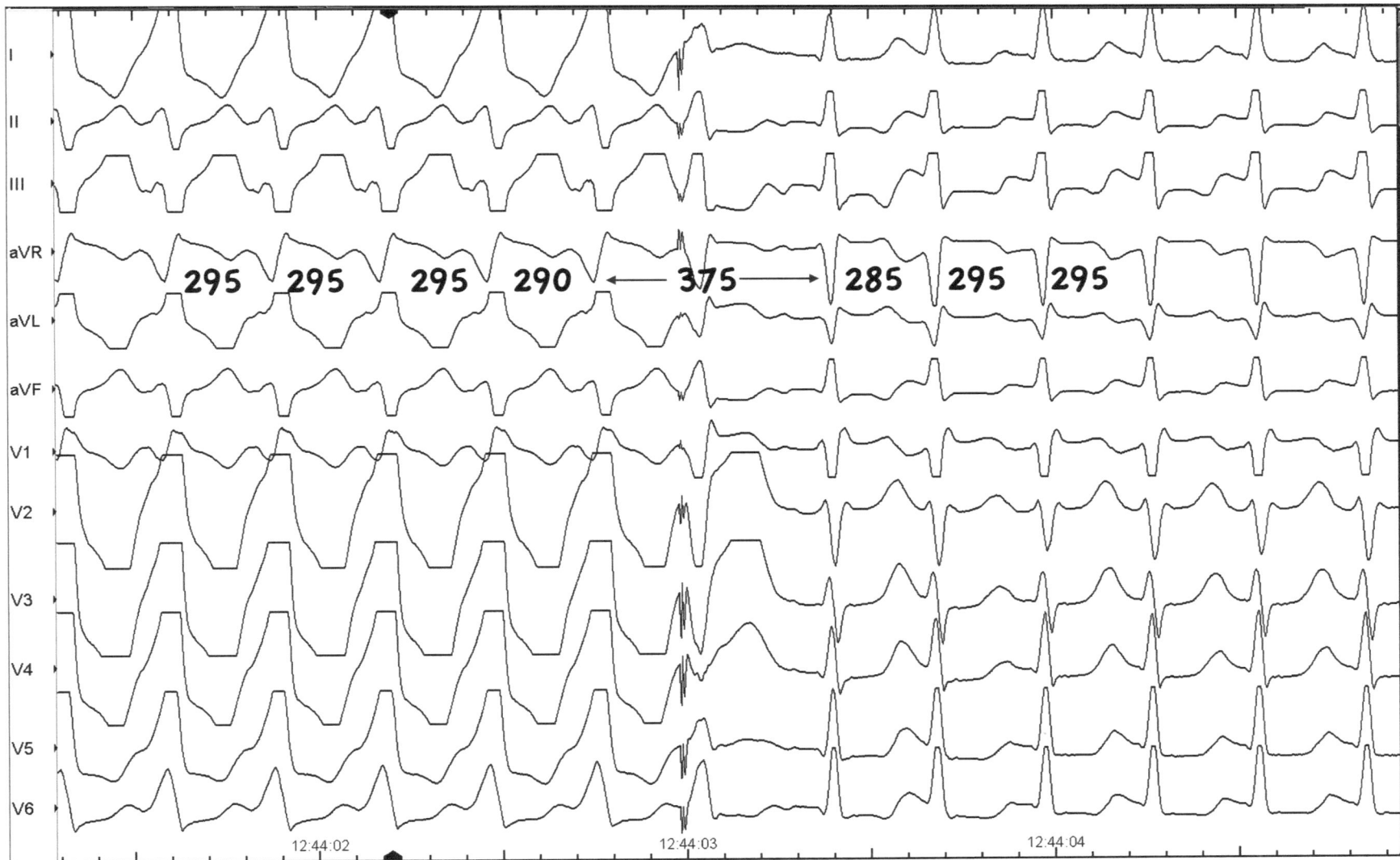

We observe that the CLs of the WCT and the NCT are identical, i.e., 295 ms. For all practical purposes, this means that we are dealing with one tachycardia mechanism. Otherwise, we are in the predicament of assigning the patient tachycardias of 2 mechanisms with an identical CL—certainly known to happen, but highly unlikely.

Working on this hypothesis, the WCT can now *only* be SVT. It can only be one of the following:

1. SVT with aberrancy. The bundle that is blocked during SVT is *not* involved in the mechanism. This leaves AT, AVNRT, and AVRT with the AP contralateral to the side of the bundle branch block during SVT.
2. SVT with a bystander AP not involved in the SVT mechanism.

If we focus on the 3 zones one at a time starting with the NCT, there is no convincingly visible P wave during SVT. The mechanism of SVT awaits further analysis. The WCT is more helpful. The QRS morphology is simply not compatible with a bundle branch block pattern. The QRS complexes show a basal pattern of origin with high positive voltage right across the precordial leads ("concordance"), and this can ONLY be preexcited or VT. We have already essentially ruled out VT (if we accept that it is all one tachycardia) so the WCT must be preexcited! In this particular example, the transition zone itself, frequently critical to understanding the tracing, doesn't add anything. Concealed retrograde conduction into the bystander AP is a reasonable explanation for normalization with repetitive concealment resulting into continued normalization after the tachycardia normalized with the PVC.

We can now move to the tracings (**Figure 4.2C**) with the ECG having narrowed our problem to a bystander AP during an unknown SVT dropping out after the PVC.

In the analysis, I have divided the tracing into 3 zones and indicated such in **Figure 4.2D**.

Figure 4.2C

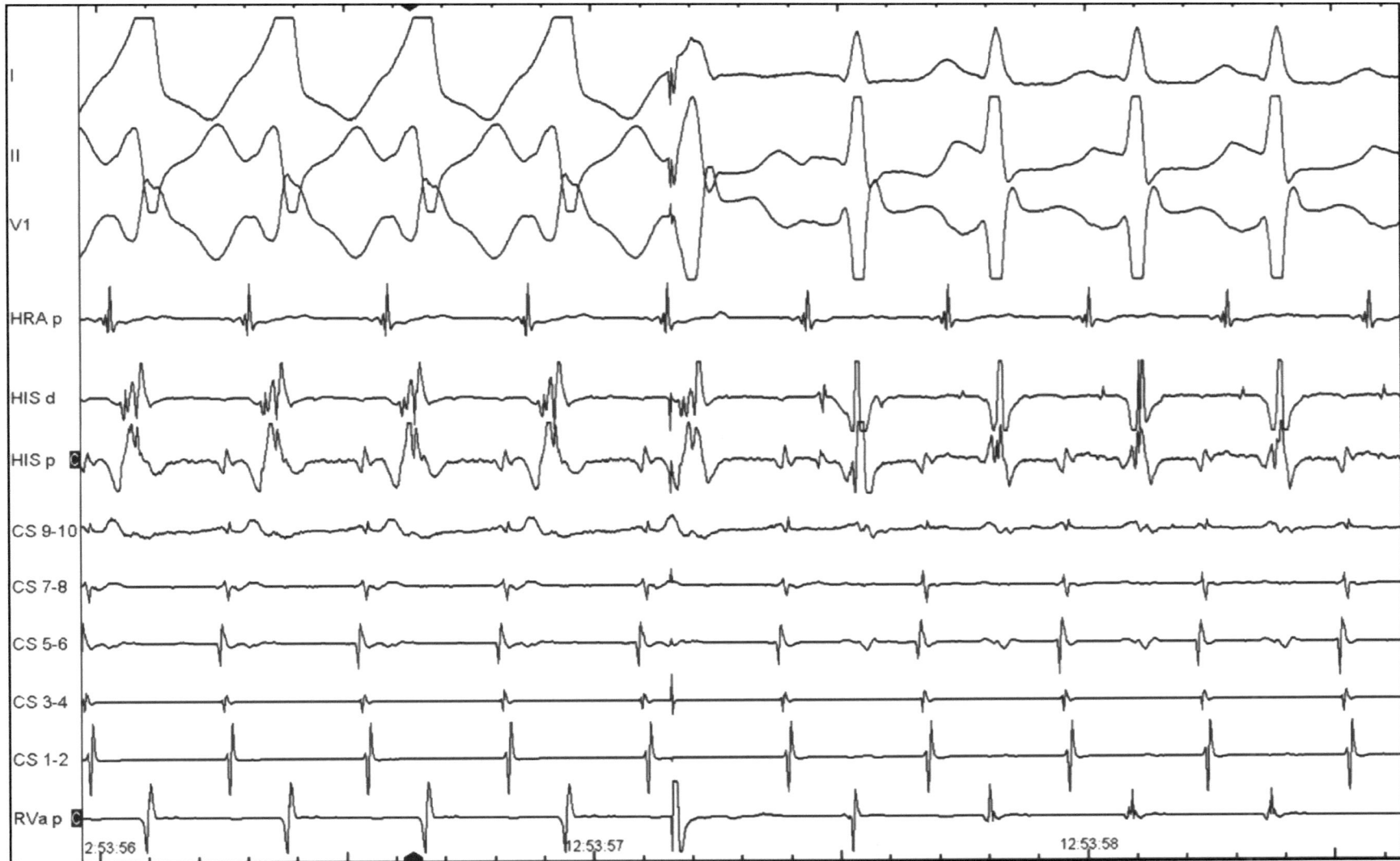

Figure 4.2D

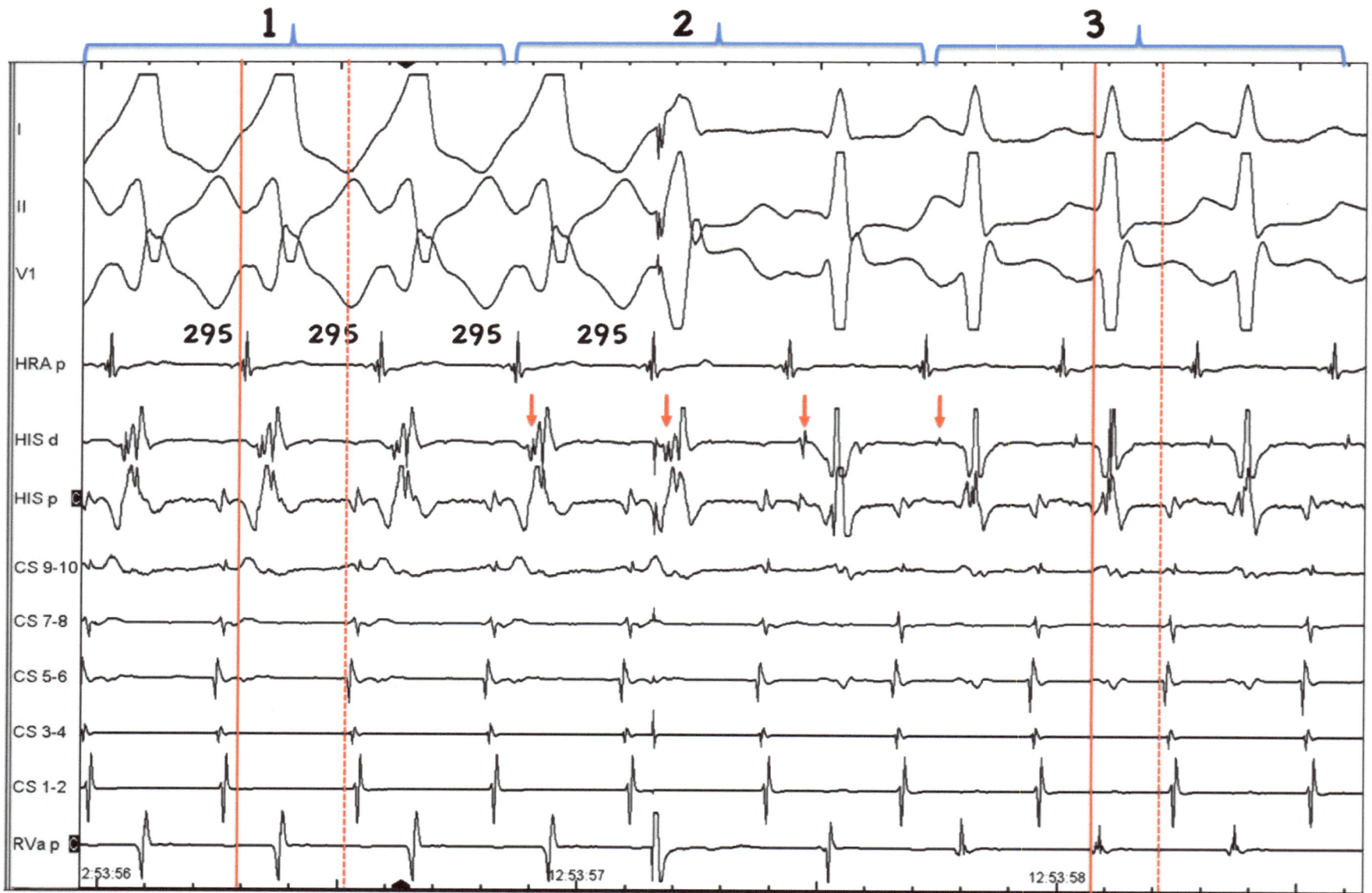

I start with the NCT, zone 3, since that might be the most straightforward segment to analyze and build from. Vertical lines are drawn at point of QRS onset and onset of earliest A EGM to facilitate interval measurement and activation sequence. We note that earliest atrial activation is at the mid-CS EGM, 5–6, which is slightly eccentric if we accept that the CS is well positioned with 9–10 near the CS ostium (Os). This would suggest a posteroseptal or perhaps left paraseptal AP but does not entirely rule out conduction over a retrograde slow AVN pathway.

Moving over to the WCT zone 1, we note that there is no H potential preceding the QRS. The His is very evident from zone 3 indicating reasonable catheter position and accordingly, we would expect to see one prior to the QRS onset if it were there. A sharp deflection within the QRS (**red arrows**) is in all likelihood the H but we have noted that the WCT can only be VT or preexcited tachycardia by its QRS morphology and hypothesized that VT was not tenable if it is all the same tachycardia. We further note from **Figure 4.2D** that the atrial activation is identical to that of the SVT in zone 3.

Finally, we look at the transition zone—zone 2. We note that the transition occurs *without any influence* of either the atrial EGM timing or the HB timing (**arrows**).

What have the intracardiac tracings contributed so far? We really have not much more information than provided by the ECG tracings, namely an unknown SVT with and without a bystander AP. We obviously need a maneuver to do this and we move on to the usual "go-to" maneuver—namely, overdrive ventricular pacing (**Figure 4.2E**).

Figure 4.2E

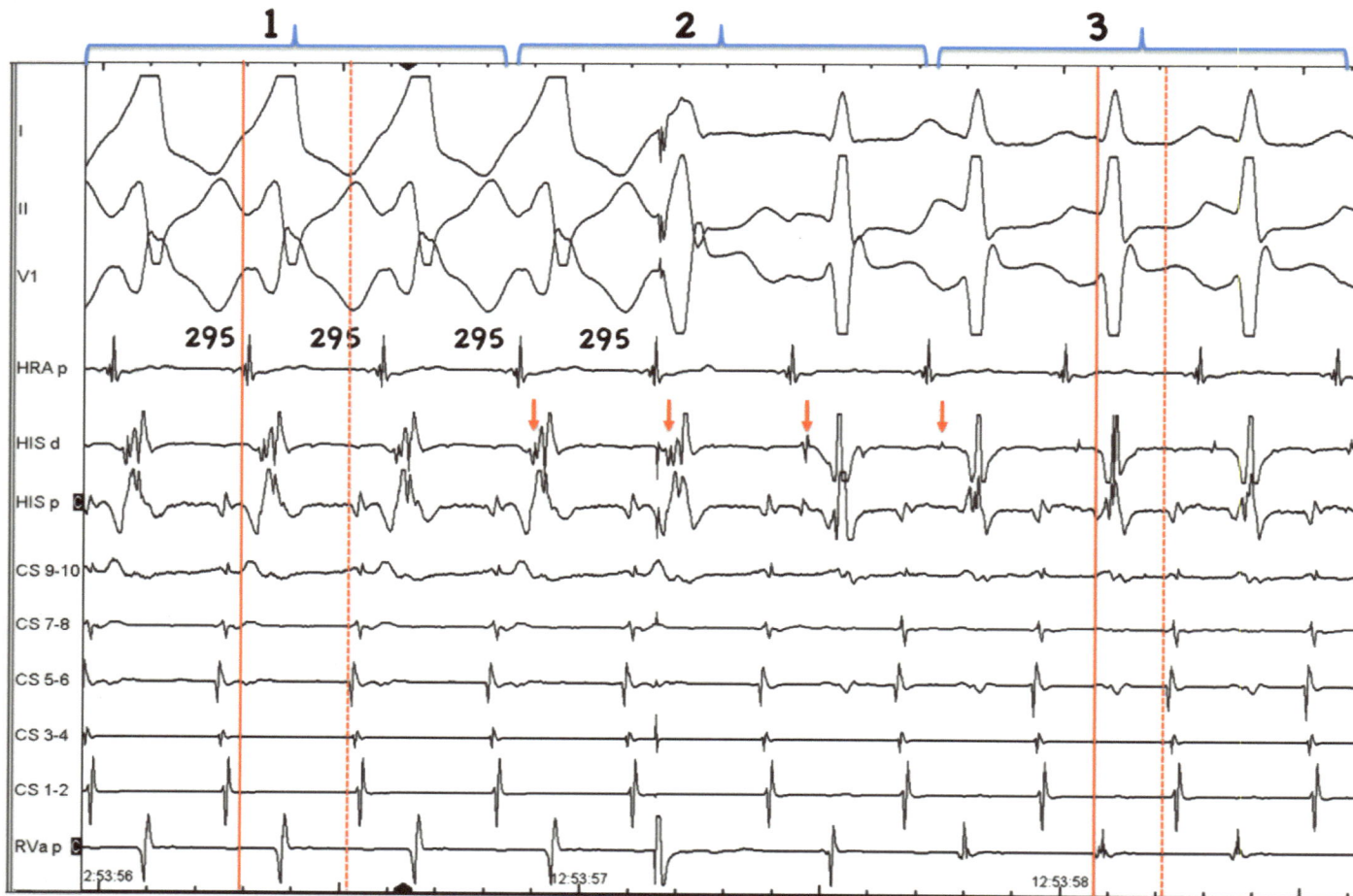

The annotated **Figure 4.2F** shows overdrive pacing from the high RV, a more basal position that is generally more discriminating for distinguishing AVRT from AVNRT. Pacing is done just modestly faster than the tachycardia rate (CL 250 vs. CL 260) to minimize prolongation of conduction time of part of the circuit that might confound the utility of the maneuver. We note that the tachycardia rate has sped up to the pacing rate. The critical step is to move the calipers along one of the atrial EGMs and *identify the last atrial EGM accelerated to the pacing rate* (**red arrow**). It is now apparent that this is a "VAV" response, indicating entrainment (versus just overdrive acceleration) allowing a diagnosis of AVNRT or AVRT and ruling out AT.

The PPI is 310 ms and the PPI–TCL = 60 ms, indicating AVRT (versus AVNRT). That is, the RV electrogram is "in" the circuit. Similar information is provided by the Stimulus-A minus the VA interval (240 − 165 = 75 ms).

We have now "solved" our problem. We have one tachycardia, AVRT with retrograde conduction over a left paraseptal AP, with and without the presence of an additional "bystander" AP.

Figure 4.2F

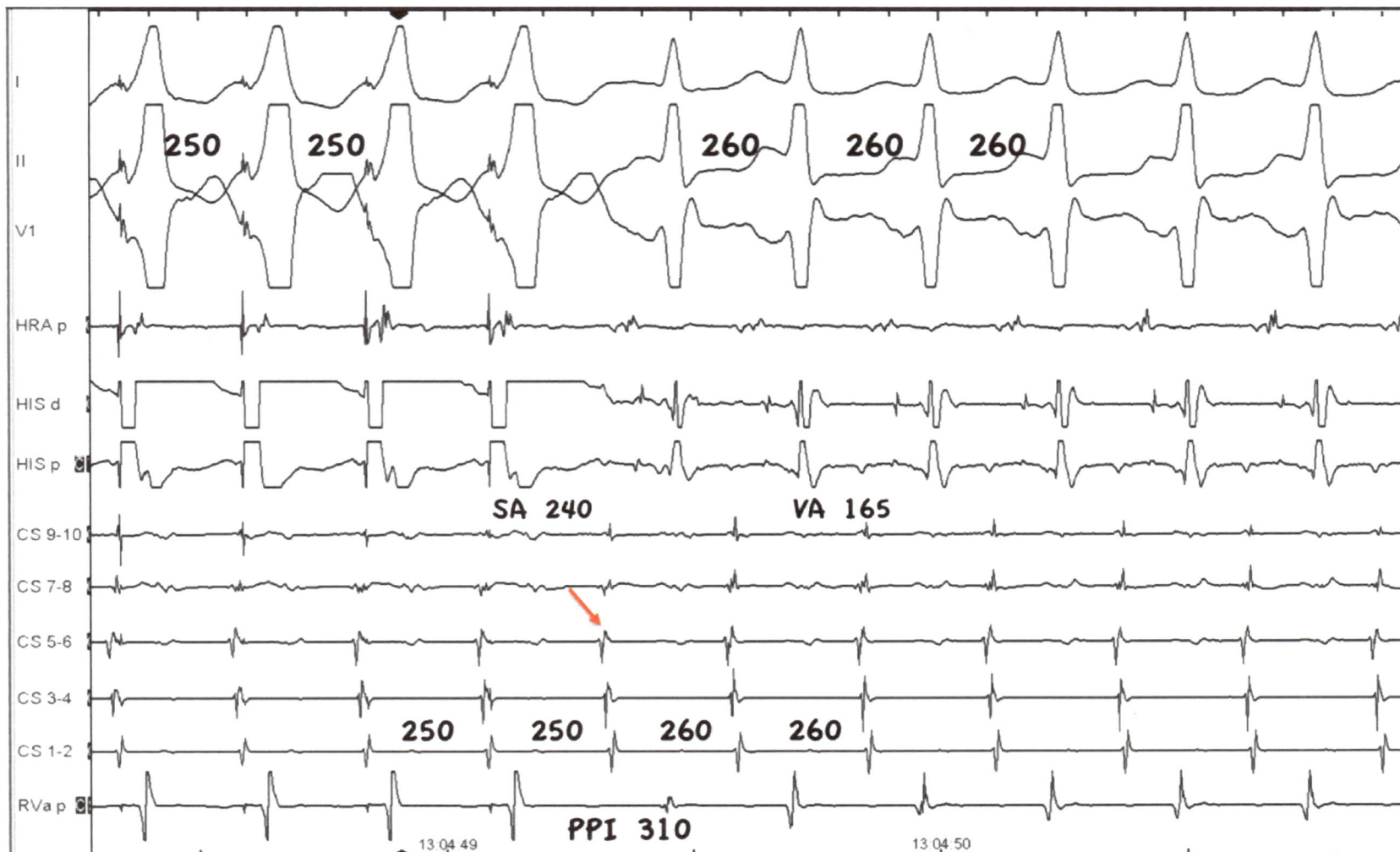

Problem 4.3

Figures 4.3A to **4.3E** come from the same patient and admittedly constitute a more advanced exercise. Try to get as much possible from the ECG in **Figure 4.3A** before moving on to the intracardiac part in **Figure 4.3D**. Use all the cognitive "tools," measuring with calipers, magnifying when appropriate, and concentrating on zones of transition.

Figure 4.3A

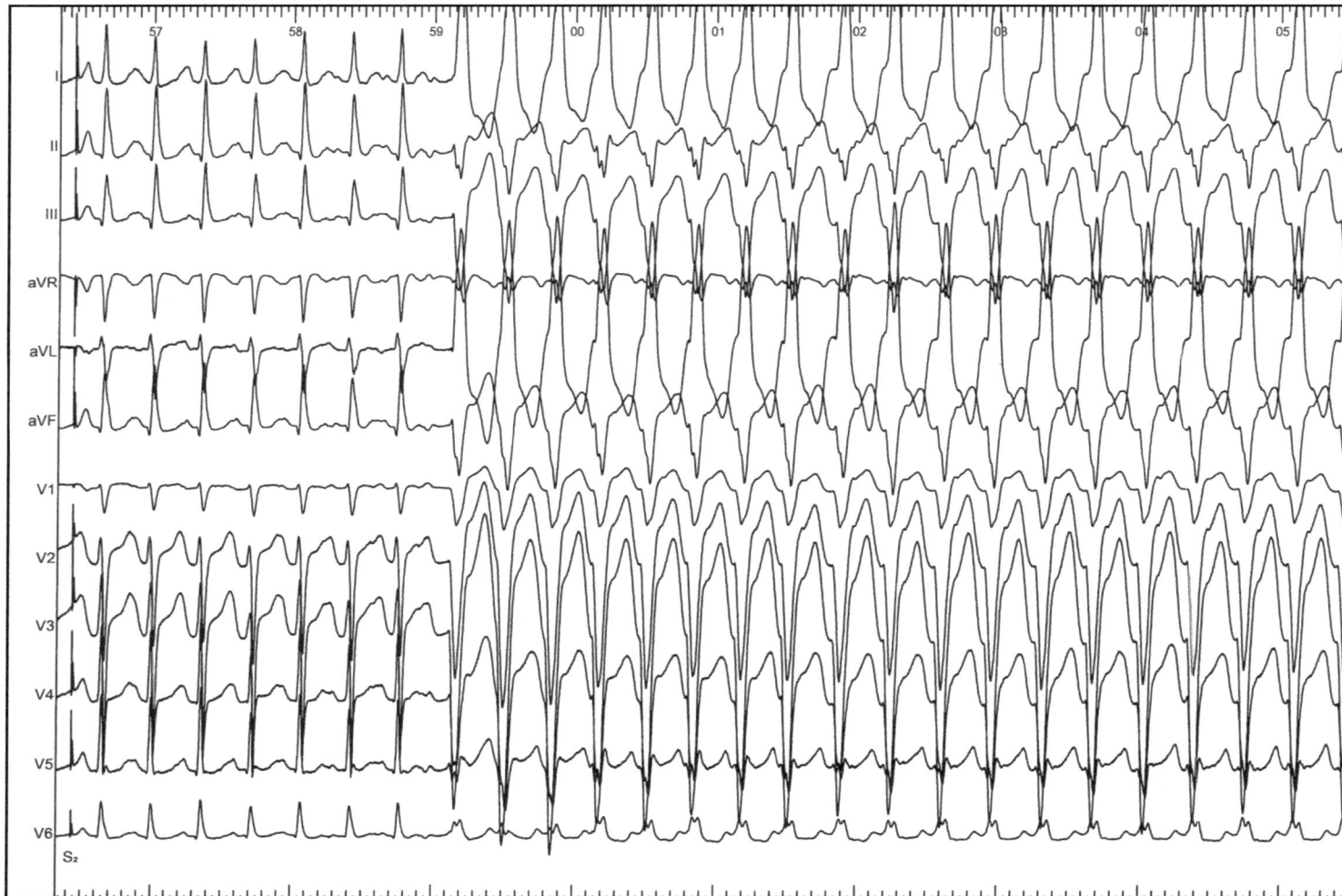

There are 2 obvious zones, namely a narrow QRS tachycardia and a WCT separated by a transition zone. I will start by simply magnifying the transition zone for reasons that should be immediately obvious by inspection of **Figure 4.3B**.

Figure 4.3B

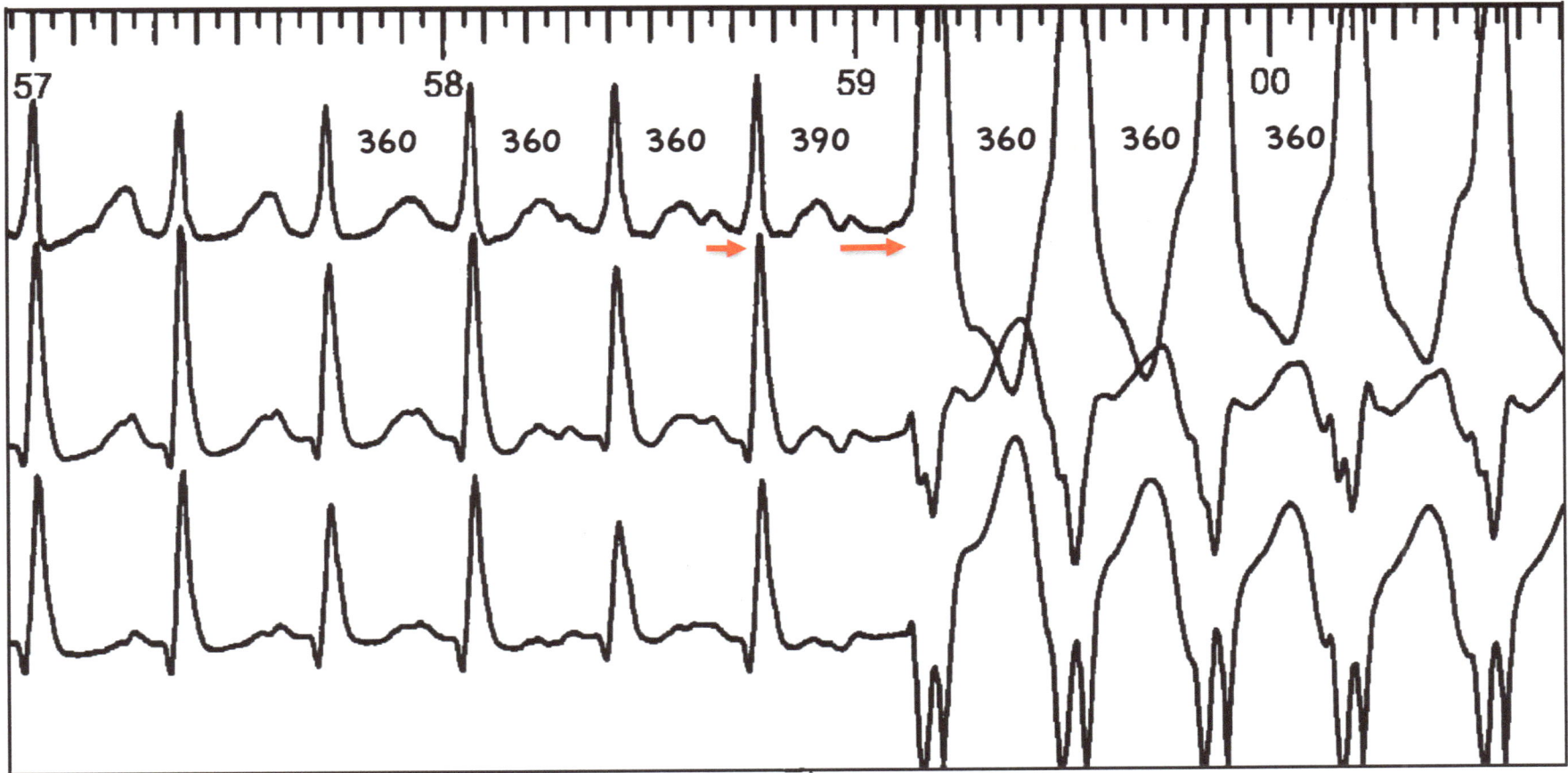

The SVT has a CL of 360 ms prior to the transition. The P waves "emerge" from the T waves and are positive in the limb leads (high to low activation). This is not compatible with AVNRT or AVRT and must be AT or possibly sinus tachycardia and the first part of our mystery is solved.

The next observation is at the transition to the WCT. It would be a huge coincidence if the WCT were VT and just happened to start simultaneously with PR prolongation of the previous beat! For all practical purposes, we have ruled out VT for the WCT, especially if the same were observed on more than one occasion.

Having run our calipers along the tachycardia, we note the CL of the WCT is exactly the same as the SVT. Although it is possible that the WCT has an entirely different mechanism, it is far more likely that they share the same fundamental mechanism. *It is most probable at this point that the WCT is AT with bundle branch*

block or bystander preexcitation. The QRS morphology would be reasonable for either of the above.

We then go back to **Figure 4.3A** and continue to run our calipers through the WCT. We note that there is an abrupt change in cycle and enlarge the region of interest in **Figure 4.3C**. A change in CL of this tachycardia after a transition can only mean some change in tachycardia mechanism. Prior to the transition, AT was determined to be AT with either bundle branch block or AT with bystander accessory pathway conduction. At this point, a critical observation is a relatively "sharp" deflection in early repolarization that changes in timing at the transition (**blue** and **red arrows**). This can reasonably be considered to be a P wave. We now note that the P-wave change *precedes* the change in the next QRS arrival, linking the next QRS to this P wave and again mitigating against ventricular tachycardia.

Figure 4.3C

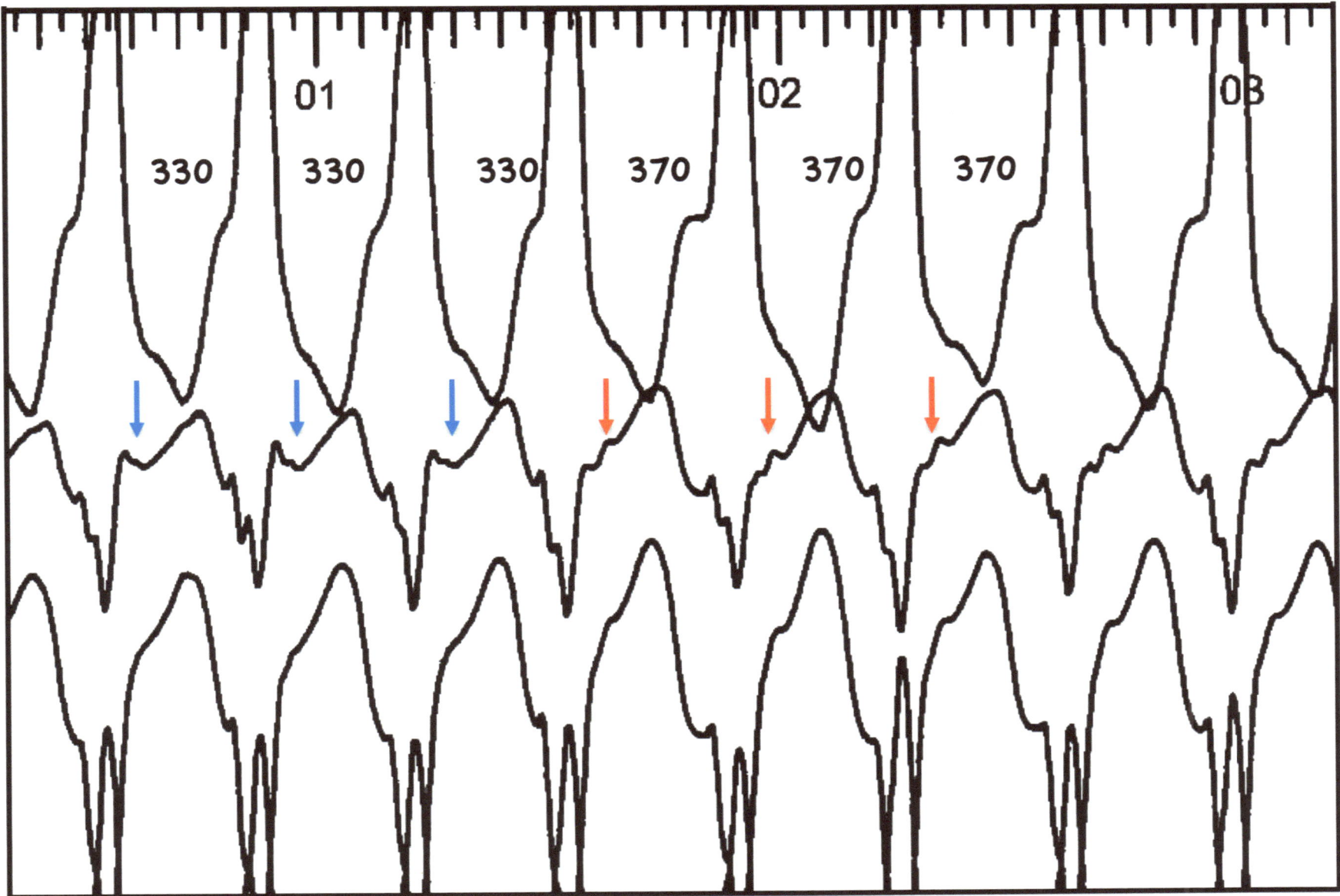

At this juncture, we (and certainly I) have probably reached the limit of what we can glean from the surface ECG. We can conclude that AT with a narrow QRS transitions into the same AT but with a wide QRS, either due to bundle branch block or due to a bystander AP. The WCT then slows with a different associated P wave, with a slightly longer RP interval. This can theoretically be any SVT mechanism and we now can move to the intracardiacs for further enlightenment, **Figure 4.3D**. Before you move to the annotated version, focus on the following:

1. Is a His deflection discernible?
2. What is the ventricular activation sequence?
3. What is the atrial activation sequence for each tachycardia before and after the transition zone?
4. Create hypotheses to explain the transition.

Figure 4.3D

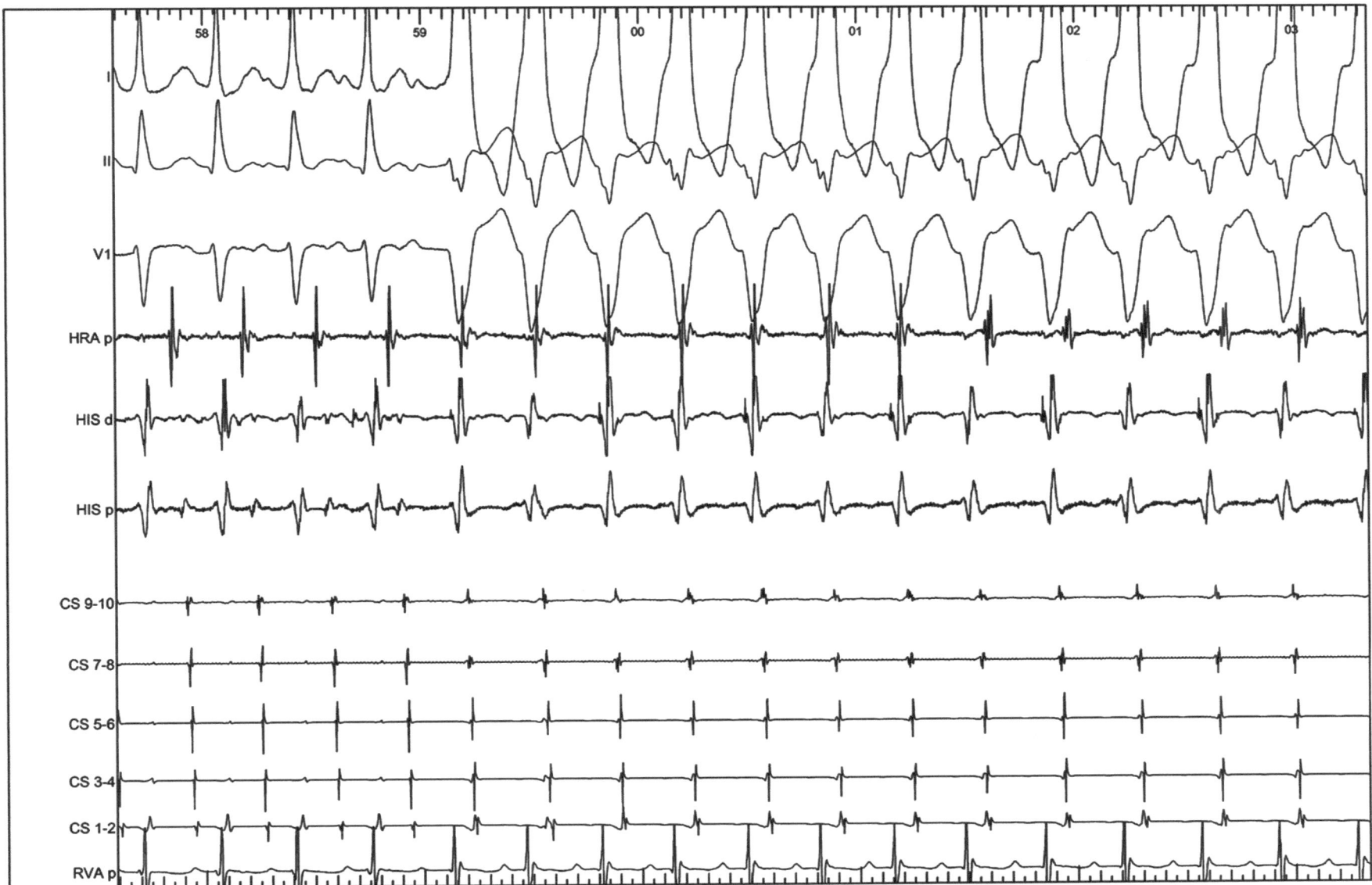

The annotated version, **Figure 4.3E**, enlarges this transition zone and we will try to answer our questions. First, A His deflection is indeed visible at the onset of QRS (HV interval is approximately 0) for each of the tachycardias that I will designate as WCT right and WCT left. This must then be *preexcited* for each of WCT right and left. Second, we note that the RV apical electrogram "leads the pack" (**red line**) for ventricular activation (RV to onset QRS approximately 0). This is not compatible with the more common AV accessory pathway and is characteristic of the atriofascicular pathway. Third, we note that the RA EGM is earliest for WCT left (**green dashed line**). The CS orifice (CS 9–10) is earliest for WCT right with the HB atrial EGM not clearly seen, i.e., central retrograde activation sequence.

We have now established that WCT left is a right AT with anterograde conduction over an atriofascicular pathway. WCT right can only be an AT or AV reentry with the retrograde limb being either the normal AVCS or another septal AP. Unfortunately, the transition doesn't help us with this distinction, although it validates our ECG observations that the change in P wave preceded the change in QRS timing.

Among our 3 options for WCT right, the most common mechanism by far for preexcited atriofascicular tachycardia with a central retrograde activation sequence would be AV reentry with the anterograde limb being the atriofascicular pathway and the retrograde limb being the normal AVCS and this is what it turned out to be. Consider how you would go about proving this, by demonstrating that both the atrium and the ventricle must be part of the circuit and that retrograde conduction is proceeding over the normal AVCS rather than a septal pathway.

As a final exercise, we can consider a thought experiment where the more rapid right AT of WCT left is actually entraining AV reentry on the right. Consider spontaneous termination of right AT as analogous to discontinuation of right atrial pacing and you can then measure the PPI at the RA pacing site. You note that the PPI–TCL is 50 ms, which suggests that the atrium is "in" the circuit. Of course, this doesn't help us directly with our short list of diagnoses for WCT right but does rule out entities where the atrium is not part of the circuit (such as AVNRT with bystander preexcitation).

Figure 4.3E

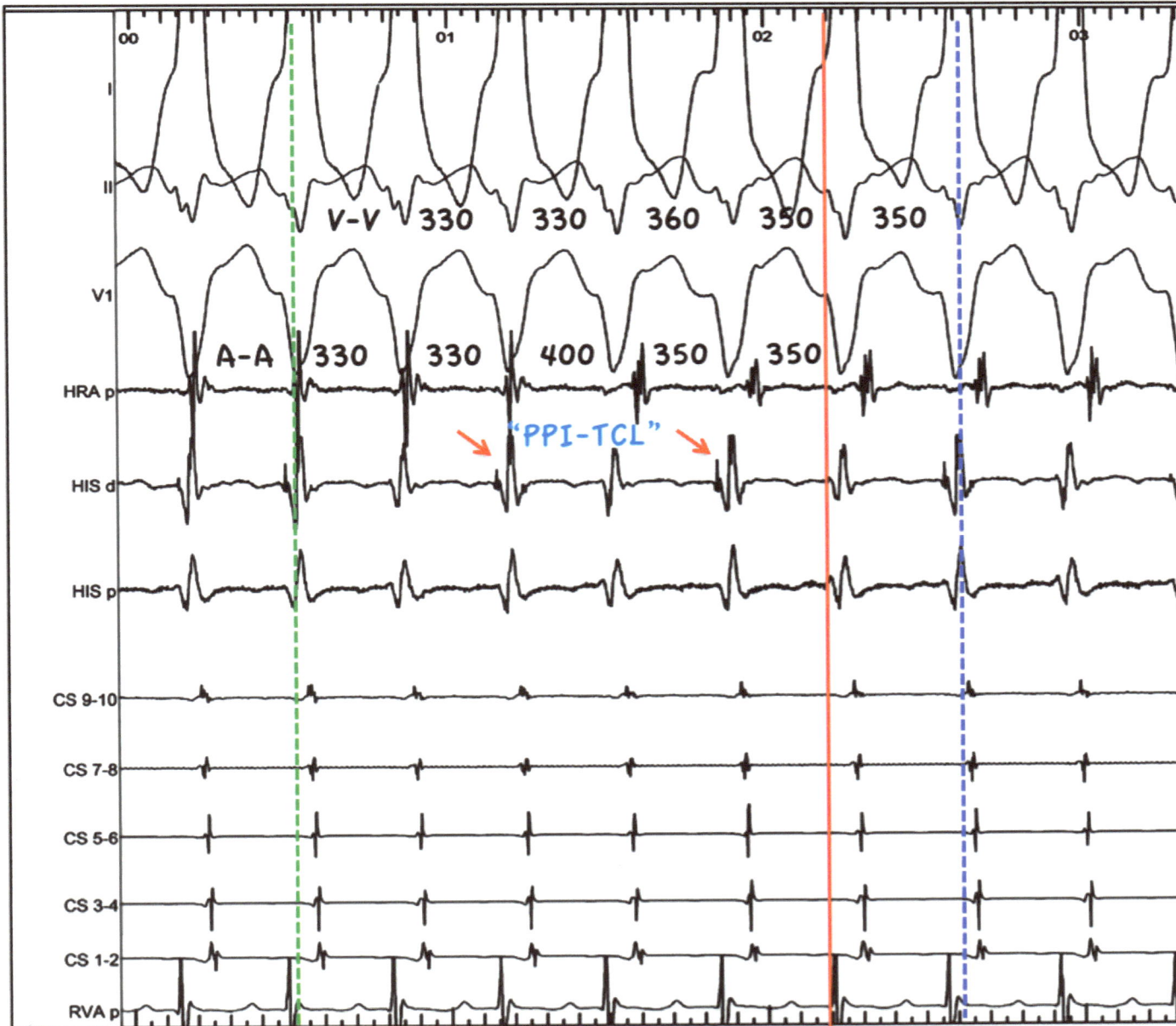

Problem 4.4

An overview of **Figure 4.4A** allows us to frame the problem as a WCT with a 1-to-1 AV relationship. We also observe an abrupt acceleration of the rate without obvious change in the QRS and a shorter VA interval after the transition. Finally, we note that the QRS morphology would be quite unusual for aberrant conduction. In addition, the earliest *ventricular* activation we observe from our limited leads occurs in the LV base, signaled by the far-field V EGM at the CS catheter (**red line**). This would not be compatible with bundle branch block, where activation at the LV base would be late. Without a His EGM preceding the QRS and the QRS pattern and ventricular activation not compatible with bundle branch block, we are moving to a short list of diagnoses, namely preexcited tachycardia versus VT.

Figure 4.4A

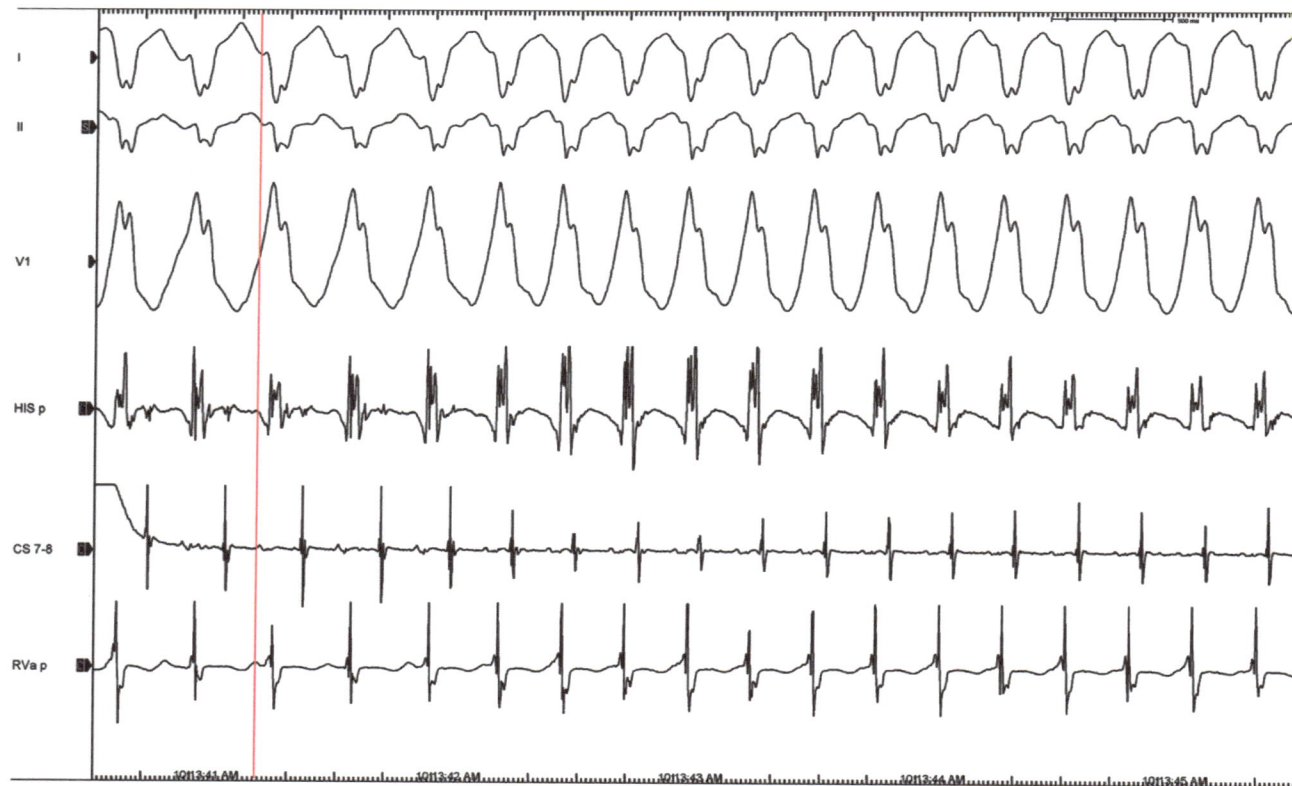

We now focus on the transition zone by enlarging the area of interest and removing some redundant leads, **Figure 4.4B**.

The first question I ask myself at a "transition zone" or change in tachycardia is, *which electrogram moves first?*—meaning, which one leads the change. In this case, the A suddenly advances (shorter AA) and the VV only shortens AFTER the previous AA becomes shorter. This might be expected with acceleration of an AT or shortening of the VA interval but would NOT be compatible with VT where any change in the A could only *follow* the V.

Figure 4.4B

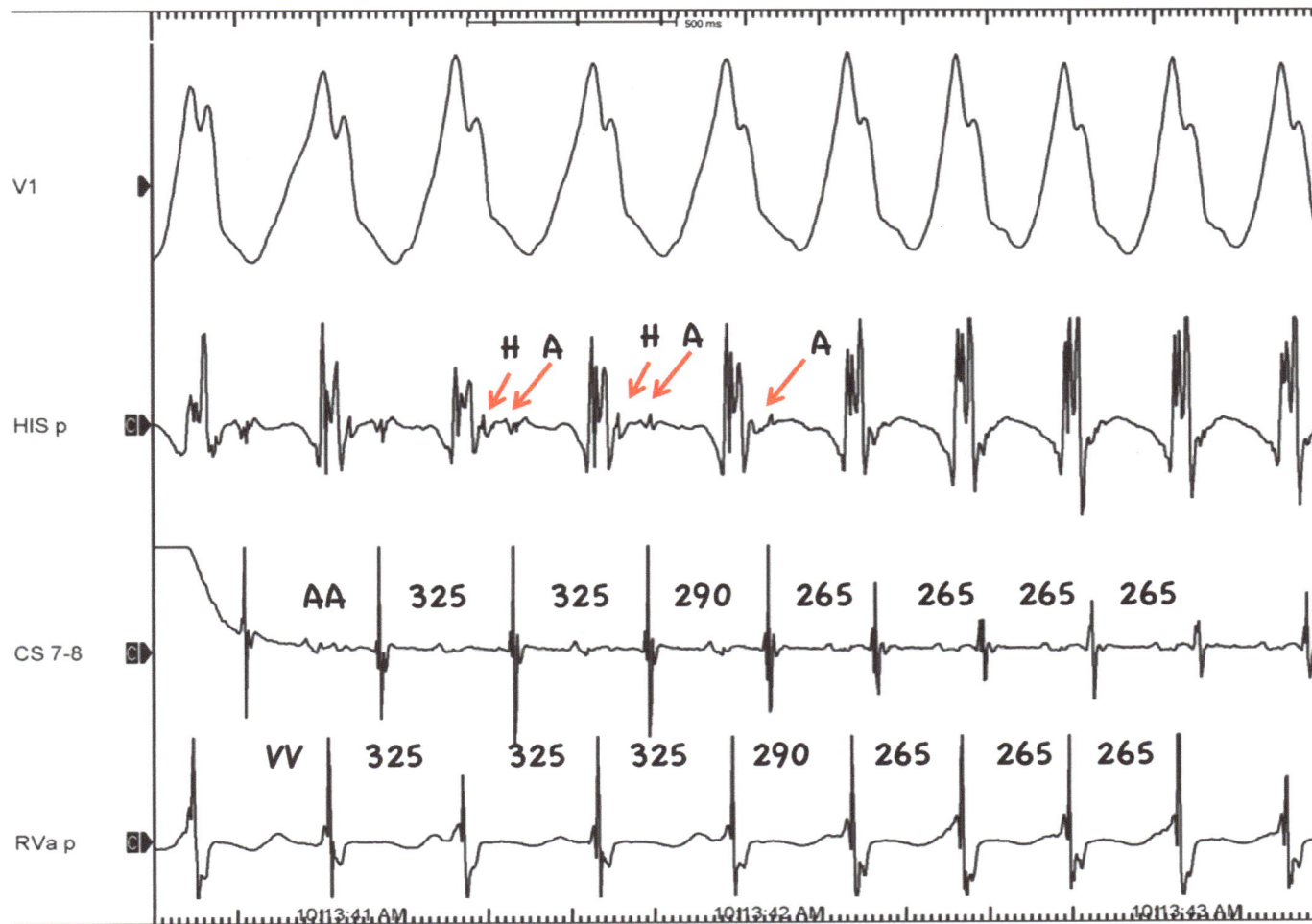

Now we need some signal recognition skills. The deflection designated as H (His) falls within the QRS boundary and may theoretically just be part of ventricular activation. However, this deflection disappears when the VA interval shortens without change in the QRS itself. Thus, the shortening of the AA is *preceded* by disappearance of our putative His deflection, making AT untenable.

Thus, we have a preexcited tachycardia with shortening of the VH and VA intervals causing CL shortening. This is readily explained by retrograde conduction over the normal AV-conduction system (antidromic tachycardia) with initial retrograde LBBB. With spontaneous resolution of retrograde LBBB, shortening of the circuit caused both a shorter VH and VA. This is illustrated schematically in **Figure 4.4C**.

Figure 4.4C

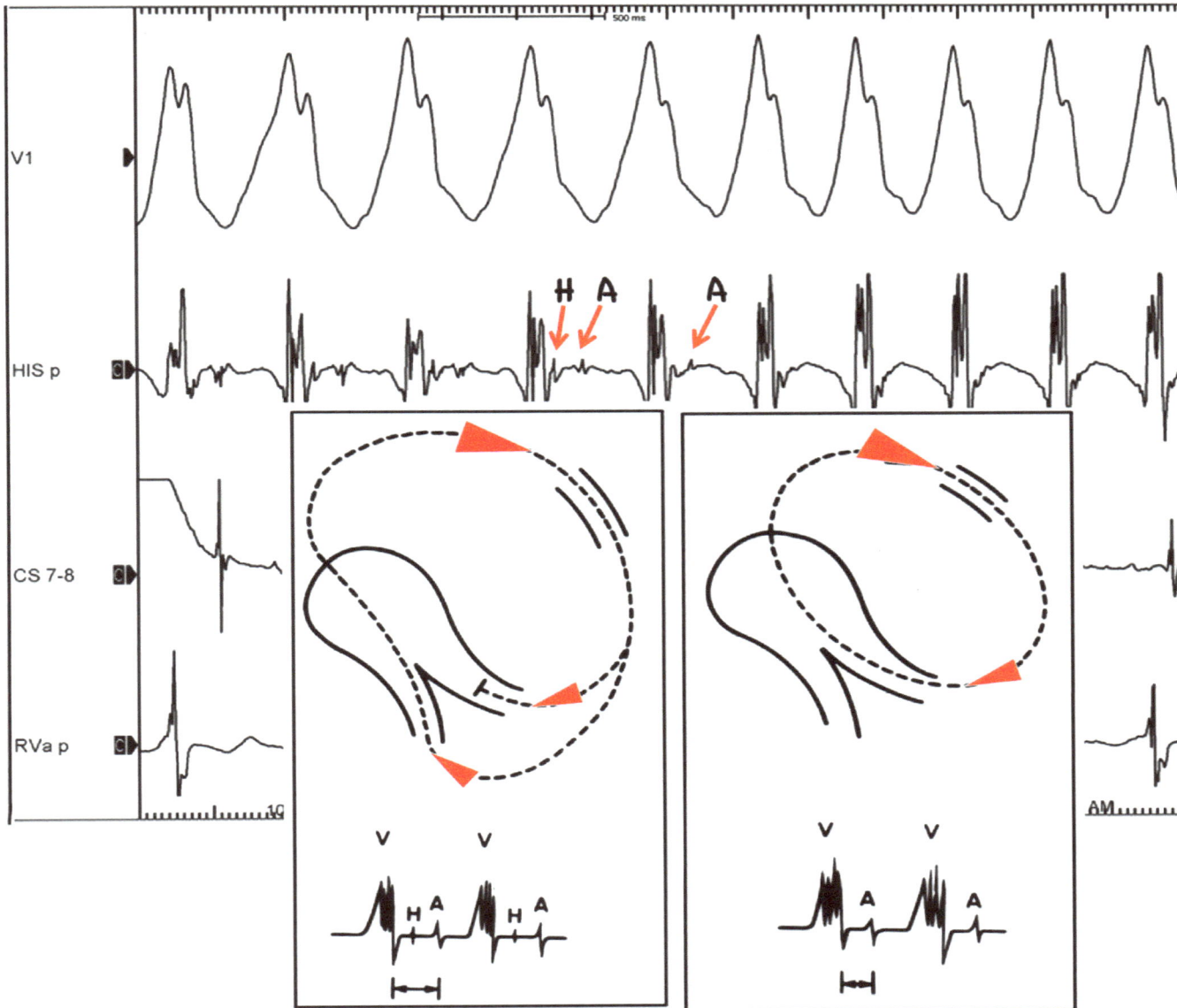

Problem 4.5

The patient originally had WPW surgery for an anteroseptal AP about 30 years previously and was well until he developed this tachycardia (**Figure 4.5A**). The multipole catheter is positioned in our standard RA location for a tricuspid-caval isthmus ablation with the distal poles 1–2 just lateral to the isthmus and the proximal poles more septal and the presumptive diagnosis was AT. Atrial electrograms span 280 ms of the cardiac cycle of 380 ms.

This is most consistent with atrial macroreentry but is also possible with a focal tachycardia and secondary conduction slowing. Virtually all of the conduction delay is evident in the RA catheters, suggesting a right atrial origin of tachycardia. However, the tracing can't definitively distinguish a right or left atrial origin of tachycardia. This is addressed by RA overdrive pacing from the mid RA septal region (**Figure 4.5B**).

Figure 4.5A

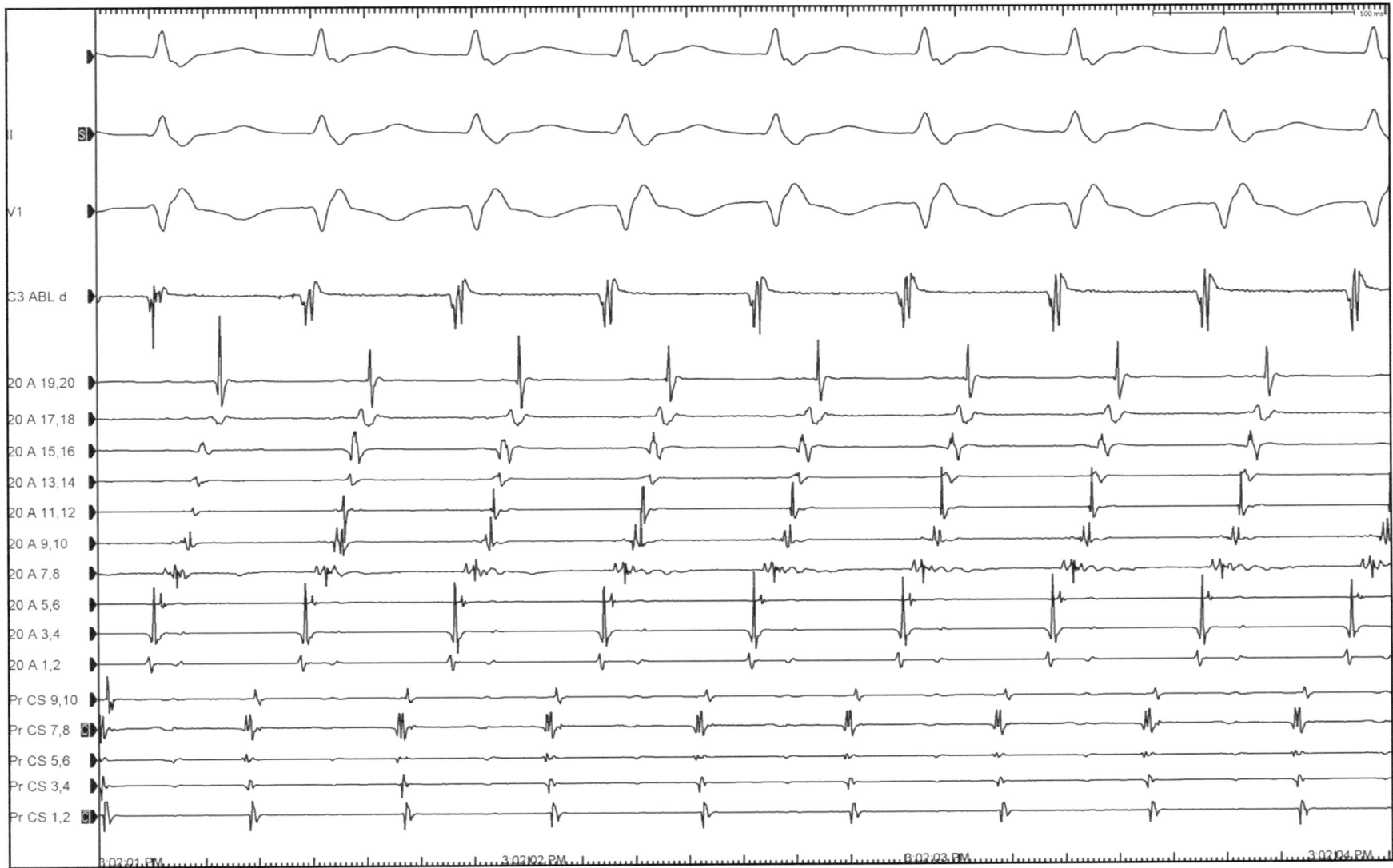

Figure 4.5B

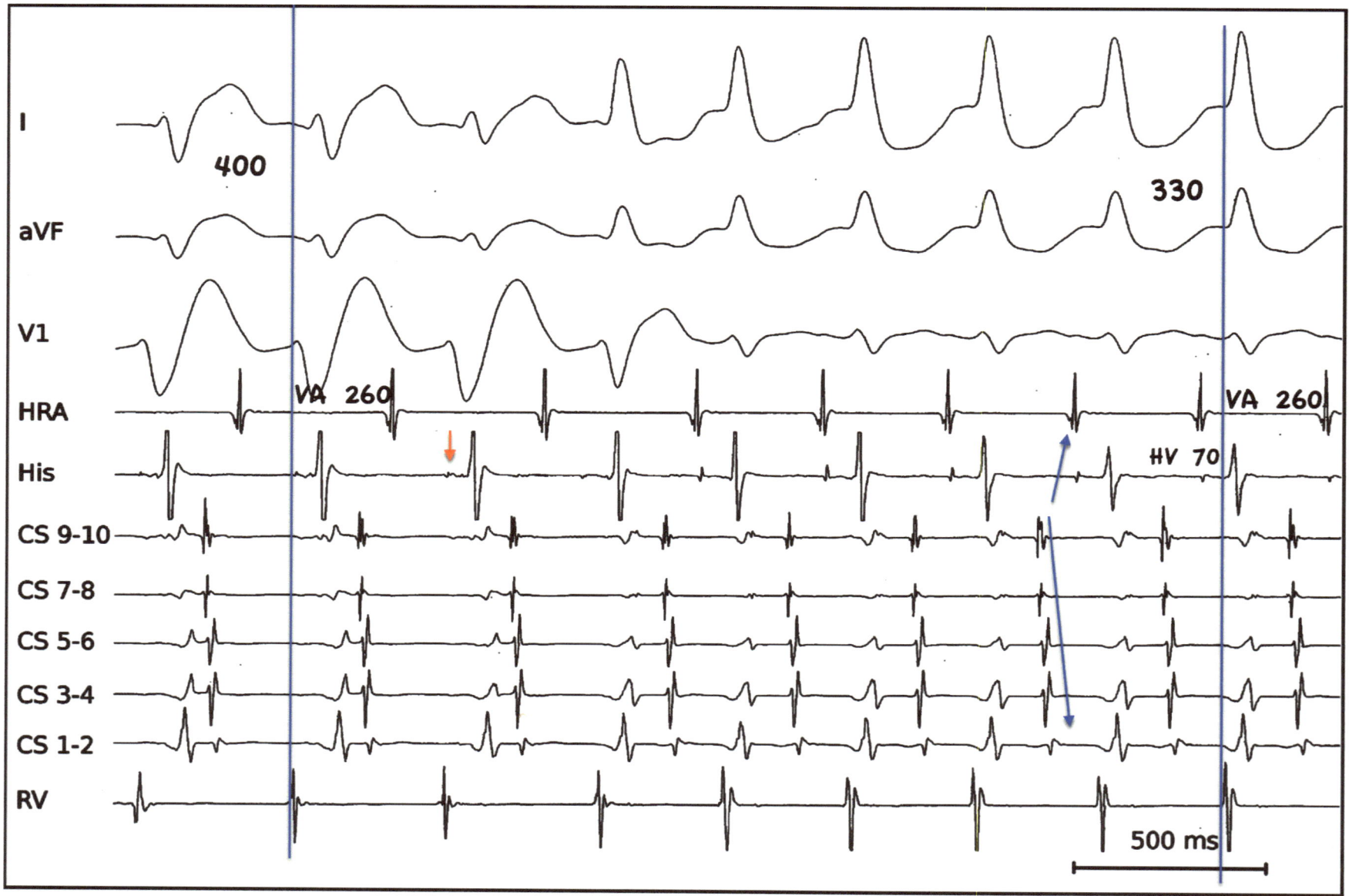

The PPI at the pacing catheter does not need fine measurement and is obviously considerably "out" of the circuit, but there is considerable more information to be gleaned from this figure.

For this we will use "classical" entrainment concepts and move to the annotated version of **Figure 4.5C**.

Figure 4.5C

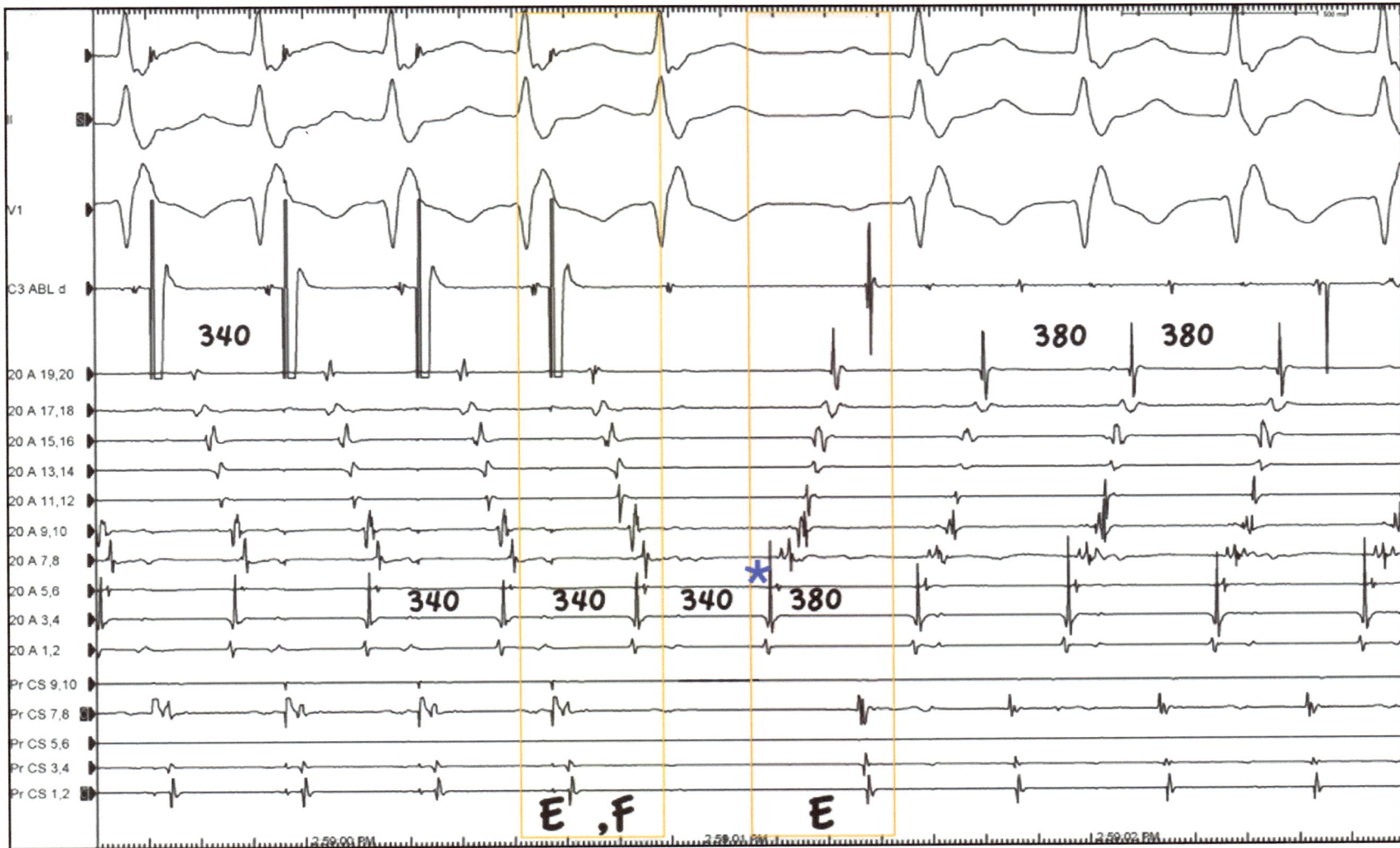

The first step after verifying that the tachycardia has been accelerated is to *identify the last atrial EGM accelerated to the CL of pacing*. This is indicated by the **blue asterisk** and informs us that this site is *still entrained* BUT no longer fusing with the paced beat. We now identify the cluster of EGMs that is the last one both fused and entrained (**F, E, yellow shading**) as well as the cluster entrained but no longer fused (**E, pink shading**). The asterisk (*) in the EGM is a long way from the pacing stimulus that has advanced it to the CL of pacing.

We also note that the fused beat has an entirely different pattern than the tachycardia beat, that is, it is mainly captured *antidromically*, also supporting the observation that the pacing site is a long way from the breakout site of the tachycardia from its slow conduction zone. Remember that "long way" means electrophysiological long way and may be close anatomically but with tremendous conduction delay to the breakout site.

Identifying the cluster of electrograms that represents the first wave breaking out of the slow conduction zone now allows us to see the "head" of the wave and we readily see that the *LA (CS electrodes) is trailing the activation and not leading it*. Knowing the region of the critical slow conduction area allows us to use our mapping systems in a more focused way and indeed "late meets early" was very close to our asterisked zone.

You may try to relate the EGMs in **Figure 4.5C** to the schematic of classical reentry with an anatomic slow conduction zone in **Figure 4.5D**. The slow conduction area is represented by the black cylinder. At a slower pacing rate, you may see more balanced fusion with a contribution of both the orthodromic wave going "against the current" of the tachycardia wave emerging from the slow conduction zone (**Fusion 1, *not* represented by our tracing**). At a faster rate, the antidromic wave has virtually taken over the circuit but has not penetrated the area around the exit site (**Fusion 2**), allowing the tachycardia to be accelerated and continued and this is reasonably what is happening in our figure. With further acceleration of the pacing rate, the slow conduction area is invaded from both directions and the tachycardia will not be present when pacing stops (broke).

Figure 4.5D

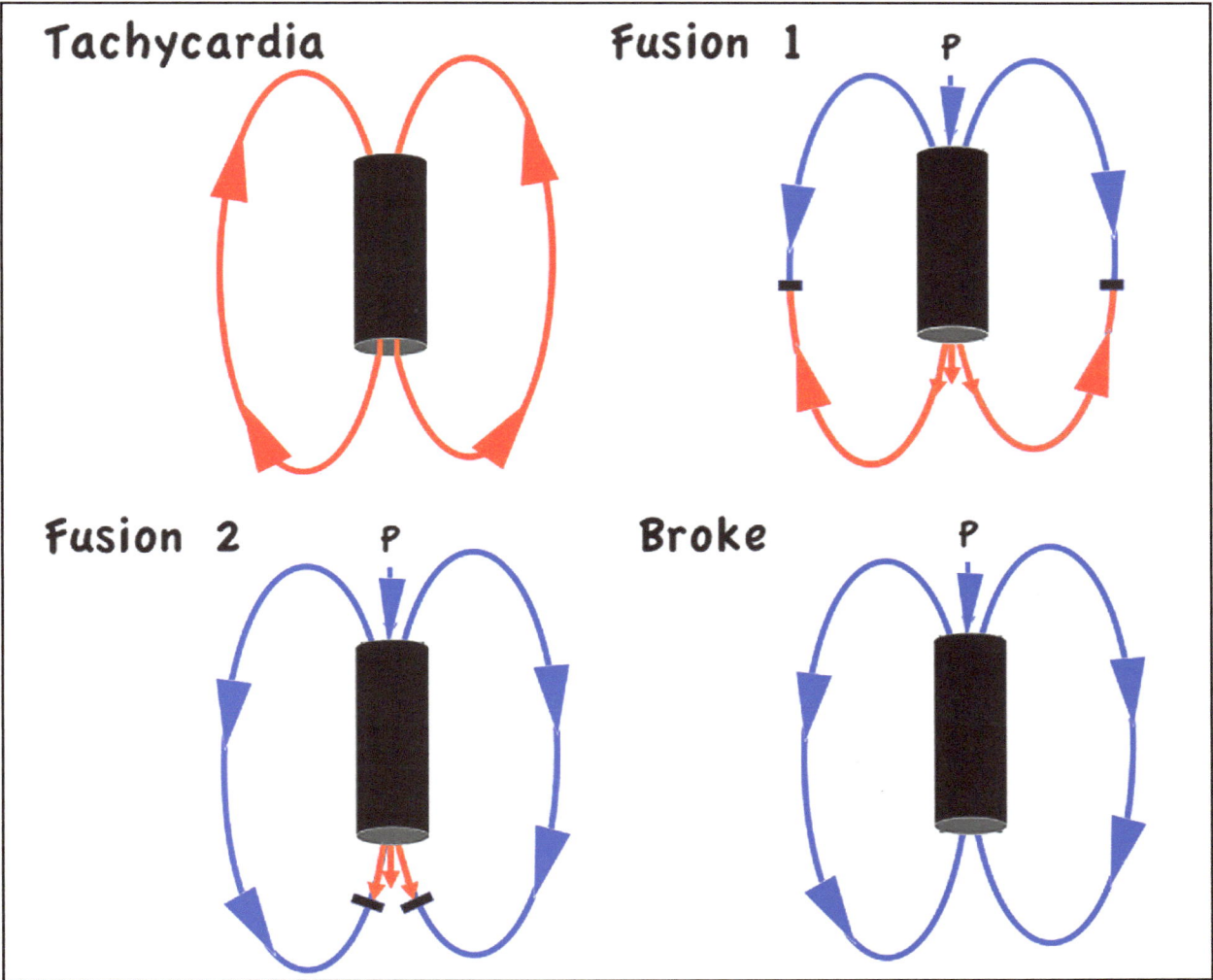

Problem 4.6

An overview of this tracing shows a relatively regular tachycardia, starting as a relatively narrow QRS tachycardia and transitioning to a WCT in the middle of the tracing. The WCT is clearly slower than the NCT, informing us that we are dealing with 2 distinct tachycardia mechanisms or at least a change in the circuit if it is one mechanism (**Figure 4.6A**).

Starting with these obvious factors, we begin to analyze. The "traditional" way is to start at the beginning and proceed to the right, beat by beat. I find it preferable to start analyzing a complex tracing by starting with something I consider the easier part of the tracing and then build on my conclusions as I move on.

Figure 4.6A

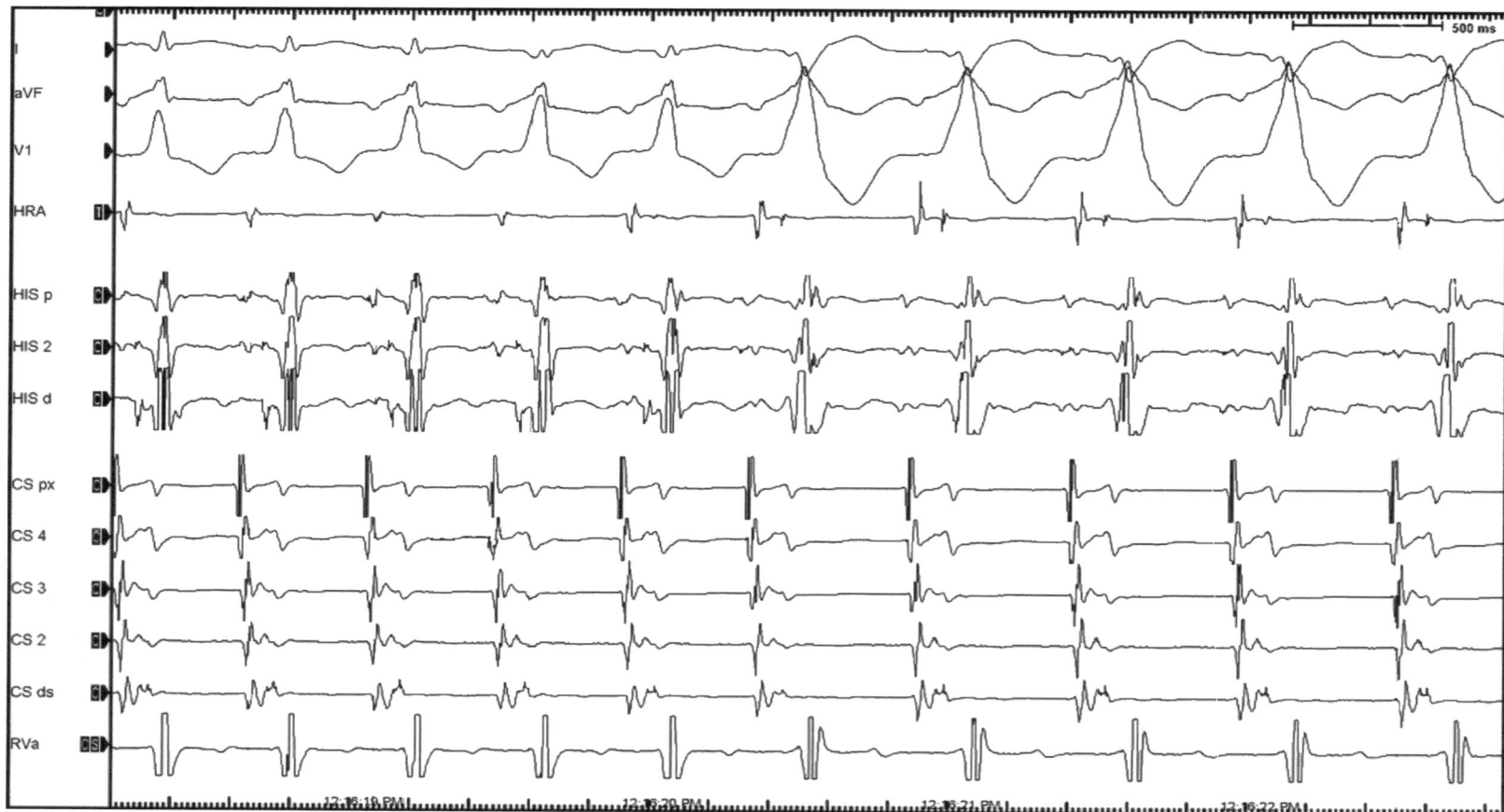

I have divided this tracing into 3 segments or zones as labeled in **Figure 4.6B**. The reader is urged to focus on one zone at a time before trying to put it all together.

I have elected to start with the WCT (zone 3), which appears relatively straightforward. The ECG leads show a QRS pattern that would not be expected with a BBB pattern and is more compatible with LV preexcitation or VT. This is verified by identifying the ventricular activation sequence (**dashed red line**), which shows ventricular activation earliest in the distal CS leads and proceeding to the RV and HB. The atrial activation sequence is "central," with the His A activated earliest (**solid red line**). *This tachycardia can only be a preexcited tachycardia or VT.*

Figure 4.6B

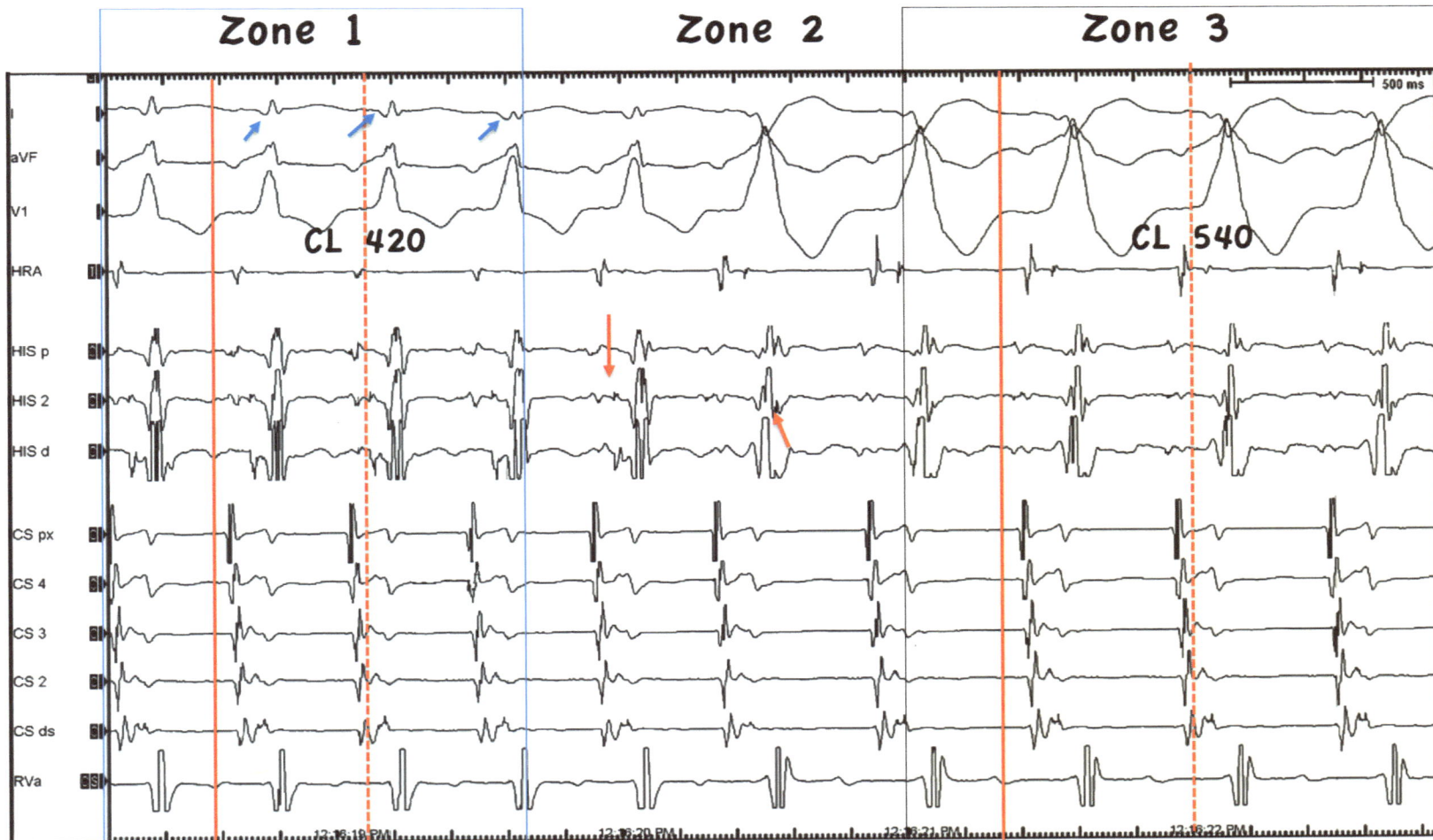

We then move on to the relatively narrow QRS tachycardia (zone 1). We note the small change in QRS morphology from beat to beat, **blue arrows**, with a tall R in V_1, definitely not normal and compatible with variable fusion. The initial QRS vector is negative in lead 1 (**from left to right**) and positive in V_1 (**back to front**) again indicating LV origin, either VT or left AP. The atrial (**solid red lines**) and ventricular activation sequences (**dashed red lines**) are noted and are essentially identical to that of the tachycardia in zone 3. The H is visible with an HV = 0 or less and this tachycardia to can only be preexcited or VT. If VT, it has to be isorhythmic with the supraventricular rhythm in zone 1, providing the slight variable fusion noted in these beats. *VT can now be reasonably eliminated from the diagnosis since the identical VT would have to have two different CL, as per zone 1 and 3. We are dealing with preexcitation over a left AP. Furthermore, the CL doesn't change in zone 1 while the fusion is* **variable***, informing us the AP is a bystander in zone 1.*

To recap before moving on to the transition, zone 1 is an SVT with a bystander left P. Zone 3 is an SVT with anterograde conduction over the same left AP (identical ventricular activation).

We move on to the transition zone 2 and note an abrupt transition to the WCT with a longer CL. The following is the question I always ask myself during these abrupt transitions, namely which electrogram indicates the change first, *i.e., who moves first?* The *first event in our transition is loss of the His EGM,* which subsequently reappears after the first WCT beat (**red arrows**). This key observation informs us that the AVN *must be part of the circuit* since block in the AVN changed the tachycardia. This transition effectively excluded AT from either tachycardia. We can conclude that the atrial activation indicates the retrograde limb of each of the circuits in zones 1 and 3. This must be a slow retrograde AVN pathway since the VA prolonged with loss of the His and block in the AVN. An AP as the retrograde limb should not be affected by block in the AVN.

We have simplified a relatively complicated tracing by breaking it into zones and building on our observations as we went from zone to zone. The most probable explanation for the tracings is summarized pictorially in **Figure 4.6C**, namely atypical AVNRT with a bystander left AP on the left transitioning to antidromic SVT on the right after spontaneous anterograde block in the AVN.

Problem 4.6 is based on a tracing, compliments of Dr. Hongshen Guo and Dr. Arjun Sharma.

Figure 4.6C

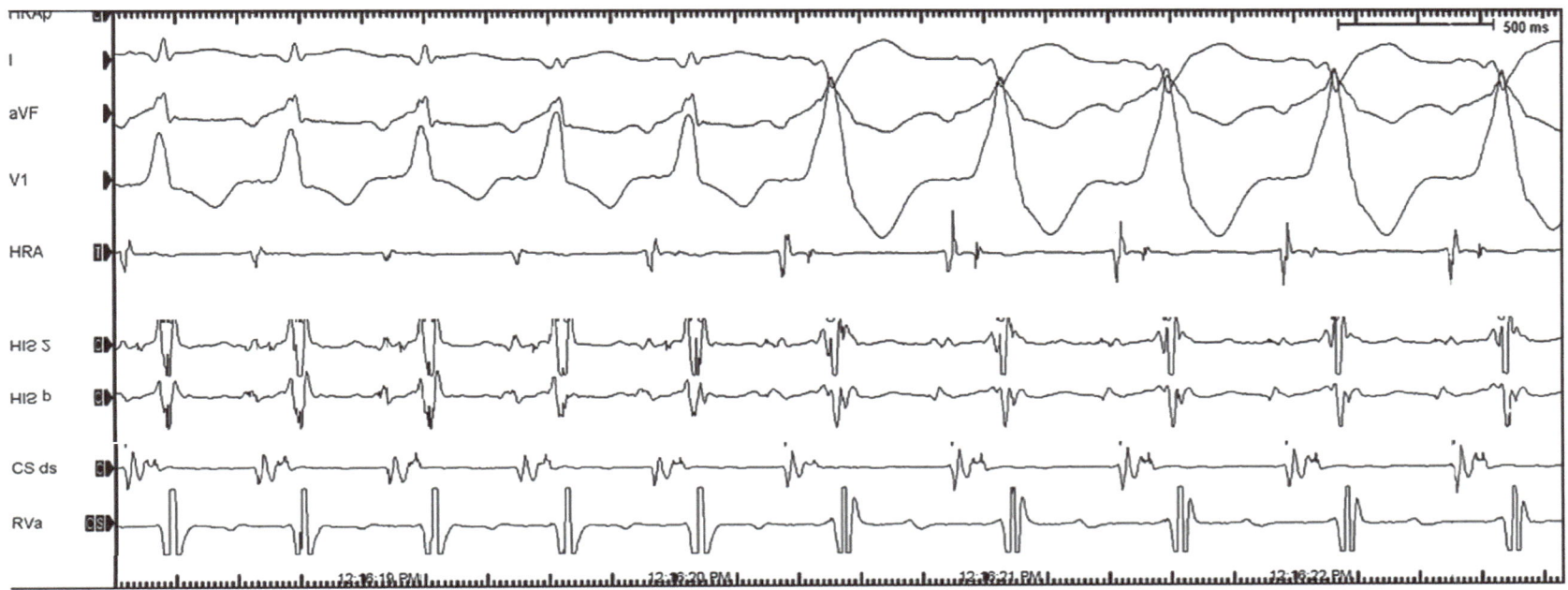

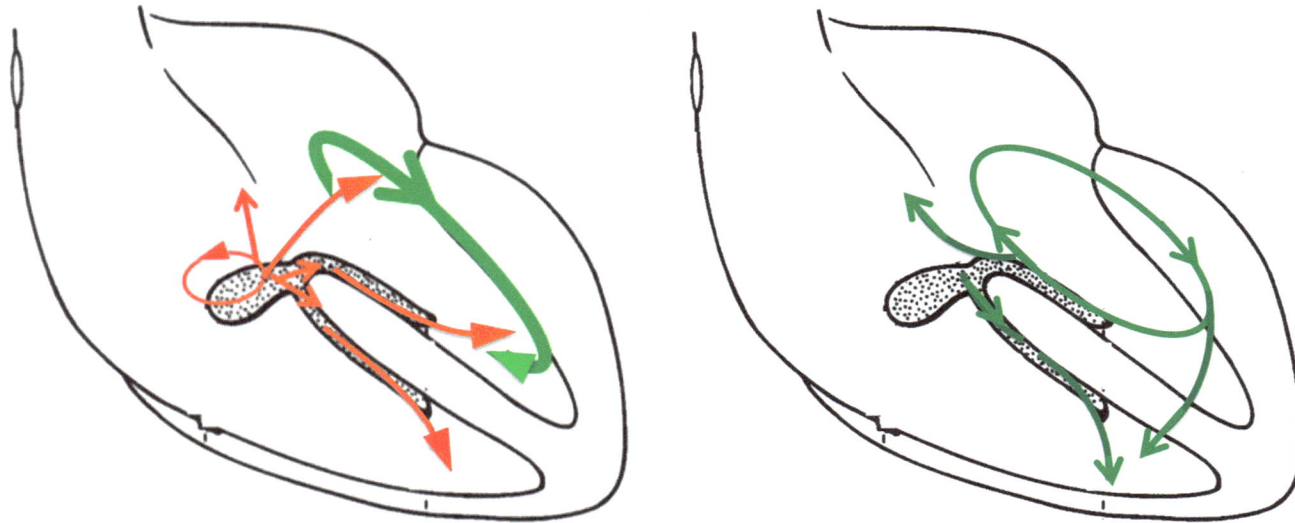

Problem 4.7

The tracing, **Figure 4.7A**, is broadly framed as a WCT with an apparent seamless transition to a NCT. The WCT has alternating long and short cycles while the NCT is relatively regular after the first 2 cycles. *A fundamental initial question in such a tracing is whether we are dealing with one tachycardia or 2 tachycardias.* By 2 tachycardias, I mean either entirely different or at least changing a component of the circuit to create a new one. The CL is obviously different, so we are dealing with the latter. As with previous examples, this tracing lends itself to being divided into 3 zones, a WCT zone, a NCT zone, and the transition.

Figure 4.7A

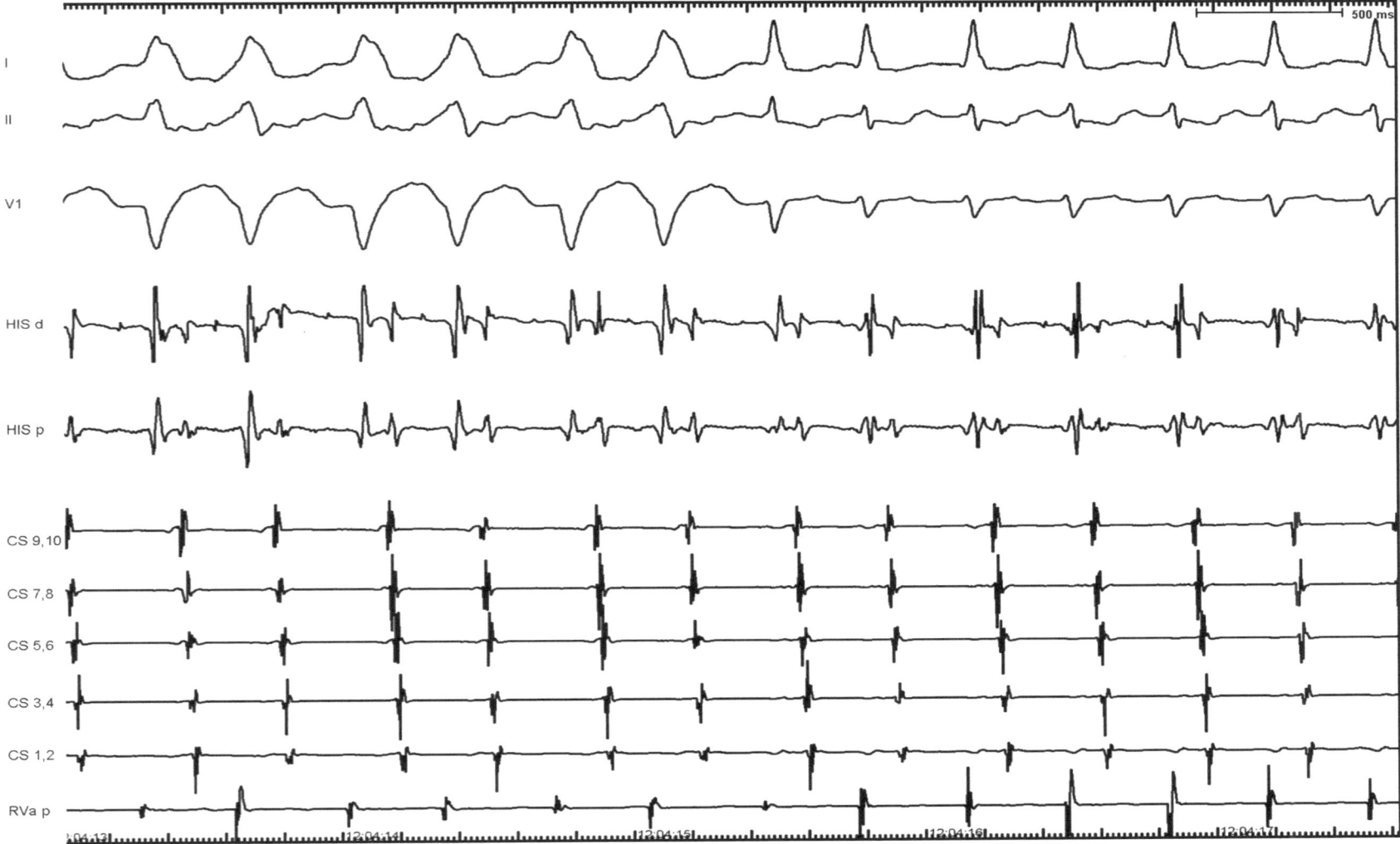

Try to focus on one zone at a time in the annotated version (**Figure 4.7B**) as if it were in isolation. Start with one that looks most straightforward to you and then build on your conclusions. We will start on the narrow QRS zone at the end of the tracing. The CL stabilizes at 340 ms. The onset of QRS is indicated by the **red line** and earliest A is indicated by the **blue line**. The HV is normal and the VA interval is constant. Atrial activation is central (septal) with earliest activation in the CS orifice (**CS 9–10**) and the HB atrial activation slightly later. The VA interval at the HB EGM is 135 ms.

At this point, the differential diagnosis includes the usual range of SVT mechanisms. We are drawn to the CL change at the onset where the CL increases from 310 to 360 abruptly. The change in the HH interval precedes change both in the VV interval and also the AA interval (VA remains linked). This indicates that the AH is part of the circuit, i.e., prolongation of the AH prolongs the next QRS. AT is definitively excluded.

The NCT is then either AVRT or AVNRT (atypical by definition).

Figure 4.7B

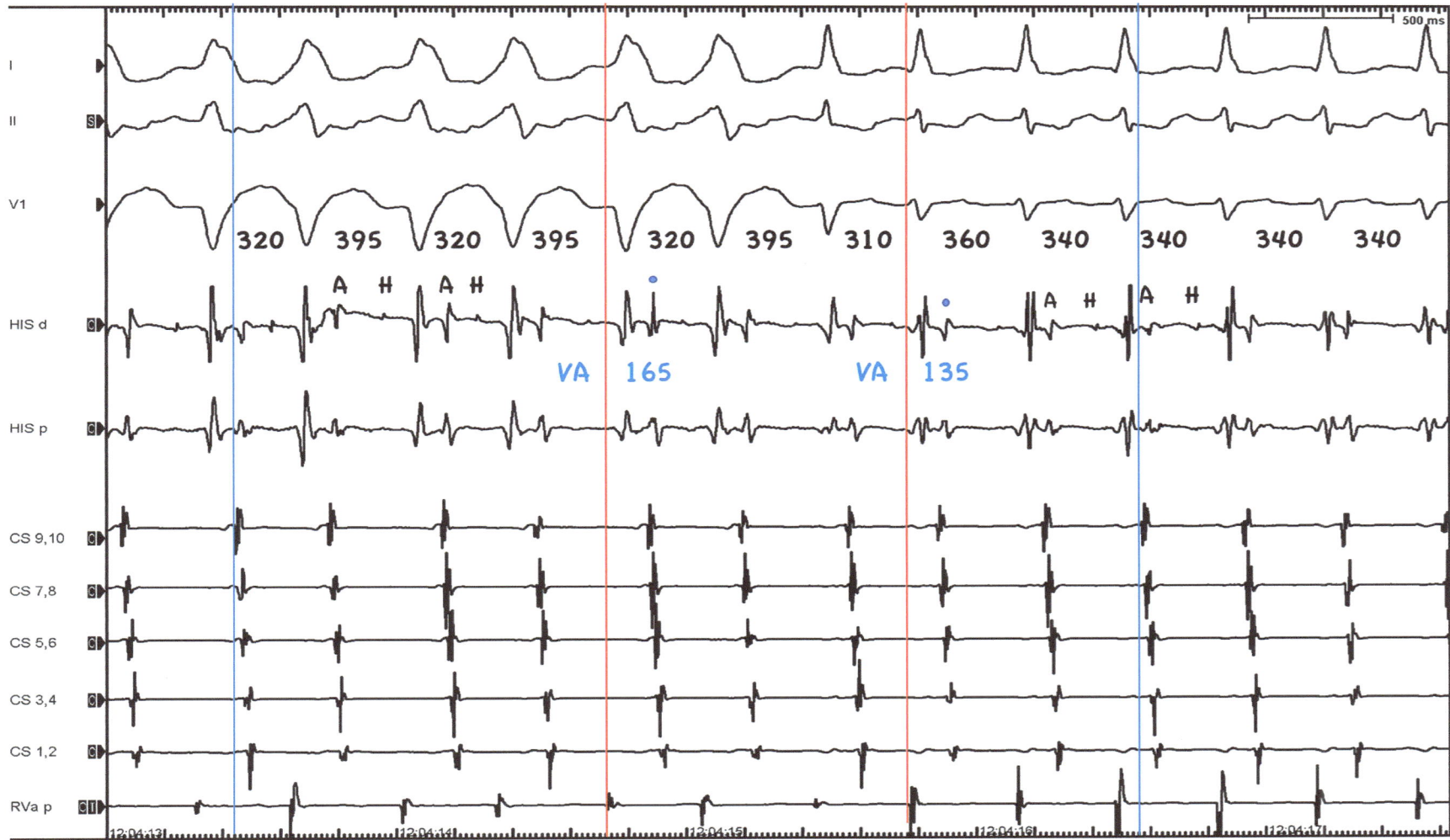

We then move over to the WCT zone. The QRS morphology is relatively typical for LBBB and earliest ventricular depolarization occurs at the RV apex and the HV is in the normal range, all of this making LBBB aberrancy a safe bet. We note that the alternation of CL is related to alternation in the AH interval, indicating that the AV node must be part of the circuit, again ruling out AT.

We are still left with a diagnosis of either AVRT or AVNRT for the WCT and can move over to the transition zone, which I have enlarged for clarity (**Figure 4.7C**).

At any transition, the key task is to identify the EGM that moves or changes first. In this example, you observe that the H, RV apex, and *onset* of QRS are not perturbed just prior to the transition but the initial event that is evident is the normalization of the QRS (resolution of LBBB). This results in shortening of the VA interval. Thus, the *LBB must be part of the circuit*, ruling out AVNRT. Restoration of the LBB allows the AVRT circuit to become shorter. This is obvious when you examine the relationship in a diagram, **Figure 4.7D**. The AVRT circuit with a left lateral AP includes the LBB. Consequently, LBBB forces a larger circuit via the RBB.

We can conclude by saying our tachycardia is AVRT over a left AP as the retrograde limb, with and without LBBB aberrancy. The AP is relatively close to the septum, resulting in earliest atrial activation relatively central and VA change of only 30 ms.

Figure 4.7C

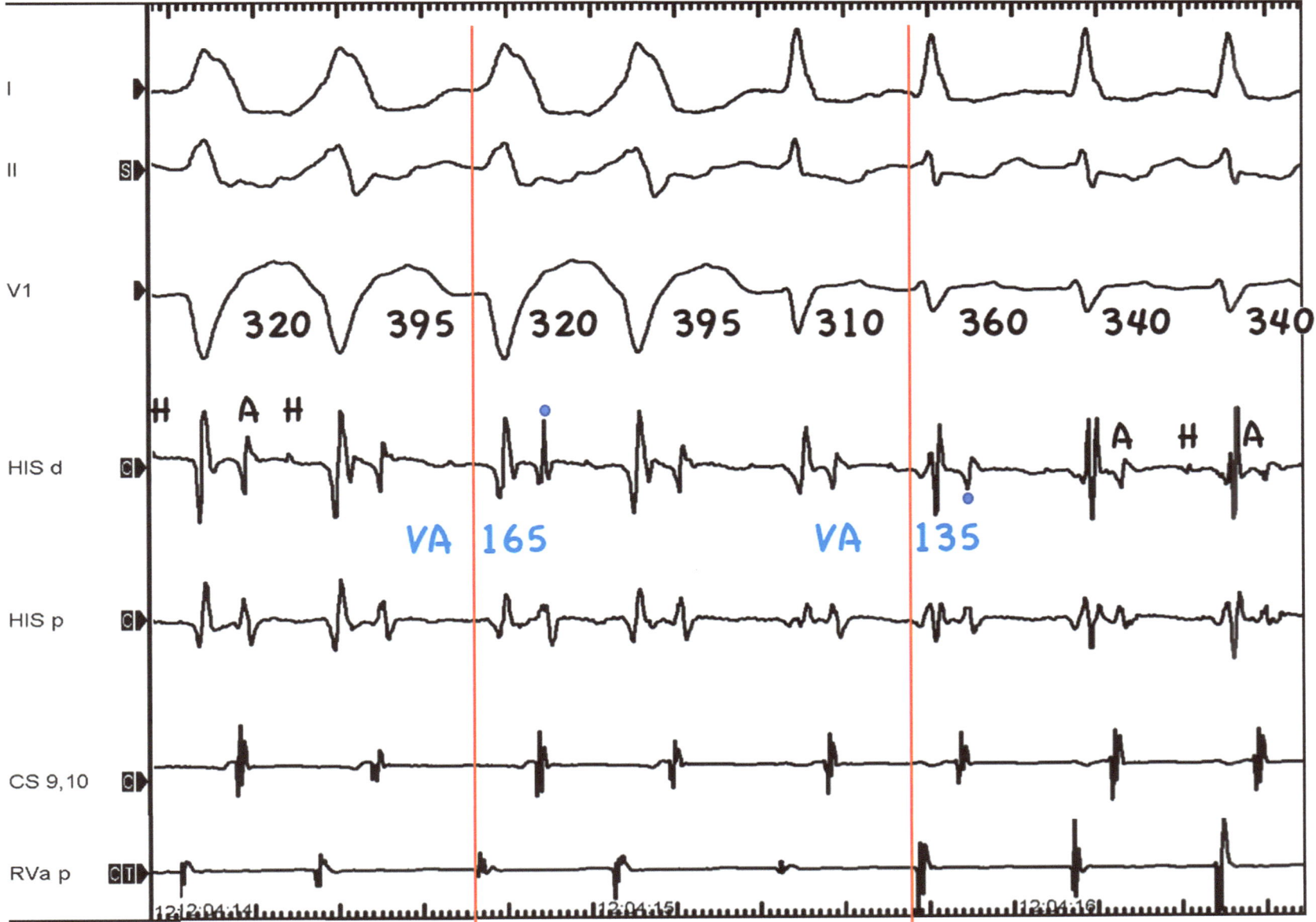

Figure 4.7D

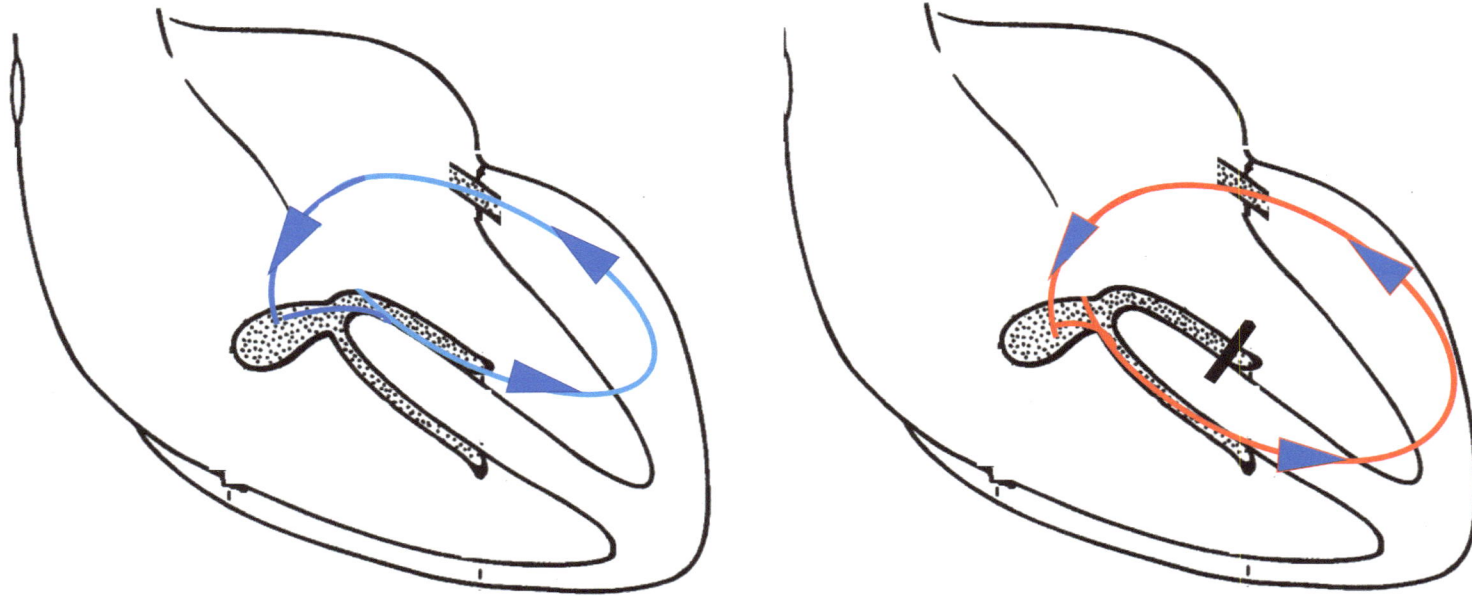

Chapter 5

Transition Zones: Importance of the Onset and Termination of Tachycardia

Problem 5.1

Figure 5.1A should not be difficult for most readers but does illustrate some important principles. The question posed is the mechanism of the WCT, which can reasonably be SVT, VT, or preexcited SVT. Which mental "tools" will help?

The QRS morphology is not really helpful in this 3-channel rhythm strip. Atrial activity can be reasonably guessed at, but even if seen, may not distinguish whether it is the driver of tachycardia or the result of retrograde conduction from VT.

The first beat of the WCT is different and arguably a "fusion" beat of sinus and ventricular. One must be very cautious with "intermediate" beats as fusion may be difficult to distinguish from "incomplete" bundle branch block aberration.

Figure 5.1A

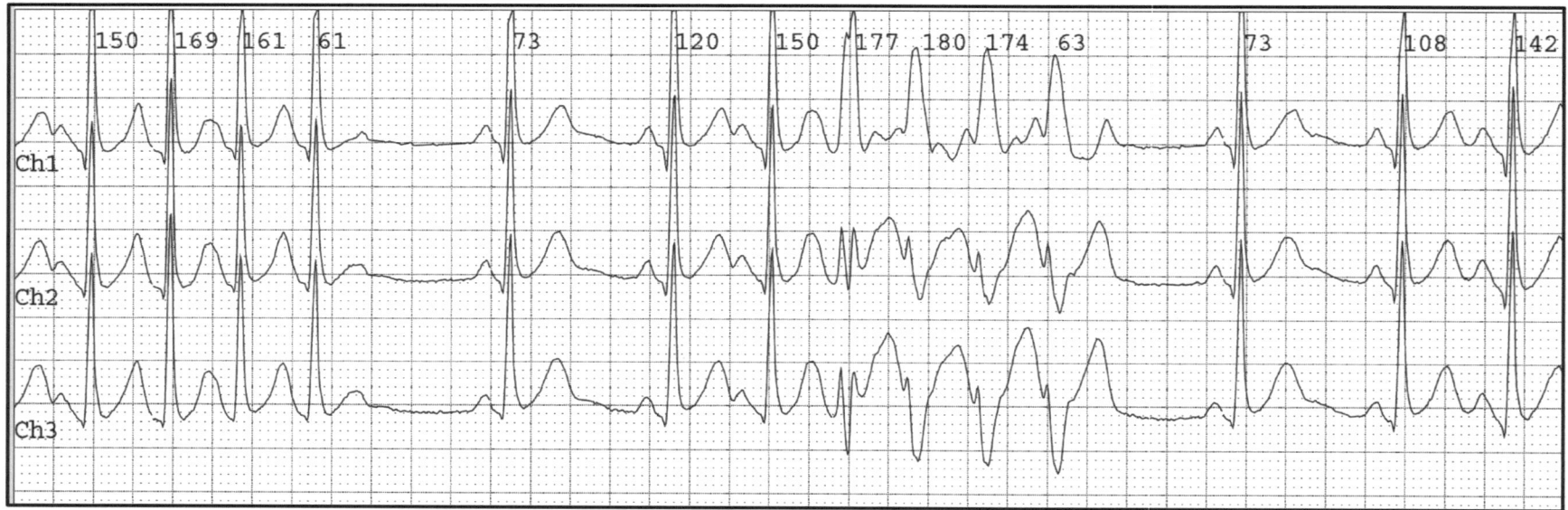

An overview at this point makes it obvious that there are 2 brief runs of tachycardia, one narrow QRS and one WCT. Running the calipers through the tracing shows a very similar if not identical CL for the 2 tachycardias (**Figure 5.1B**). This of course makes it highly probable that they share a mechanism, either SVT with and without aberrancy or SVT with and without a bystander AP.

Figure 5.1B

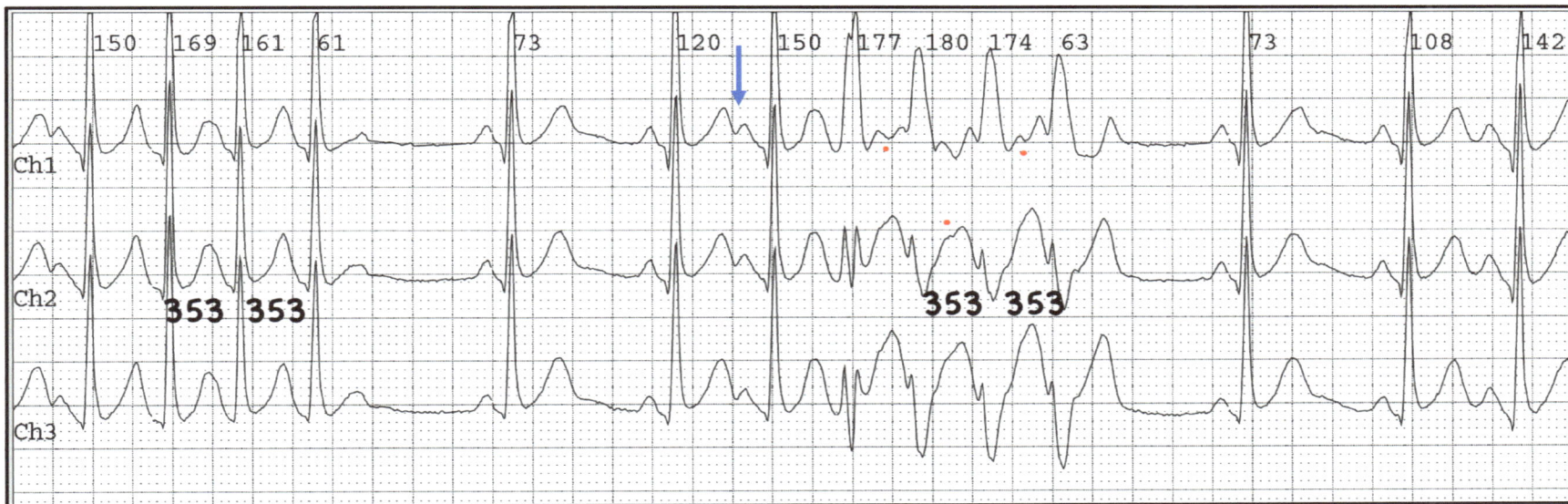

If we examine the onset of the WCT, we observe that it begins with a PAC (**arrow**). This would be highly unusual for VT. In addition, the PAC would in general show some degree of preexcitation at this coupling interval if an AP was present but in the final analysis, we have not ruled out SVT with a bystander AP. The latter, of course, would be statistically considerably less likely than SVT with aberration.

Lastly, I believe I see P waves (admittedly not a bulletproof observation) during the WCT (**red dots**) but NOT after the last WCT cycle. This is also against the diagnosis of VT, which would not be expected to terminate and coincidentally block to the atrium.

All of this makes it "highly probable" that WCT is SVT with aberrancy. Our "tools" consisted of running through the tracing with calipers (measurement), enlarging the area of interest (the WCT) to look for P waves, paying attention to ALL of the tracing and focusing especially on the onset and termination of tachycardia.

Problem 5.2

This problem is readily framed as a WCT with LBBB pattern. An overview of **Figure 5.2A** quickly narrows the problem such that it can be reframed *as WCT with AV dissociation*. This now reduces the universe of possibilities to all tachycardias that don't require the atrium, namely VT, AVNRT, or NVT. A putative His deflection is seen close to mid-diastole for most cycles, but this is not too helpful in distinguishing our candidate diagnoses.

Figure 5.2A

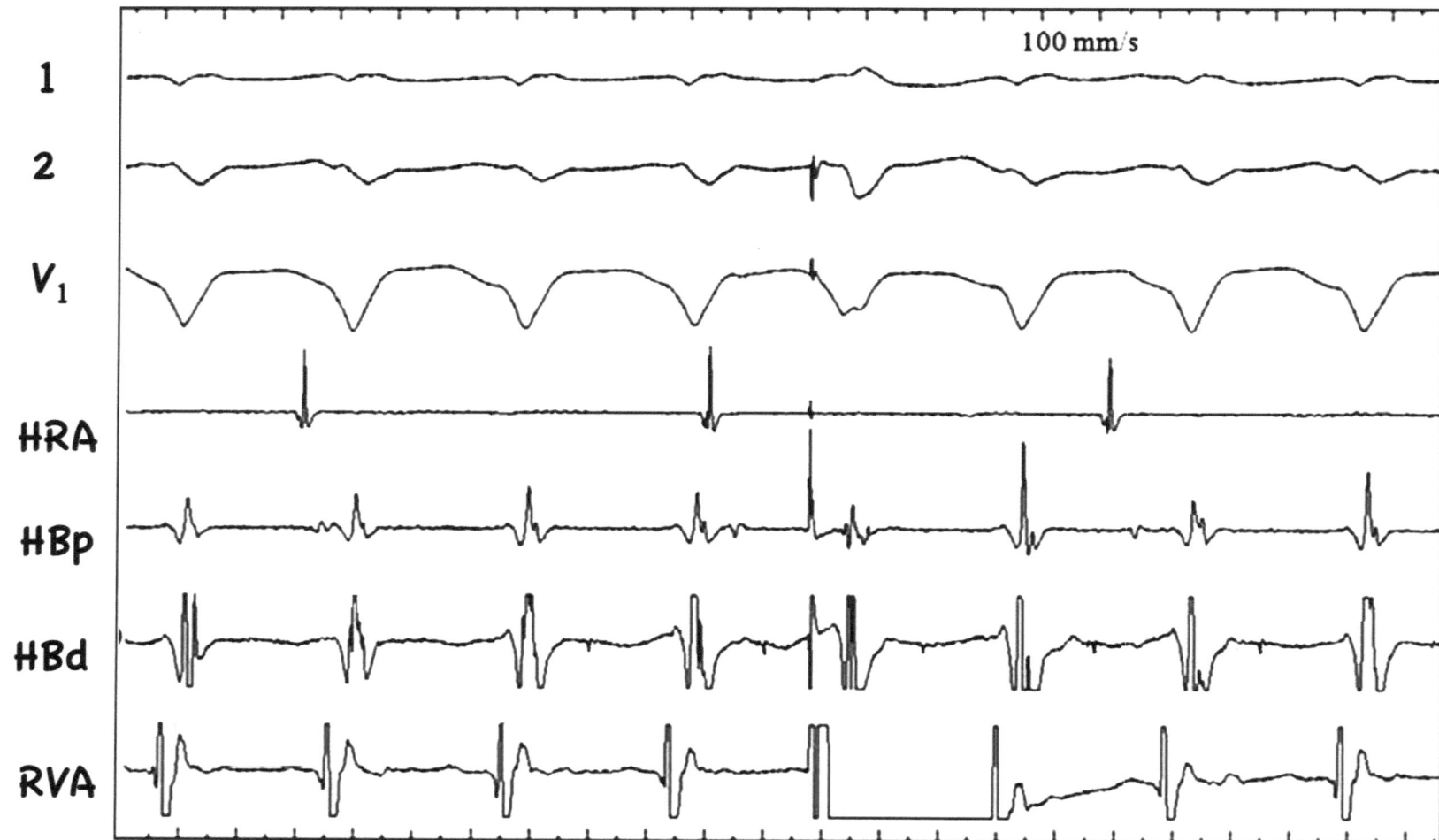

We move on to the PVC programmed into the latter third of the cardiac cycle during tachycardia (**Figure 5.2B**). Moving our calipers over V_1, we note that the VT cycle after the PVC has been advanced (**red arrow**), i.e., the tachycardia has been "reset."

We note further that the PVC is only about 40 ms premature to the expected cycle so that it is most probably also fused. This was verified readily by comparing the allegedly fused QRS to the pure paced QRS and they were indeed different (**not shown**).

Figure 5.2B

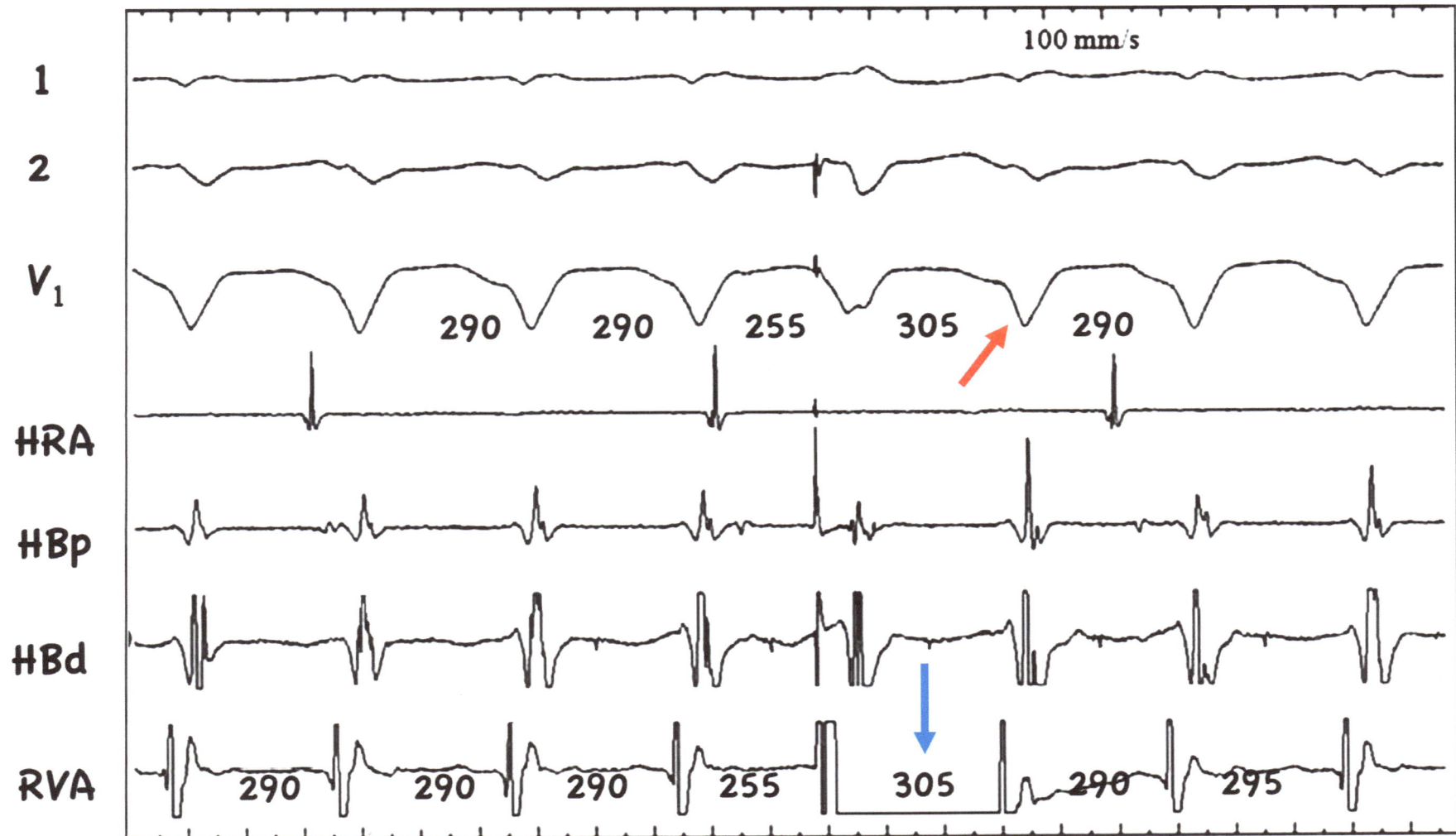

It is thus established that we have "fusion and reset," i.e., the tachycardia has been entrained for one cycle. We now note that the PPI is 305 ms, providing a PPI–TCL of only 15 ms. We have thus proved that the RV is "in" the circuit, ruling out AVNRT. This leaves only VT and the significantly more uncommon NVT as mechanisms.

A fortuitous PVC helps our cause (**Figure 5.2C**). A few observations can be made from a rapid overview as follows:

1. The PVC breaks the tachycardia
2. The PVC that breaks the tachycardia is quite late coupled and relatively narrow, most probably fused.
3. The His deflection can now be confidently identified. The HV is quite long, both during tachycardia and in the normal cycle after it breaks.

Figure 5.2C

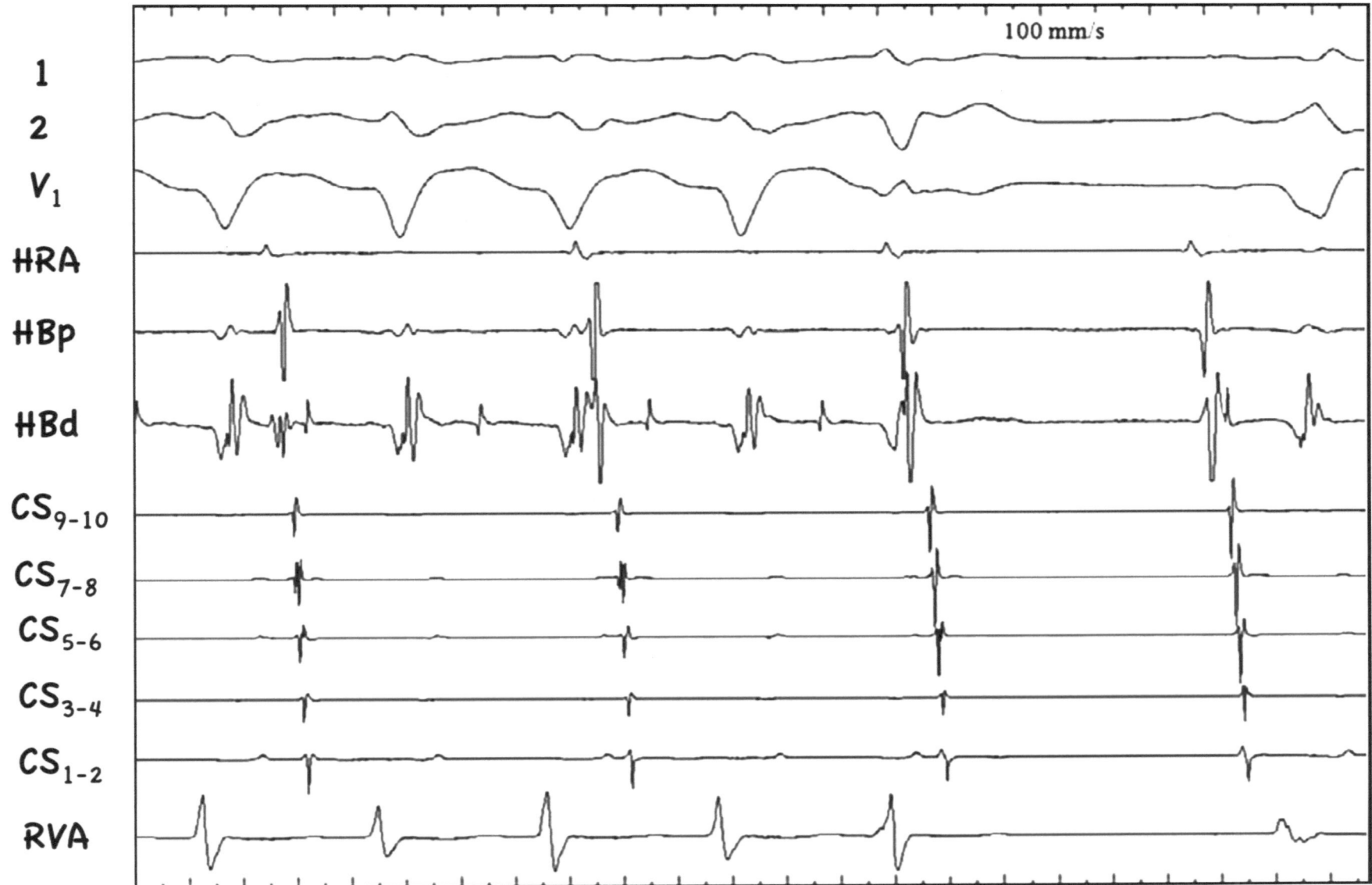

Moving on to more detailed measurements (**Figure 5.2D**) and running our calipers along the RV EGM, we note that the PVC as judged by the beginning of the far-field component of the EGM (**blue arrow**) is only 25 ms premature to the anticipated arrival of the next QRS and the terminal part of the RV EGM has not changed at all (**red vertical bars**). We have verified fusion even by looking at this one EGM.

Figure 5.2D

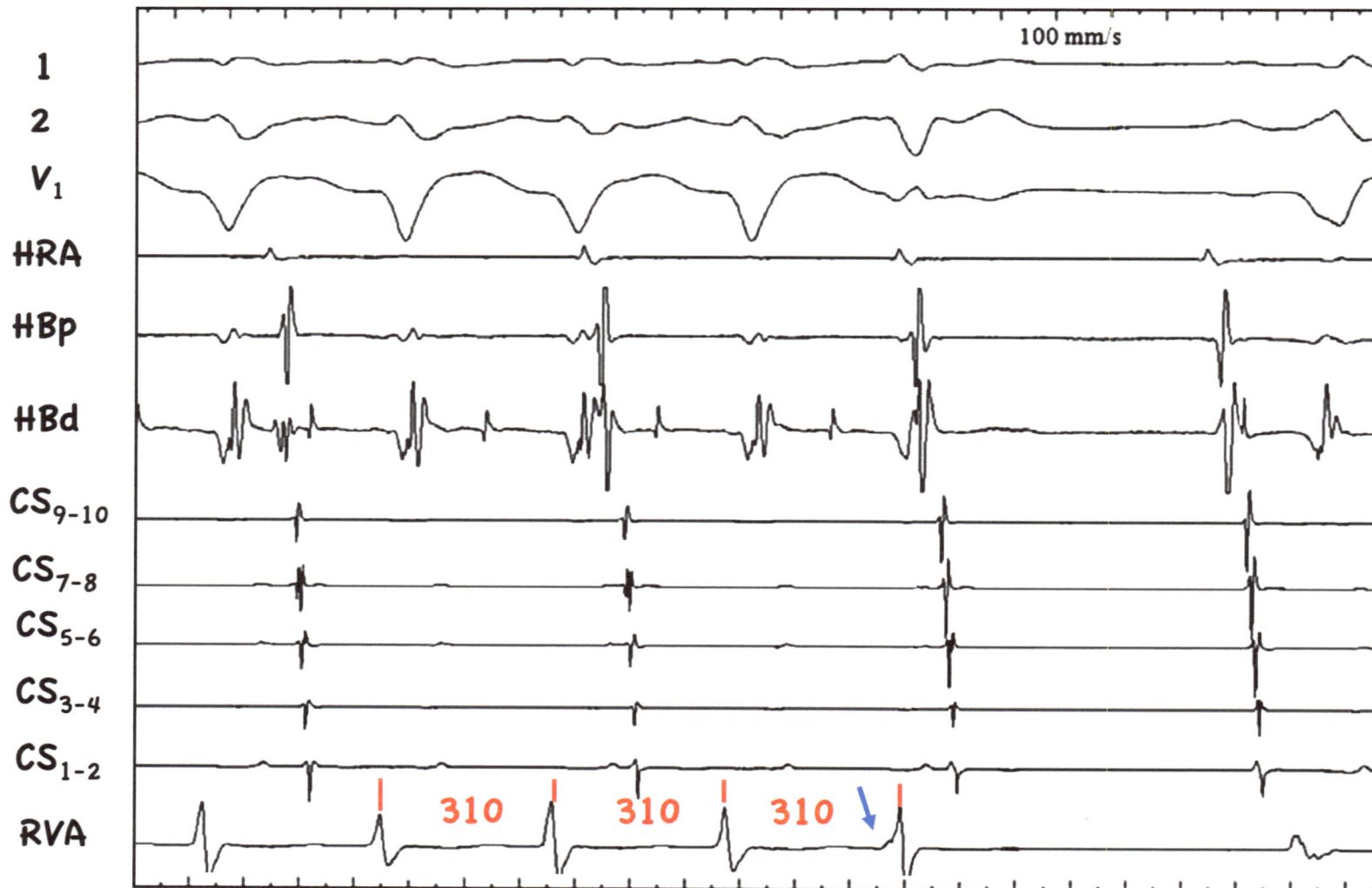

We now appreciate that the PVC has very close access to the excitable gap of the circuit and terminates the tachycardia. This PVC tends to "normalize" the LBBB QRS and must be coming from the LV. We can now reasonably conclude that the LV must be "in," i.e., part of the circuit.

Now we reframe our problem yet again to find a scenario where each of the RV and LV are within the circuit, and this provides a short list (see "Tachycardia with Both RV and LV "in"

the Circuit" in Chapter 8). This can only be either BBR VT or the much less common NV reentry utilizing a left NV pathway as the retrograde part of the circuit and coming out the RBB. The long HV both in tachycardia and SR and the relative prevalence of the 2 possibilities leads us to a diagnosis of BBR.

Case details are compliments of Dr. S. Bagga, while in the laboratory of Dr. E. N. Prystowsky.

Problem 5.3

The Holter strip in **Figure 5.3A** is readily described as a "slow" SVT with no obvious P wave and ending in spontaneous termination. The tracing is free of noise and artifact, and the QRS in sinus rhythm (SR) is unremarkable.

Figure 5.3A

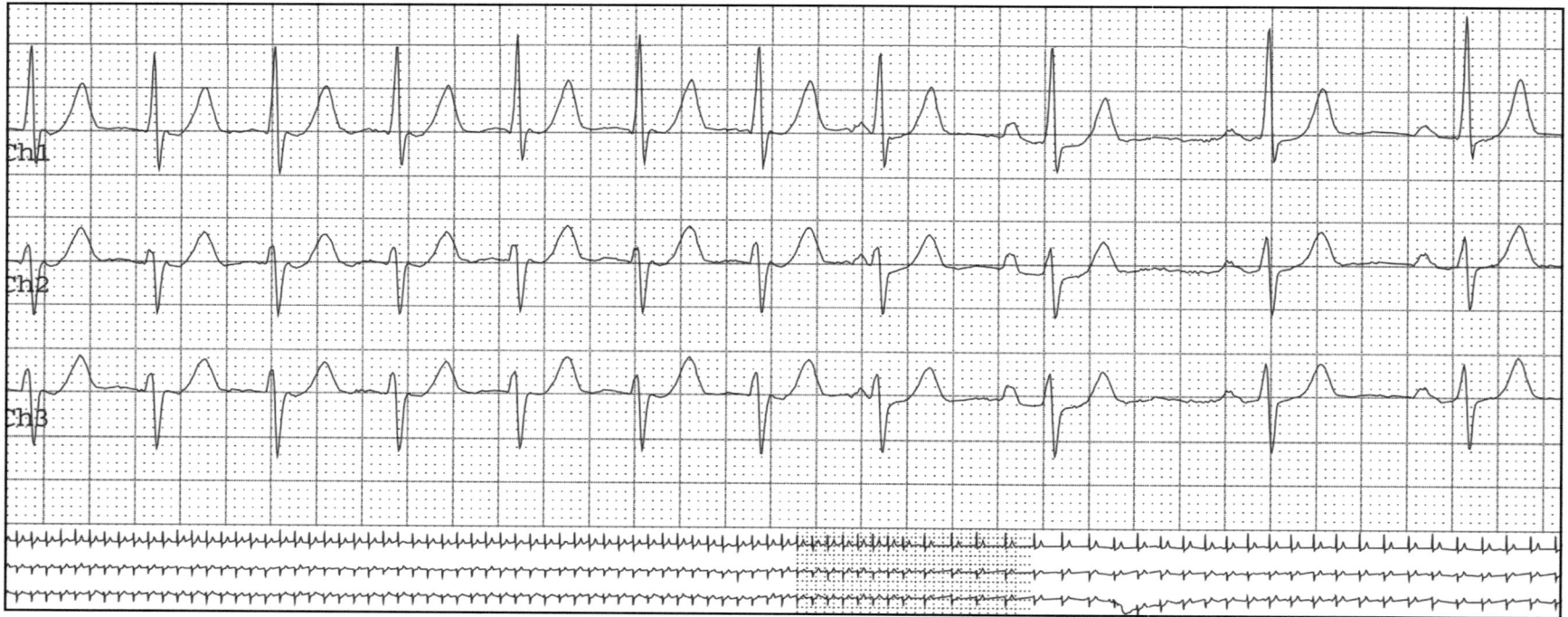

We then turn to the tachycardia (**Figure 5.3B**) and note that the tachycardia is clock regular with no obvious P wave. A relatively slow SVT with no obvious P wave over a long diastolic interval immediately suggests the presence of a slow anterograde AVN pathway, all things being equal.

The next step, when atrial activity is not readily apparent, is a very deliberate side-by-side comparison with the available ECG of sinus rhythm to help identify the "hiding" P wave. When this is done, a deflection is observed simultaneously with the end of QRS during SVT that is not present in SR (**red circles**), a P wave in all probability.

Figure 5.3B

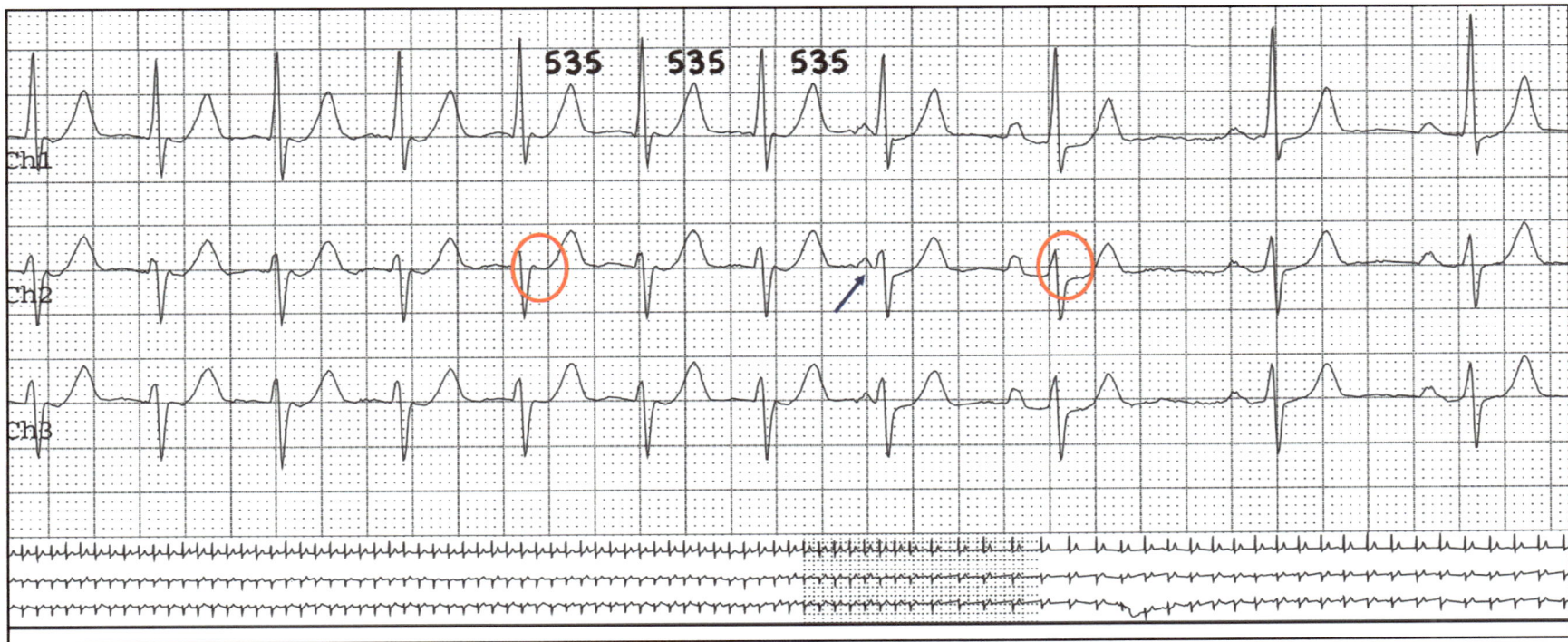

We now "reframe" our problem more specifically as SVT with a very short RP interval ("P on QRS") that can only be AVNRT, AT over a SP, JT, or rarely a nodoventricular tachycardia (see Chapter 8).

It is difficult to miss the P wave immediately prior to the last QRS of the tachycardia (**blue arrow**) and it seems highly likely this has something to do with the termination of SVT.

Our next task ("tool") is to look at the potential mechanisms on our list to see how well each fits with this pivotal observation.

AVN reentry might be stopped by a premature atrial contraction (PAC) or sinus capture beat that invades the retrograde AVN pathway and terminates reentry. Alternatively, the PAC may start to conduct over the slow pathway after it is has recovered excitability in late diastole only to block completely in the SP due to its prematurity. Thus, AVNRT fits well to explain the observation.

Nodoventricular tachycardia (anterograde conduction over a slow AVN pathway and retrograde over a nodoventricular AP) might be expected to terminate in this manner and is not ruled out by the observation.

Junctional tachycardia is unequivocally ruled out. The P wave that arrives when the QRS immediately in front of it is committed and on time. The P wave would encounter a refractory His bundle, depolarized just before the arrival of the P wave.

AT is possible, but it would seem a stretch for such a late-coupled sinus capture beat to terminate an AT. Nonetheless, AVN reentry fits well and would be the most prevalent diagnosis by far on statistical grounds alone, making it our preferred diagnosis.

Problem 5.4

The tracing in **Figure 5.4A** was obtained nearly at the beginning of the diagnostic study and was the first arrhythmia induced in this young individual with recurrent PSVT. With the safe assumption that these two beats will be the same as those induced subsequently and compatible with the clinical tachycardia, what else is required before a firm diagnosis is made?

Figure 5.4A

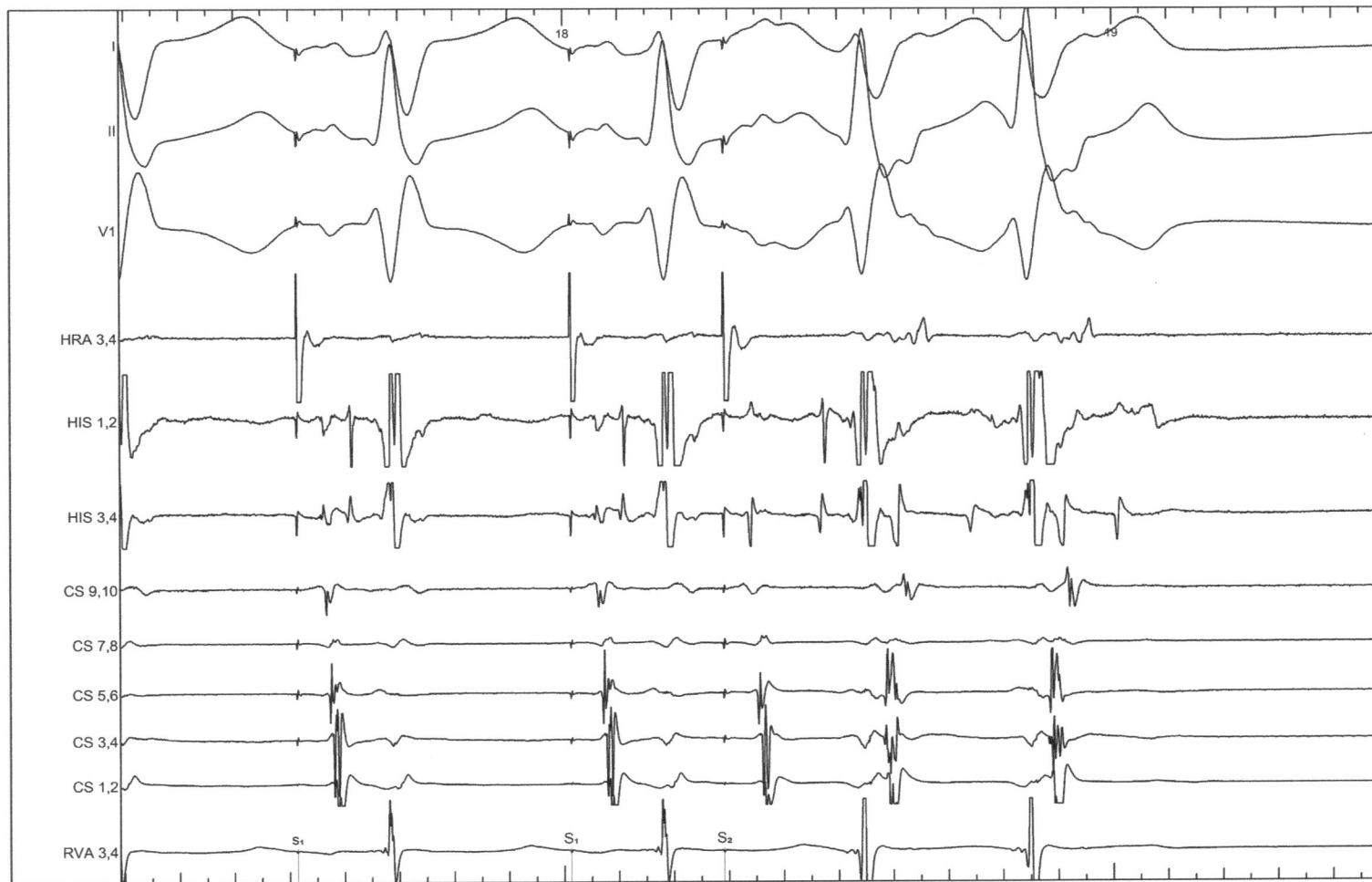

Figure 5.4B

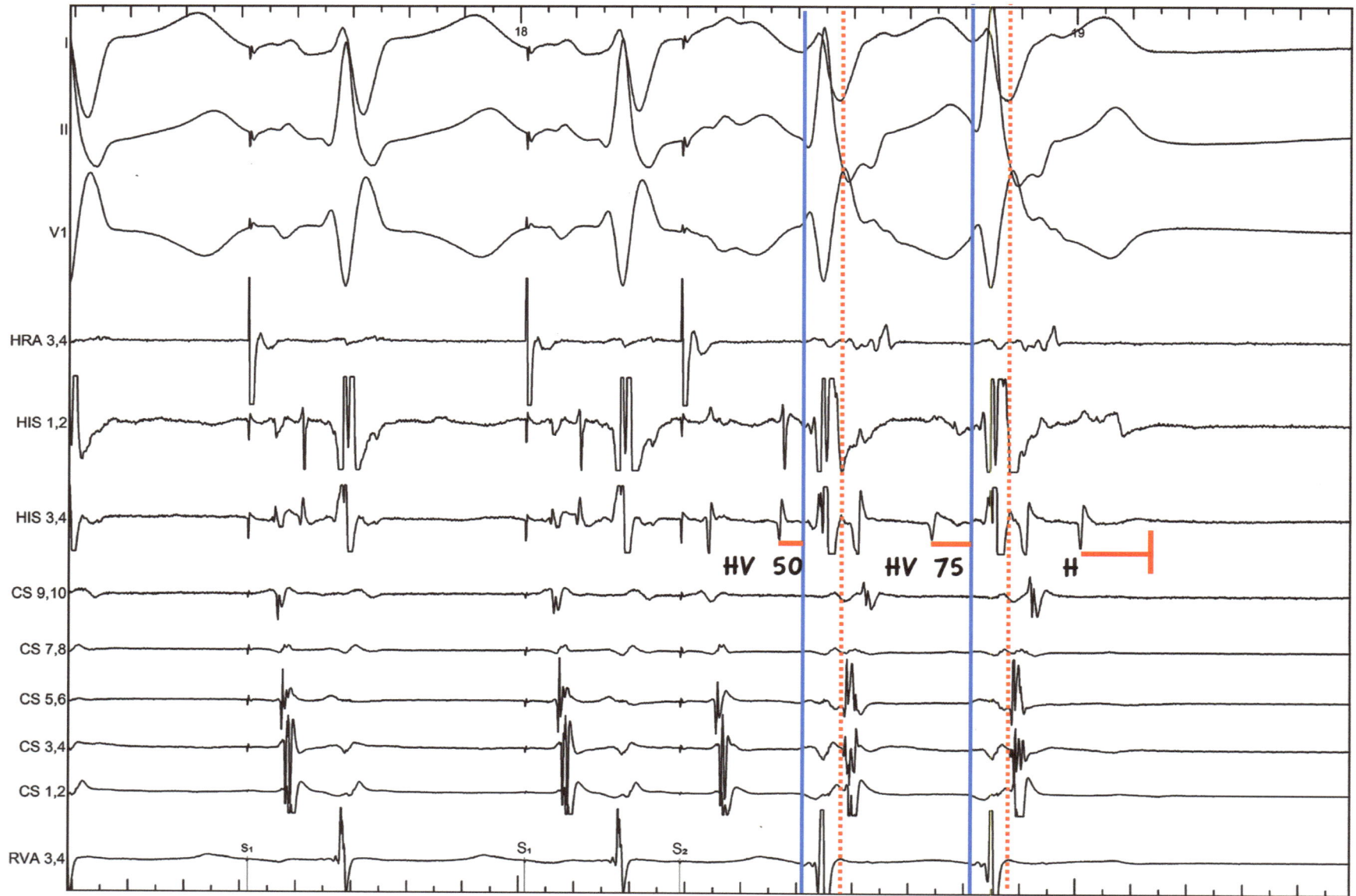

We note that the cycles after S1 show a normal AH and HV interval and the QRS shows RBBB that was preexisting. The extrastimulus S2 prolongs the AH interval, and this is followed by a couple of echo cycles.

We can now examine (annotated version, **Figure 5.4B**) the atrial activation of the echo (**dotted red line**). Earliest activation is just inside the CS (**CS 7, 8 at the orifice**) just slightly earlier than the His A. This is compatible with a "central" activation sequence and at this point may be seen with AVNRT or AVRT.

The diagnostic information comes from the method of termination. The last event is His activation (**solid red lines**), that is, block below the His and tachycardia terminates. *The His bundle therefore must be part of the circuit*, and this, of course, rules out AVNRT.

Even before this, we note that the HV prolongs in the cycle prior to the blocked beat. Prolongation of the HV does not change the VA relationship (i.e., HV prolongation results in prolongation of the HA interval) and hence, the His must be in the circuit.

This is not the case in AVNRT, where prolongation of the HV would have no direct relationship to the timing of atrial activation. Consequently, the HA relationship would surely change, with the V delayed and the A not affected, hence shortening the apparent VA interval.

The answer to our initial question is that the essential part of the diagnostic study is already available in **Figure 5.4A**.

Problem 5.5

The tracing (**Figure 5.5A**) may be described as a WCT initiated during atrial extrastimulus testing. The WCT has a right bundle branch block (RBBB), left atriofascicular block (LAFB) pattern, and AV dissociation is evident. The broad differential diagnosis for *WCT with AV dissociation* is limited and would include only VT and SVT with aberrancy (AVNRT or NVRT are the only options with AV dissociation). Many of the trainees that I have shown this to immediately suggest AVNRT, as it seems to fit well with onset during atrial extrastimulus testing and a "2-for-1" response over fast and slow AVN pathways. A more detailed look is warranted (**Figure 5.5B**).

Figure 5.5A

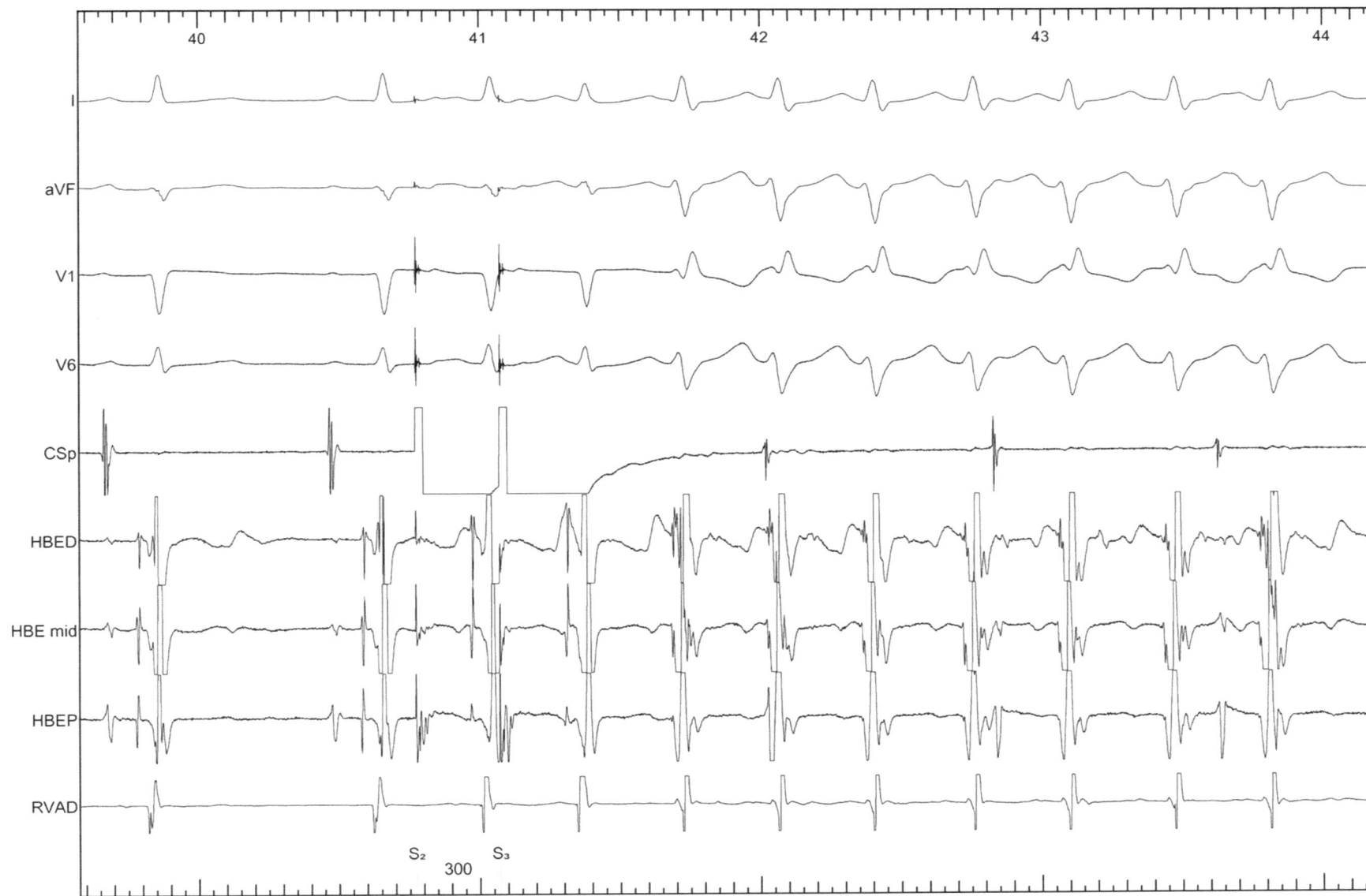

Figure 5.5B

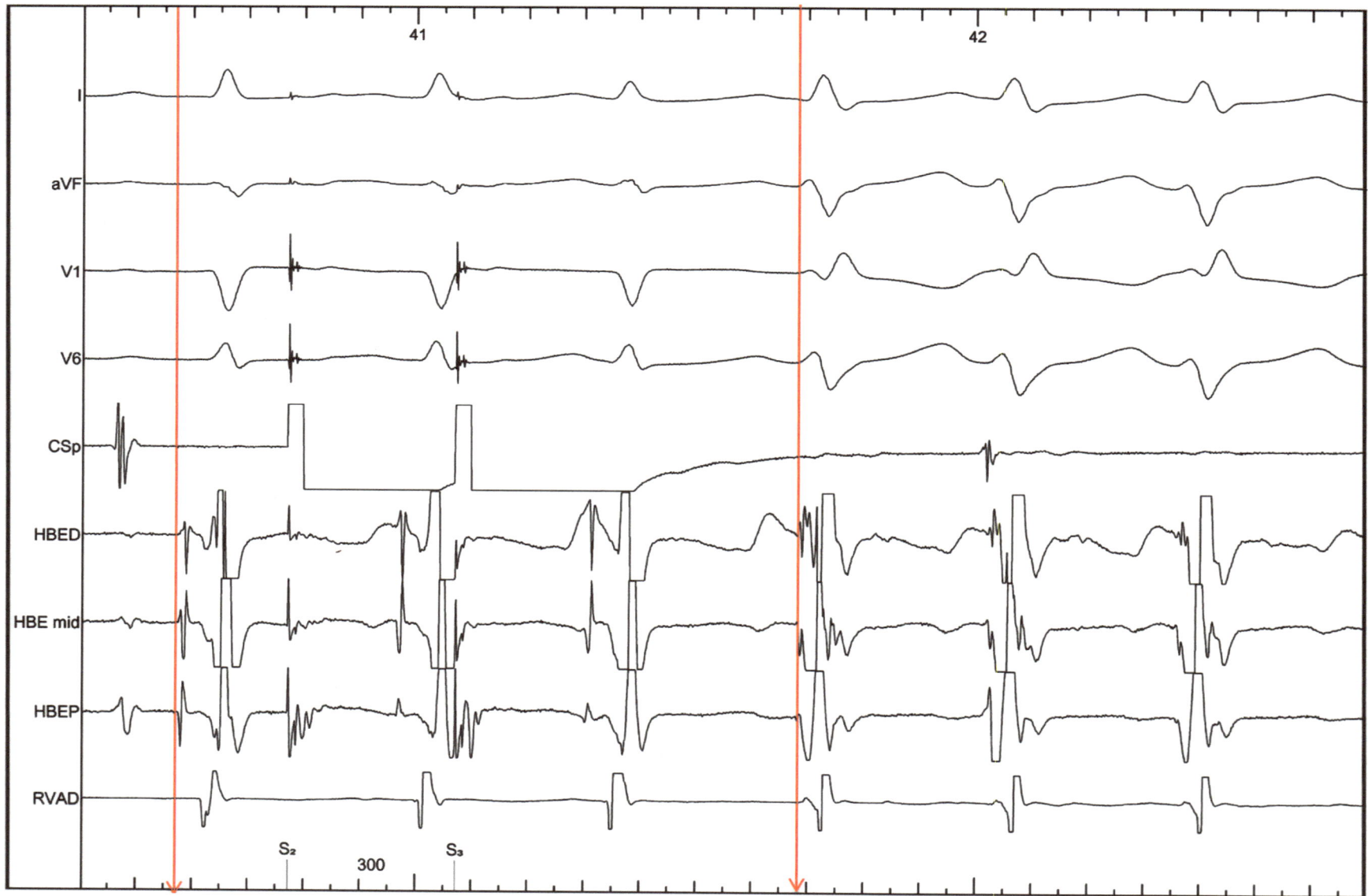

If we focus on the WCT, it is evident that the H deflection is at the onset of the QRS, and consequently, this *can only be VT or preexcited tachycardia*. However, by previously framing our problem as WCT with AV dissociation, preexcited tachycardia was **not** on our list of possibilities. This can only be VT!

We note further that the distal His (HBED) is now earlier than the proximal His (HBEP); it has moved into the QRS (**red lines**) whereas the HBEP was earliest during atrial pacing. That is, the H with the WCT is a *retrograde* H.

This type of VT characterized by RBBB, LAFB in its more common form is related to reentry, with the circuit closely related to the distal LBB area, near the posterior fascicle. Hence it is closely related to the normal His fascicular system and onset can be observed with atrial pacing and extrastimuli. In addition, retrograde conduction is rapid and retrograde His activation can be observed prior to the QRS onset.

The observation of some irregularity in the WCT (**Figure 5.5C**) indicates that the H moves before the QRS. This does not exclude a ventricular source of activation, since the His is in reality a retrograde His and only passively involved in the tachycardia.

Problem 5.5 is based on a tracing provided by Dr. Francis Murgatroyd, London, UK.

Figure 5.5C

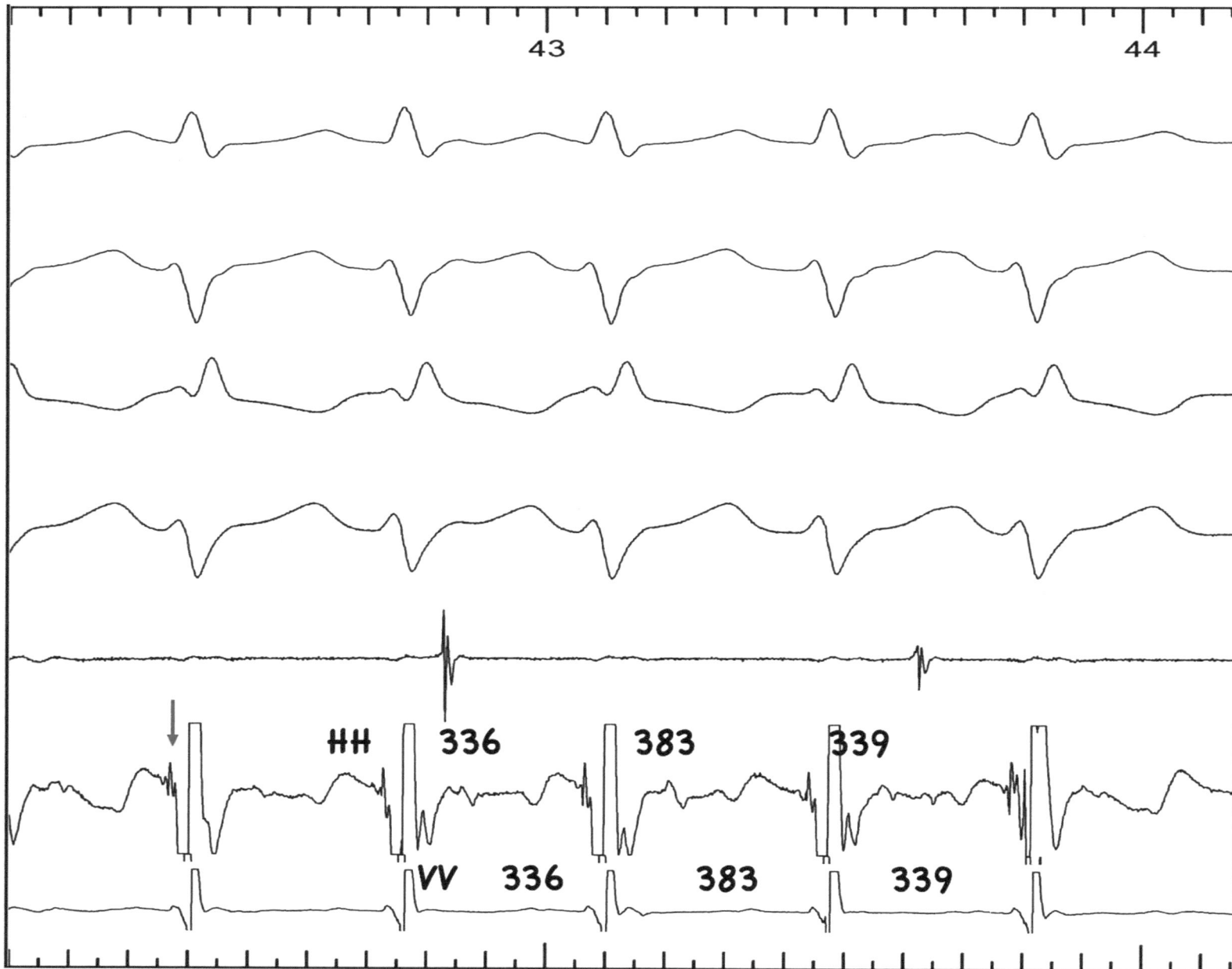

Problem 5.6

This tracing emphasizes the equivalence of approach to the ECG and electrogram tracing and how much information can be extracted from the ECG (**Figure 5.6A**). The general overview shows a normal QRS during sinus rhythm and termination of an SVT by aPVC. The P wave has low-to-high activation and follows the QRS temporally (PR > RP). The PVC is relatively late-coupled and narrow, suggesting it is likely *fused* with the last QRS of the tachycardia.

Figure 5.6A

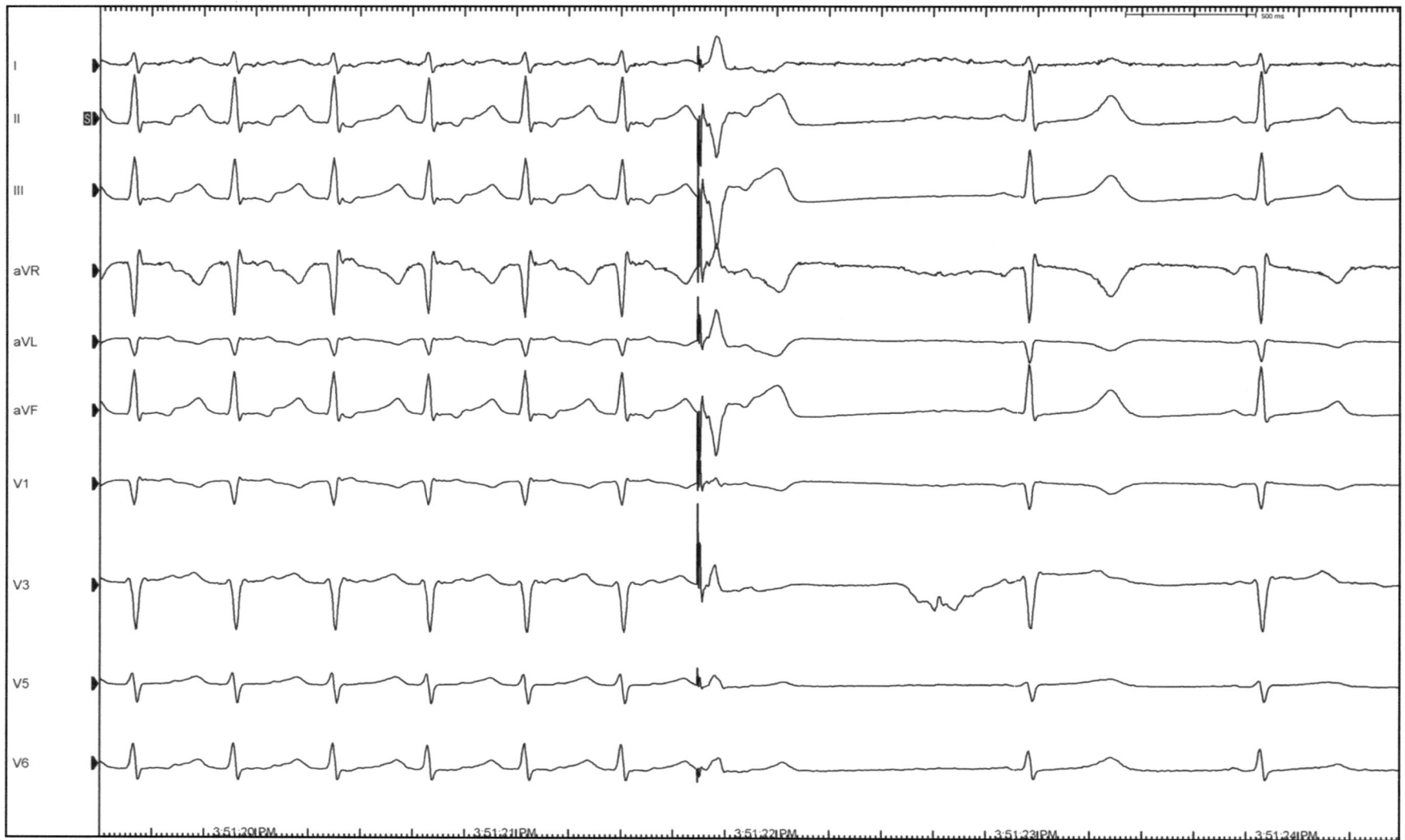

It is time to make some measurements and examine the transition zone more closely, **Figure 5.6B**. The SVT is initially a little unstable but settles in at CL 400 prior to the PVC. If the PVC is indeed fused, **it must be His refractory.** *One might illustrate this* by *"adding" a His deflection (**red arrows**) at approximately 50 ms in front of the QRS. This is generally a safe bet, especially in this individual with a normal QRS and PR interval, and is something I do frequently.*

Figure 5.6B

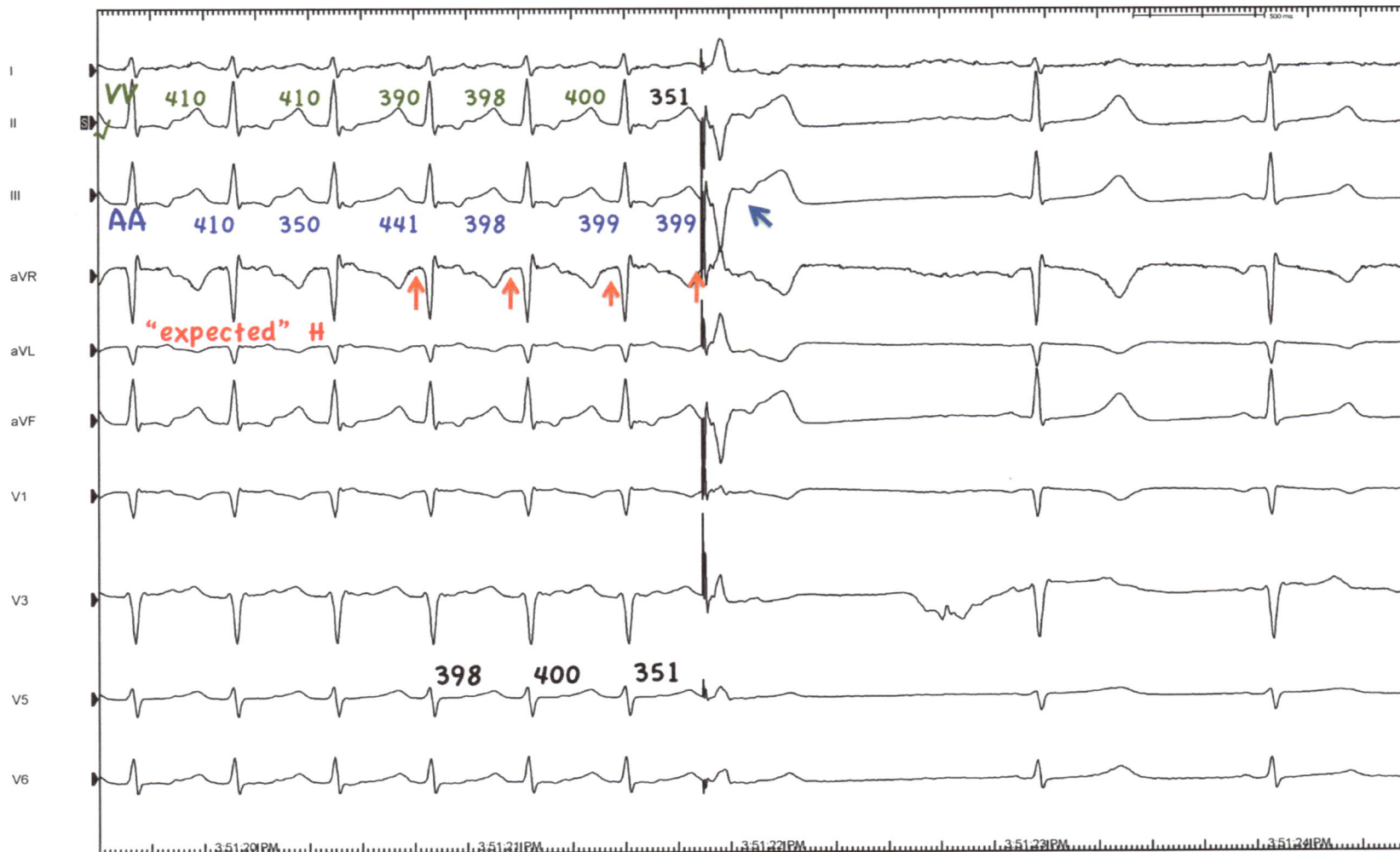

We then ask ourselves how this PVC terminated tachycardia. In AVRT, the His refractory PVC can advance the next P wave and terminate AVRT when it encounters refractoriness in the anterograde AVN limb. In this case, *the His refractory PVC does NOT move the next P*, but tachycardia still stops after the P. We have created refractoriness in the AVN, but it could not be mediated by an accessory AV pathway causing atrial activation prematurely. Thus, we are NOT dealing with AVRT. Similarly, a His-refractory PVC would not make it to the atrium with AVNRT in the absence of some other route to the atrium.

In our example, the PVC got to the AV node to render it refractory when the next P wave came around. *This can only happen with a NV pathway that inserts into the AVN.* One could envisage a NV pathway inserting into the anterograde AVN pathway in AVNRT to cause block the next time the retrograde pathway comes around. In this scenario, we would be dealing with AVNRT and a bystander NV pathway. A macroreentrant NV SVT seems less probable since it would be expected to advance the next atrial activation, much like in AV reentry, unless decrement to the atrium exactly corrected the prematurity.

We can only speculate as to what is happening at a microanatomical level, but there is little doubt that the only way the His-refractory PVC can stop the SVT by block in the AVN is using an accessory pathway inserting into the AVN.

The intracardiac EGMs really did not inform us beyond the ECG leads. The final presumptive diagnosis after the EP study was atypical AVNRT with a bystander NV pathway, and ablation in the "usual" slow pathway location was successful.

Problem 5.7

Figure 5.7A shows a WCT with termination after an apparently normalized beat, followed by sinus rhythm. It lends itself to description in 3 zones: a WCT zone, a transition zone, and a sinus zone. Focus on one zone at a time. The annotated versions (**Figure 5.7B**) and discussion follow.

Figure 5.7A

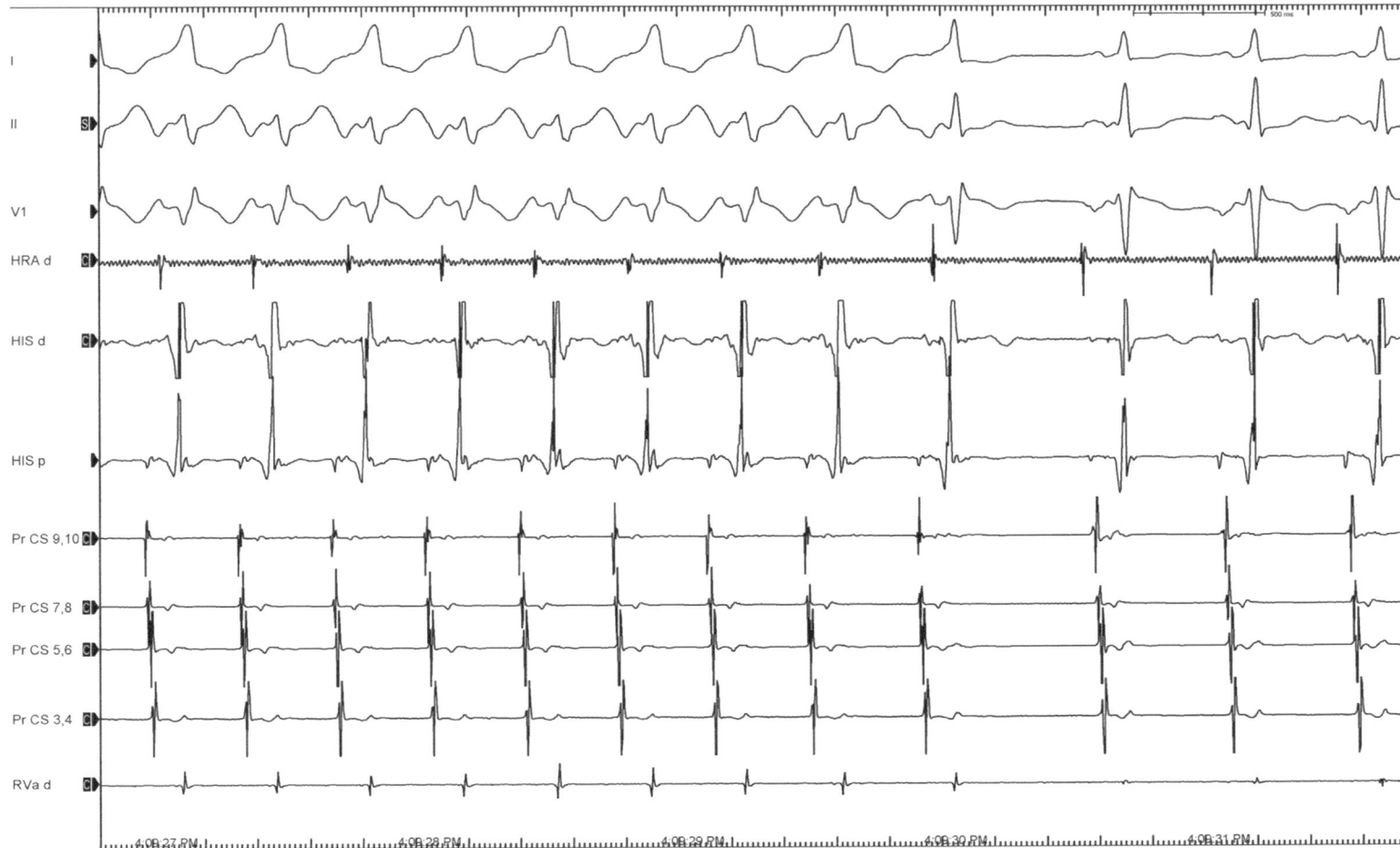

Figure 5.7B

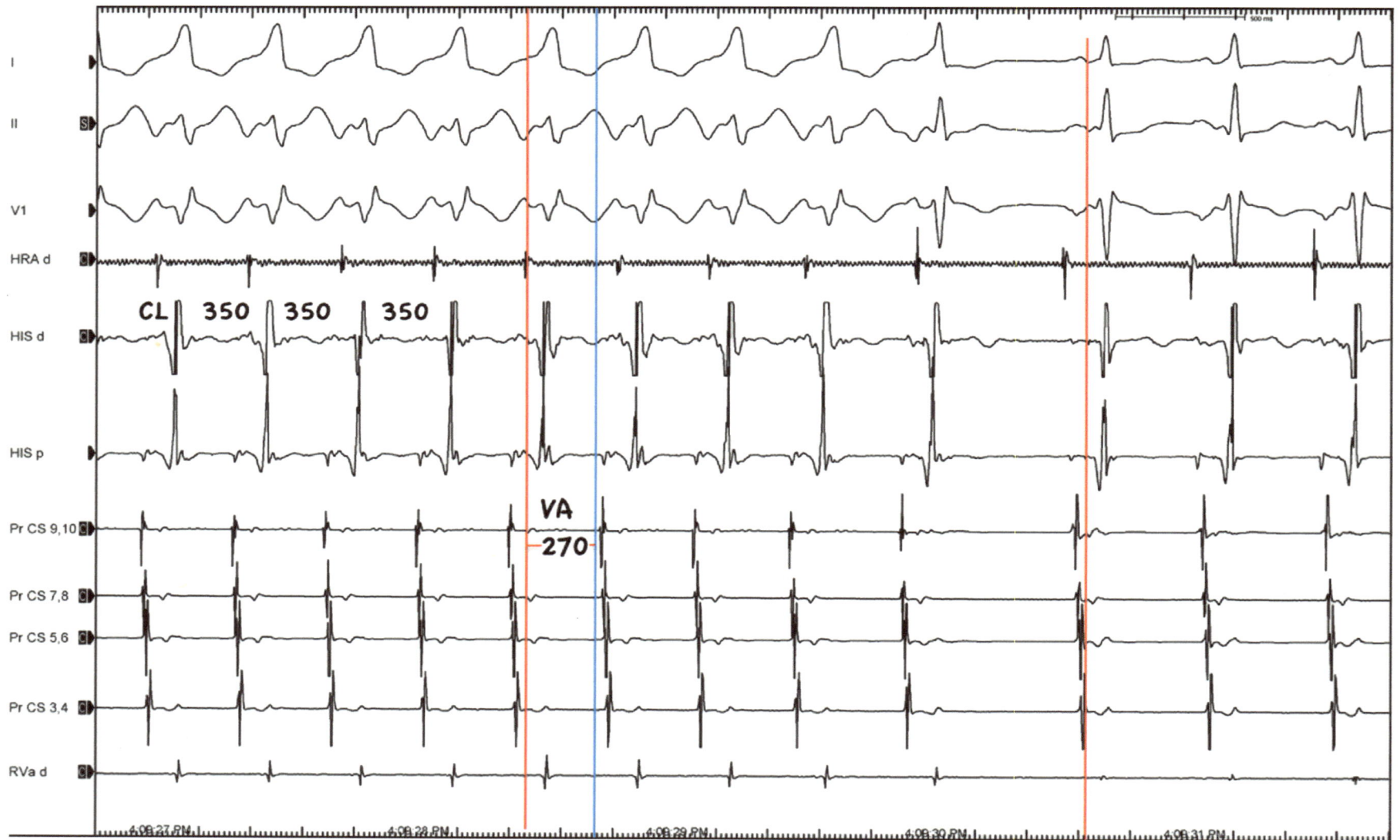

I will begin by looking at the sinus rhythm zone, obviously the easiest to understand even though it is "away from the action." There is a suggestion of preexcitation in lead 1, and this is verified by looking at the ventricular activation sequence (**red line**). The latter shows earliest ventricular activation (albeit far-field) at the proximal coronary sinus EGM CS 9–10 with the RV apical EGM following all of the CS ventricular EGMs. This is not compatible with LBBB and most compatible with preexcitation over a posteroseptal AP.

Armed with this information, we look at the WCT in zone 1. The QRS morphology resembles LBBB but is atypical (compare V_1 to that of any patient with known LBBB if you don't appreciate this). There is no visible His when such is clear albeit small in NSR. *This can only be VT or preexcited.* We note further that earliest ventricular activation (**red line**) is at the proximal CS as it is in SR and thus it is a safe bet we are dealing with a preexcited tachycardia. In comparison to SR, the QRS is wider and looks fully preexcited.

Sweeping calipers through the WCT, we note further that the tachycardia is regular and there is a late diastolic P wave. The atrial activation is septal with earliest activation at the coronary sinus orifice followed closely by that at the HB EGM. We of course can't tell whether the P is following the QRS or whether the P is leading the QRS (i.e., AT). If we pull out our knowledge of relative prevalence, the most likely mechanism would be antidromic AV reentry (antegrade conduction over the AP, retrograde conduction over the normal AVCS). We move on to the transition zone (**Figure 5.7C**) to see if it can inform us. It very often does.

Figure 5.7C

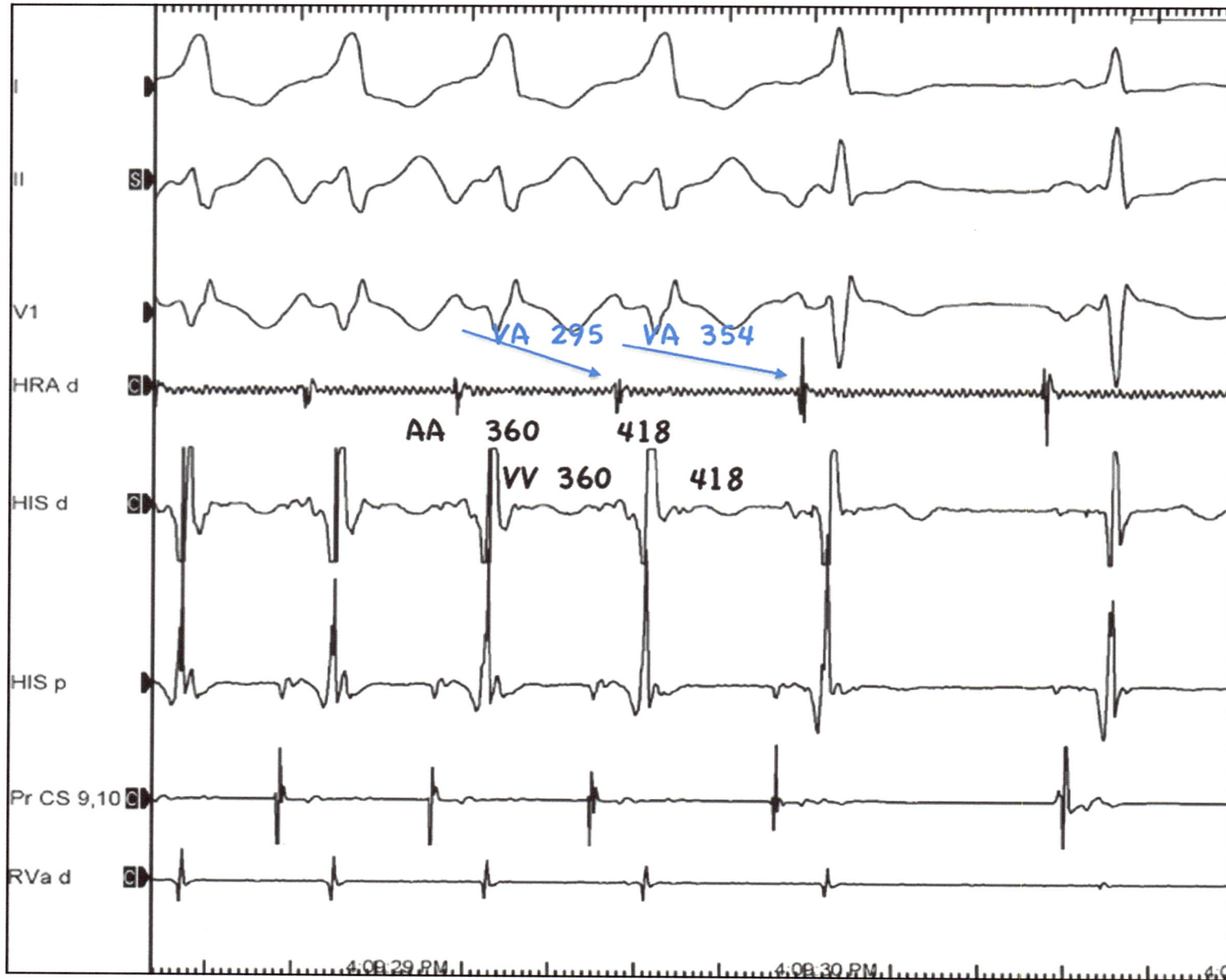

When a transition occurs, the question I ask myself is, *which EGM signals the change*, i.e., "who moves first." In this case, it is obviously the P wave with an apparent prolongation of the VA interval. This essentially seals the case for preexcited tachycardia, since there is no reason why VT should terminate coincidentally with prolongation of the VA interval.

Our next observation is the nature of the more normal-looking beat after VA prolongation. It is preceded by atrial activity with the identical activation sequence as the WCT, suggesting no change in the atrial route despite taking longer to get there. The QRS is essentially identical to that during sinus rhythm albeit with a shorter AV interval and no visible His. This is most compatible with a preexcited fusion beat.

We now have to go into a "hypothesis testing" mode, as there is no definitive proof of mechanism for the final piece of our puzzle (although AT is clearly out). In the lab, we would do a pacing maneuver of some type to clarify. In an exercise such as this one, we take the information that we have and try to find the simplest and most plausible explanation for the findings.

It is reasonable to start with the WCT being antidromic tachycardia as the best fit by prevalence and the observed data. We also keep in mind that dual AVN pathways are frequently seen in WPW. With this hypothesis, block in the retrograde fast AVN pathway occurred in AVRT. Conduction over a retrograde slow AVN pathway delayed the P wave, and an atypical AVN echo ensued with a fusion beat, signaling the end of antidromic tachycardia. The antidromic wave over the AP cannot now make it retrogradely back up the AVN, since it collides with the AVN echo conducting to the ventricle. The tachycardia must stop (**Figure 5.7D**). No further tachycardia was observed in this individual after AP ablation.

Try out some other hypothesis for yourself and see how well it fits the observed data. For example, retrograde conduction over the AVN and a second AP or retrograde conduction over 2 other AP. How about AVNRT with a bystander AP as the WCT? The more assumptions you need to make it fit, the less confidence you have in the conclusion.

Figure 5.7D

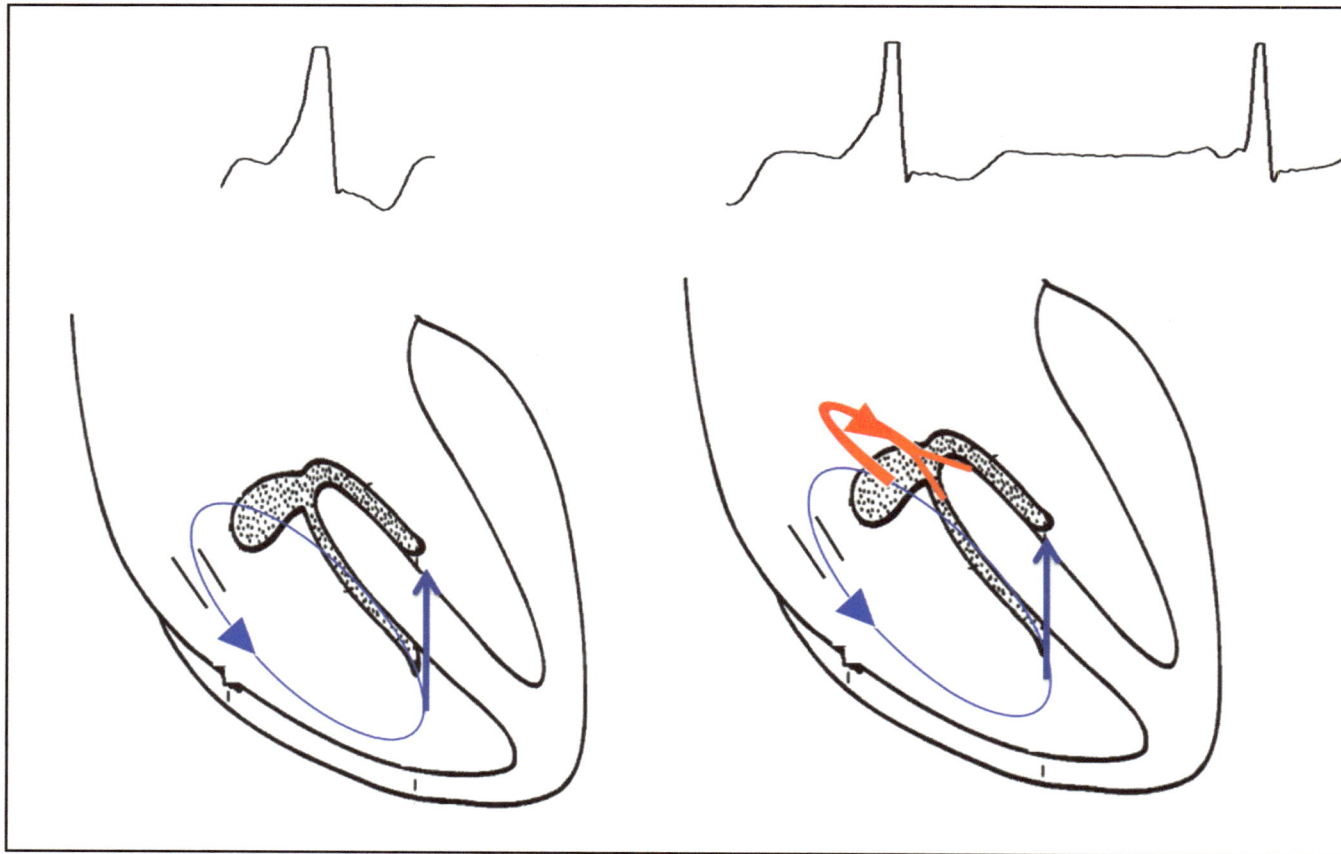

Chapter 6

Transition Zones: Ectopic Beats and Cycle Irregularity

Problem 6.1

The patient contributing this tracing was referred to us with a diagnosis of permanent junctional reciprocating tachycardia (PJRT). The permanent form of junctional reciprocating was described by Professor Philippe Coumel many years ago as an incessant or nearly incessant SVT with "low to high" P waves and with the RP interval longer than PR interval. He initially felt that it was atypical AVNRT. He and others subsequently elucidated the mechanism as being more eclectic. Patients with arrhythmia fitting this description could have one of AT, atypical AVNRT, or AVRT over an accessory pathway with long VA conduction and decremental properties. Thus, the designation PJRT is not a *mechanism* per se but a clinical presentation, and it is up to the electrophysiologist to determine which mechanism is involved with a "PJRT" presentation.

We note that our record shows SVT that terminates and reinitiates after a few sinus beats (**Figure 6.1A**).

Figure 6.1A

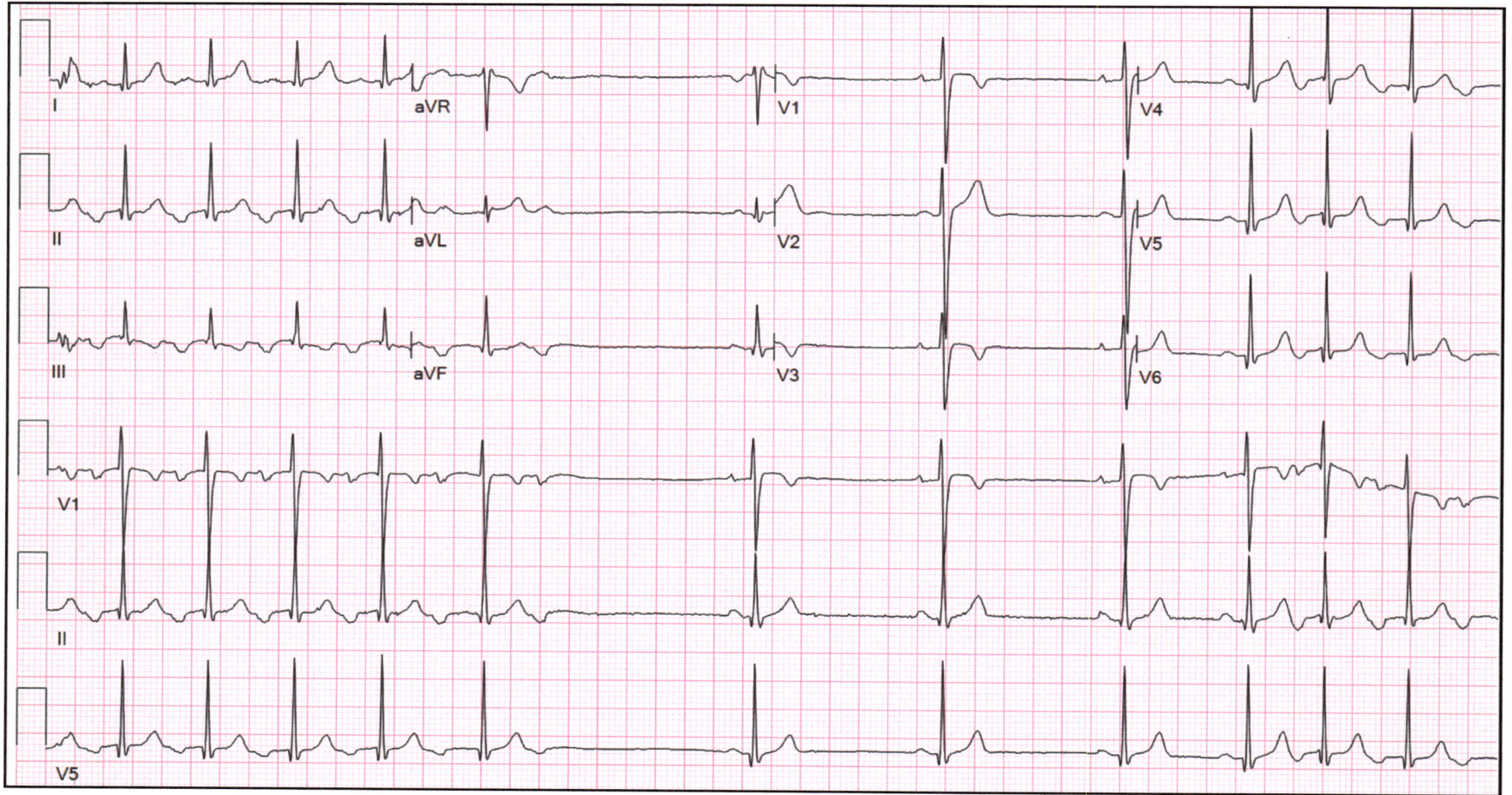

We can then focus on the two transition zones and arbitrarily start with the termination at the beginning. I enlarge this zone to facilitate measurement and to avoid distraction by the rest of the tracing at this point (**Figure 6.1B**).

Figure 6.1B

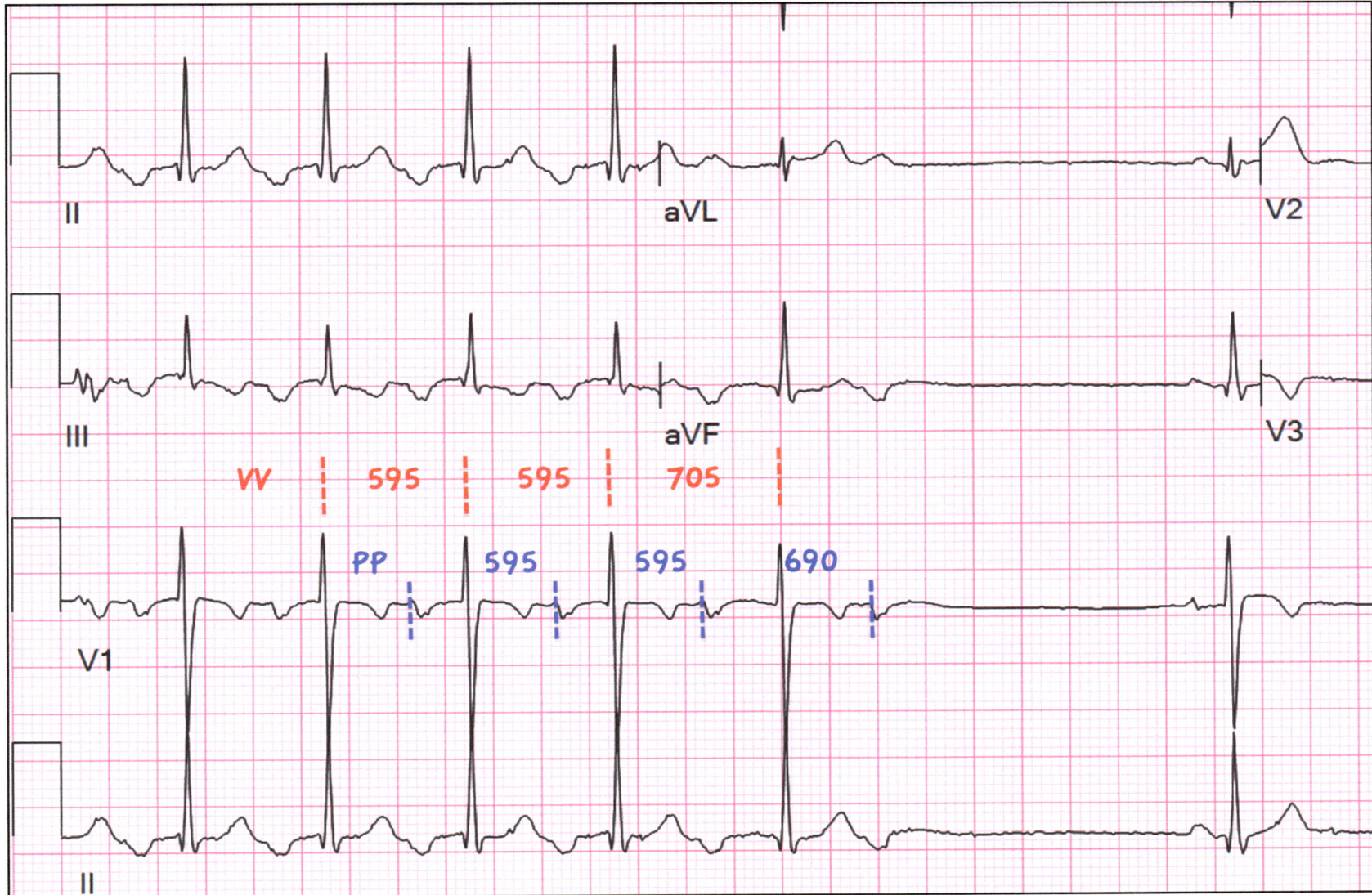

Things become obvious by simply moving calipers beat-to-beat along the tracing and measuring CL of the VV and AA intervals. One readily notes that there is an abrupt prolongation of the PR interval that is followed by atrial activation with the same VA interval. That is, the prolongation of the PR influences the circuit and hence *the AV node must be part of the circuit*. One can also look at this by saying that the change in the VV interval *precedes* the change in the AA interval, *excluding AT as mechanism*. One might also note that termination of an SVT with the last event being atrial also effectively excludes AT if consistent, since there is no reason to suspect that the AT would terminate at the exact instant that AV conduction is blocked.

We can now look at the onset of SVT later in the tracing. This is less helpful here, but if you sweep the calipers through this, you will notice that the VV prolongation precedes the AA prolongation (also excluding AT).

At this point, we have excluded AT but still can't distinguish whether this is atypical AVNRT or AVRT. This would require EP study and further maneuvers to answer whether the ventricle and/or the atrium is part of the circuit or not. In this case, the mechanism was atypical AVNRT, perhaps suggested by the long PR prior to the termination.

Problem 6.2

This patient presented with recurrent SVT and the following was recorded during an EP study. A PVC was programmed into the cardiac cycle as a diagnostic maneuver, but the tracing may just as well be thought of as a PVC occurring spontaneously during tachycardia. The presence of spontaneous ectopy during a clinically occurring tachycardia may be a gift, a spontaneous "maneuver," and should always be sought when looking at ECG records of tachycardia. In this instance, we will see how much information we get from the PVC looking initially at only the ECG component of the EP tracings (**Figure 6.2A**).

Figre 6.2A

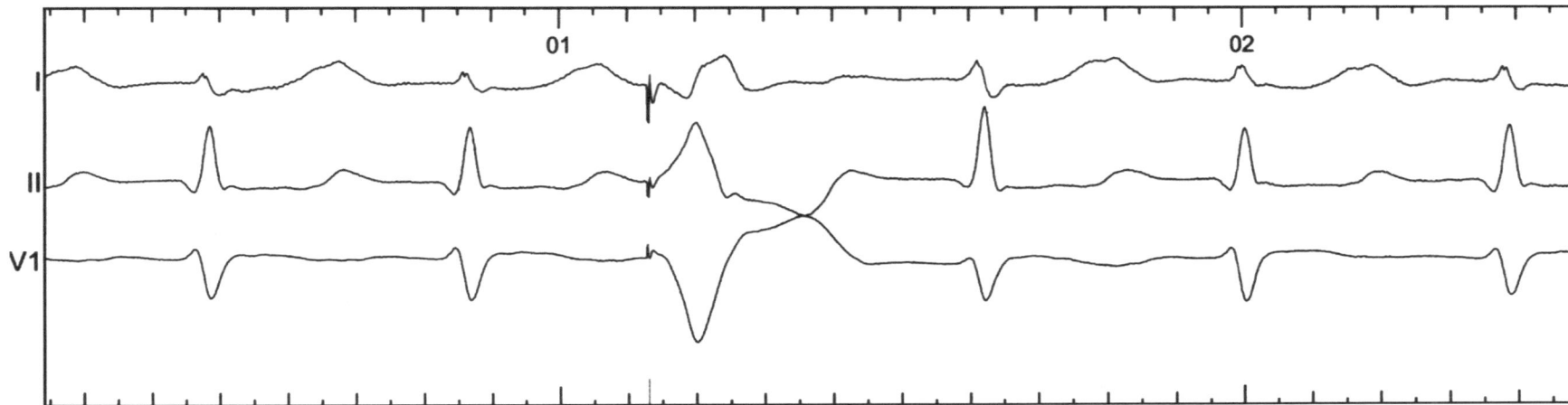

When looking at **Figure 6.2A**, I ask myself whether the SVT has changed after the PVC. Has the QRS and P relationship or the CL changed? With rare exceptions, the same CL means that the tachycardia has NOT changed. The converse is also true; that is, a change invariably means one is dealing with a different tachycardia or a change in the circuit of the initial tachycardia.

The CL in this case has not changed, 385 ms. I now ask myself whether the PVC has changed the timing or "reset" the tachycardia. This informs us on whether the PVC has access to the circuit, usually a reentrant circuit with an excitable gap such as AVRT. A simple but careful walk of the calipers through the record (**annotated Figure 6.2B**) shows that the cycle after the PVC has been advanced by 15 ms. A relatively late-coupled PVC has altered the timing of the circuit. This essentially excludes any mechanism of

SVT other than AVRT or NVRT, since the ventricle is part of the circuit in the latter. The PVC is only premature by approximately 50 ms. If one "guesstimates" a normal HV in the 50-ms rate (usually an excellent guess) and marks the ECG with their estimated H (**red lines**), it is clearly evident that the PVC is "His refractory" and we have proven, at very least, the presence of AV accessory pathway (and with rare esoteric exceptions, the participation of the AP in the circuit).

Figure 6.2B

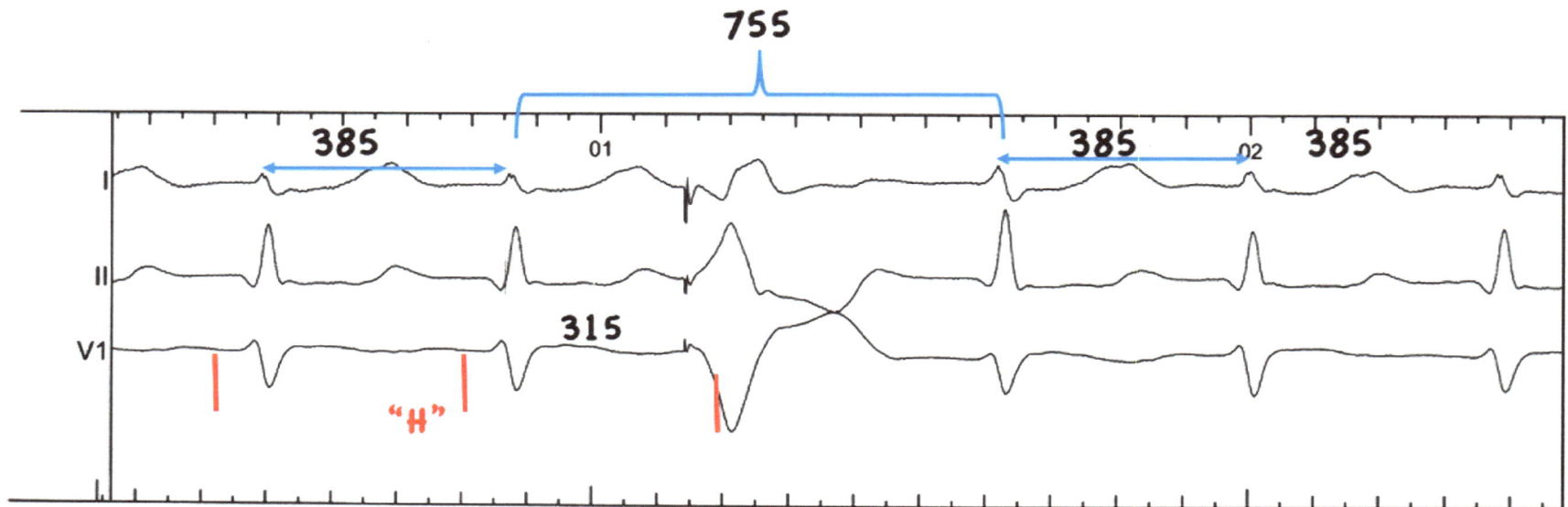

We can now examine the EP data, **Figure 6.2C**. We scan our calipers along the HRA and His EGM and verify that we have preexcited the atrium with our PVC during His refractoriness and notice that our initial estimate of where the His should be on the surface ECG was quite reasonable.

Figure 6.2C

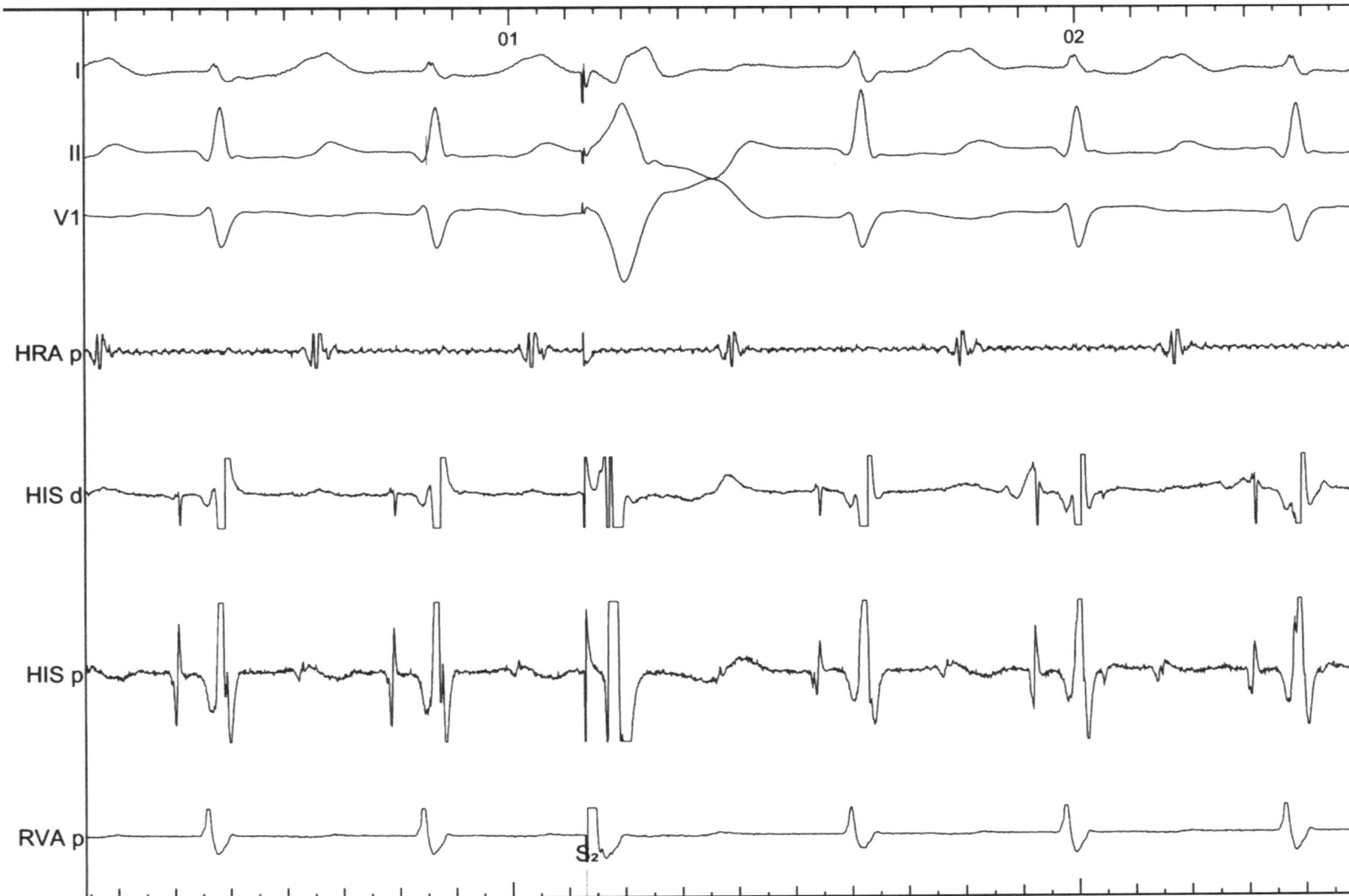

Moving to an annotated **Figure 6.2D**, I have measured the St-A and VA intervals and note that the St-A is longer than the tachycardia VA interval by only 40 ms (**blue lines**). The RV apical catheter is generally in the vicinity of the RBB breakout into the RV, close enough so that the *St-A reasonably approximates the VA during actual LBB during tachycardia.* **Thus, we have the equivalent of saying that LBBB prolongs the VA during SVT by 40 ms in this individual.** This puts the AP in the LV, probably left paraseptal or posteroseptal, to where it was mapped. (In general, the typical posteroseptal AP will prolong the VA with LBBB by 0–35 ms and VA will prolong by greater than this for a left free wall AP.)

The next concept that is very useful to understand is that the single PVC programmed into the tachycardia is essentially equivalent to overdrive ventricular pacing. *A single PVC that resets the rhythm is essentially entrainment for one cycle.* Alternatively, entrainment is merely repetitive reset by a single PVC. This means that all the measurements so useful for entrainment of SVT (notably the Michaud criteria) are applicable when single PVCs reset the rhythm. Thus, we have a delta St-A–VA < 85 ms and a PPI < 115 ms, verifying that the tachycardia is AVRT.*

---

* The initial Michaud criteria actually differentiated between AVRT over a PS pathway vs. AVNRT, but values less than their thresholds are not seen in AVNRT and can be used as indicating AVRT, whether posteroseptal or not. That is, the RV pacing site can be close enough to the circuit in AVRT (i.e., "in") to provide values less than would be seen in AVNRT.

Figure 6.2D

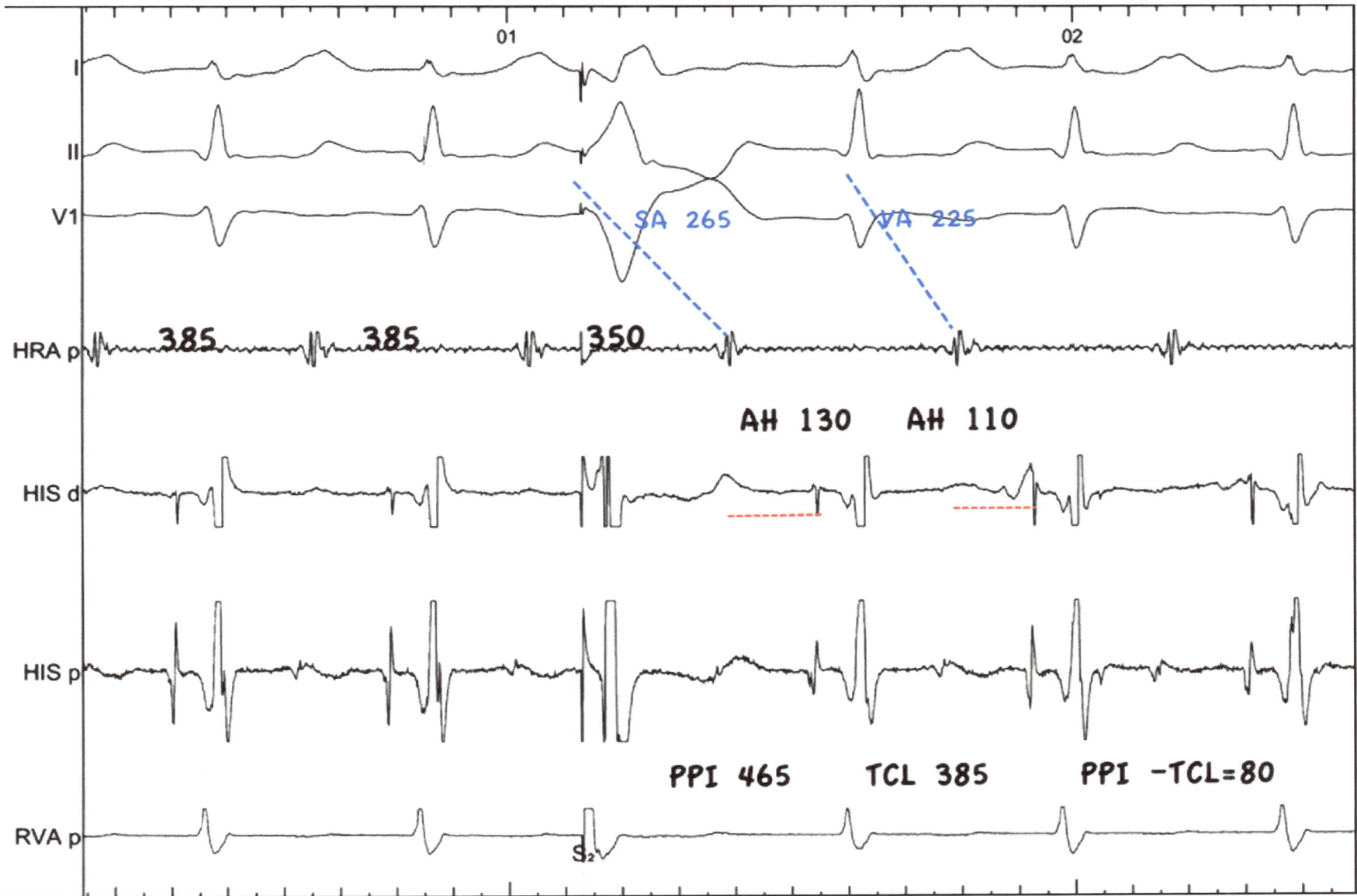

We also note that the PPI needs to be corrected for a slight AH prolonged observed after the PVC so that PPI corrected = 60 ms. For more detailed discussions of the concepts of entrainment and reset with fusion, the interested reader is referred to *Electrophysiological Maneuvers for Arrhythmia Analysis* (Cardiotext, 2014) or many other references on the subject.

Problem 6.3

This problem might at first seem difficult, but a similar approach as per Problem 6.2, it provides a solution. We again begin with examining the ECG component of the tracing recorded during programming of PVCs into the cardiac cycle during tachycardia (**Figure 6.3A**).

Figure 6.3A

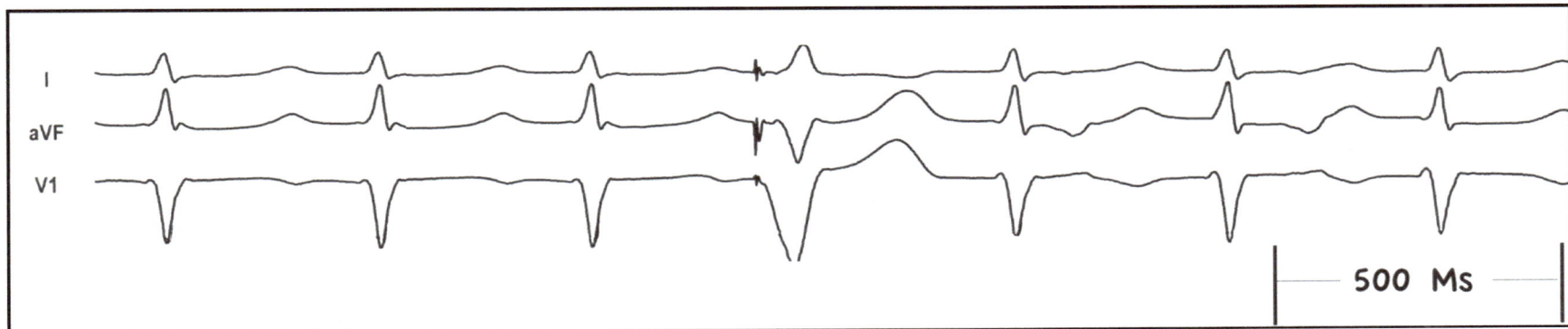

An initial scan of the tracing with calipers shows that tachycardia segments before and after the PVC have identical cycle lengths, making it highly probable that the tachycardia mechanism is the same before and after the PVC. We then focus on the transition zone and observe that the PVC does not perturb the timing of the subsequent QRS (**Figure 6.3B**). Finally, we look for P waves and see deflections only *after* the PVC, but not before (without substantive doubt retrograde P waves, set as **solid red arrows**).

This is very useful, since the SVT preceding the PVC has a wide-open differential diagnosis whereas ongoing SVT *without* atrial participation (retrograde block to A) has a very limited differential diagnosis including only AVNRT, JT, or NVRT. Furthermore, the SVT tracings before and after the PVC share a mechanism within all reasonable probability having exactly the same CL.

Figure 6.3B

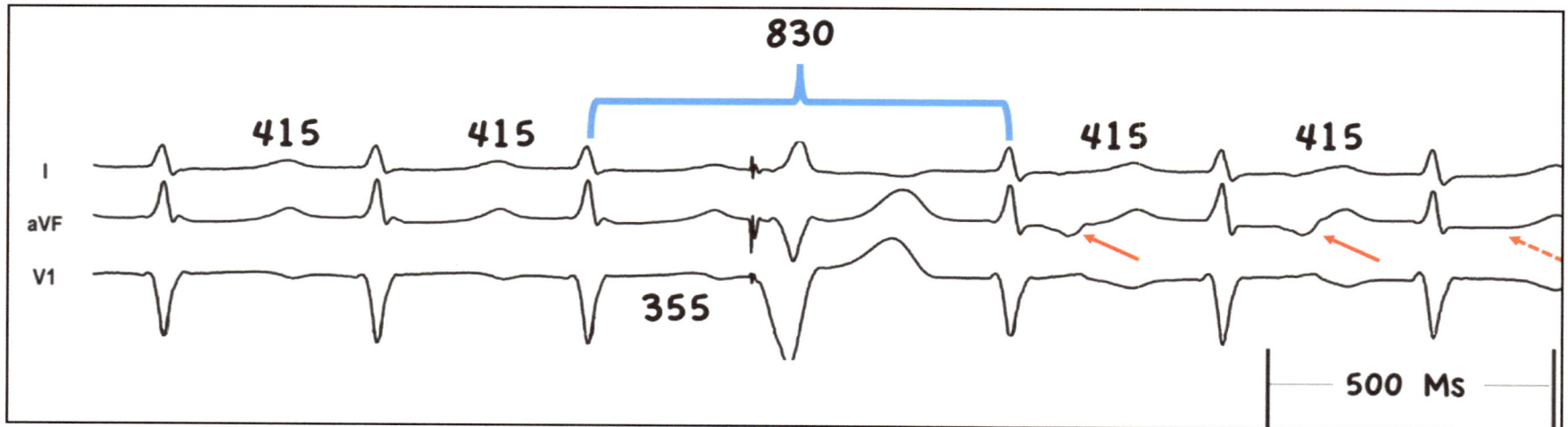

We now ask ourselves why the PVC changed retrograde conduction *without* resetting the tachycardia and will move on the intracardiac tracings in **Figure 6.3C** and subsequently the annotated version of **Figure 6.3D**.

Figure 6.3C

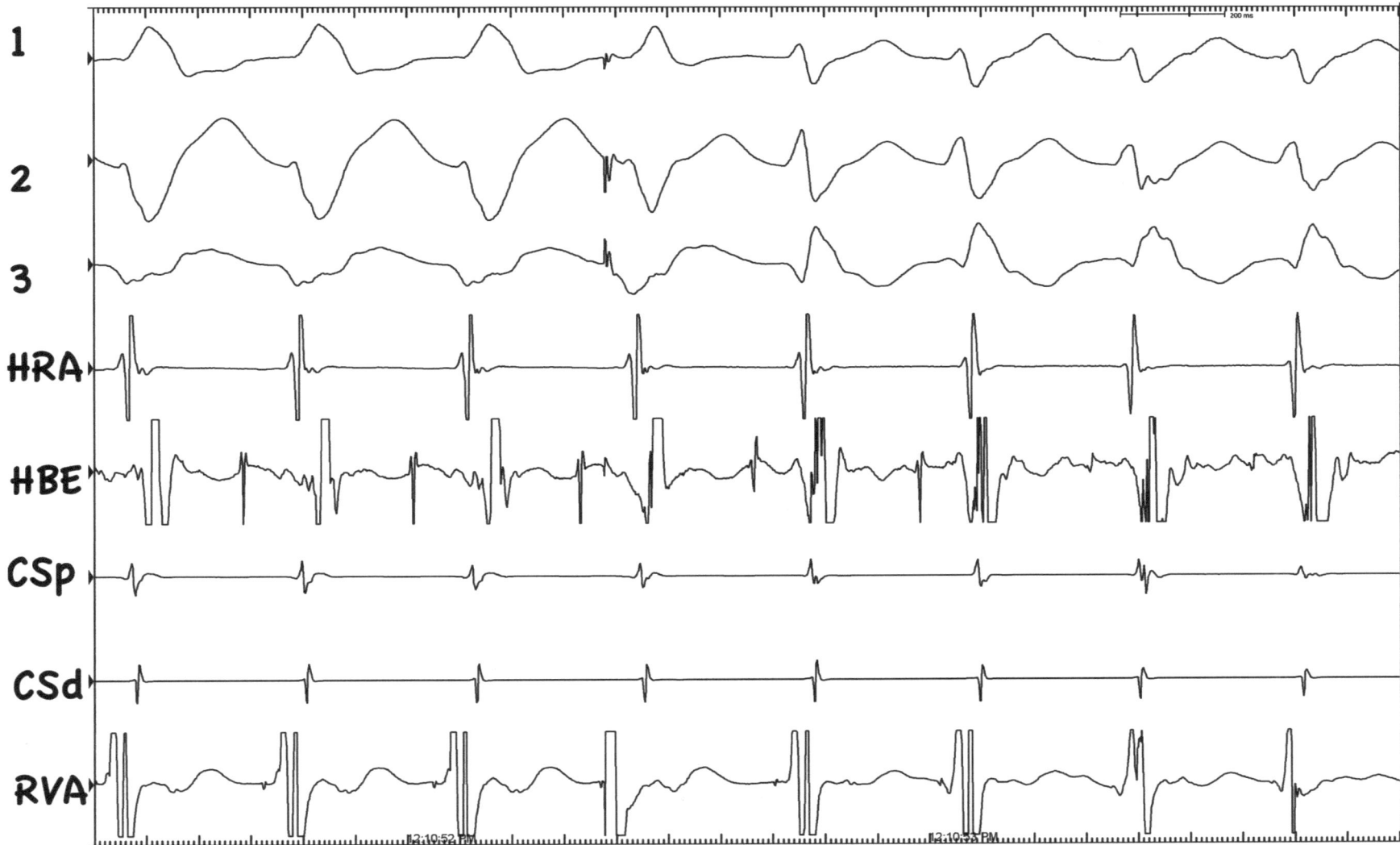

Figure 6.3D

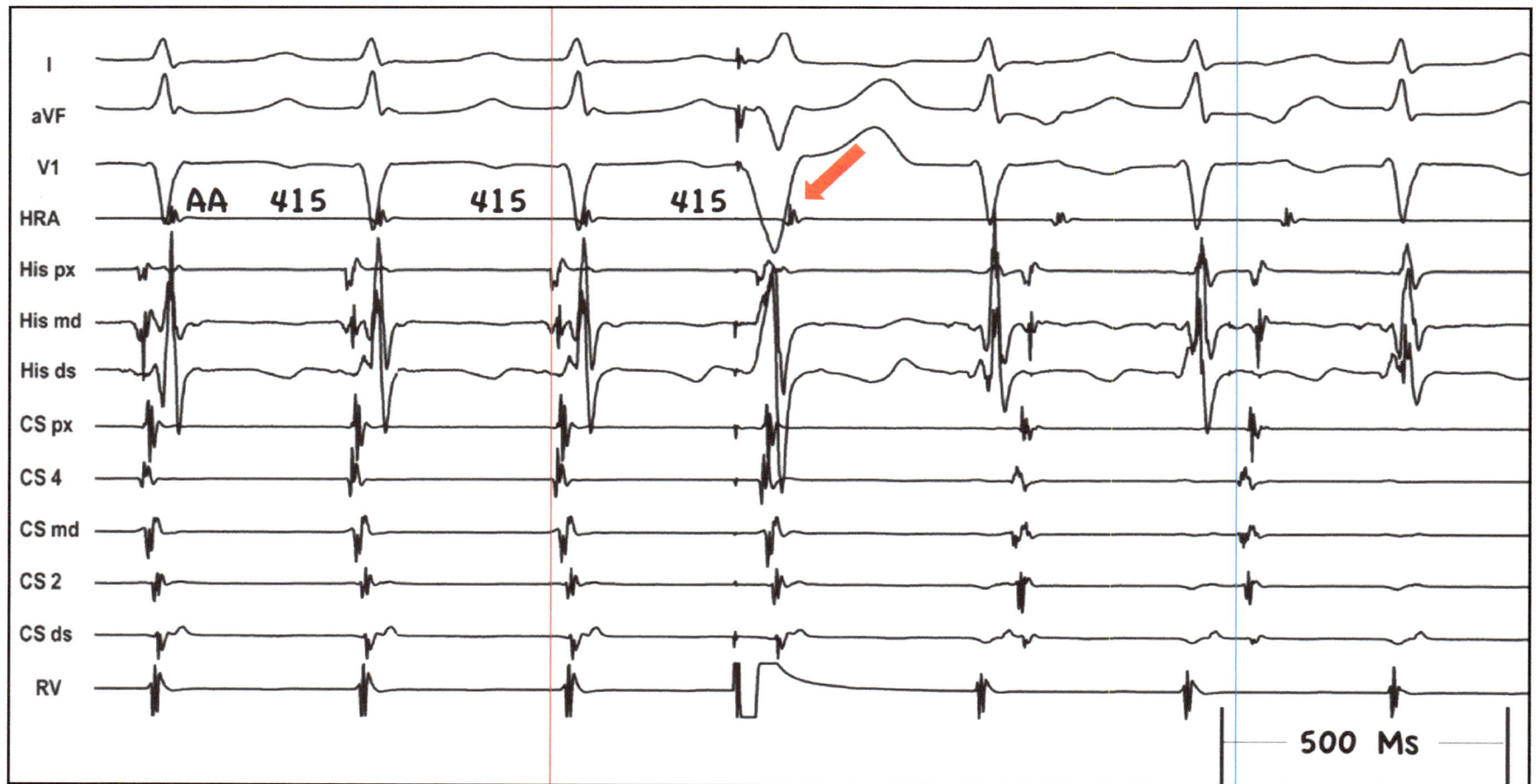

We note first that the atrial electrograms verify our diagnosis of retrograde block to the A during SVT after the PVC. We look next at the atrial sequence before and after the PVC and note that they are both somewhat central (**septal leads earliest**) but not quite the same. We draw lines (**red** and **blue**) to help us compare the atrial sequences and verify that they are different. Next, we verify that atrial activation immediately after the PVC is "on time." Finally, we determine whether the PVC is "His refractory." Although the His signal is a little challenging especially prior to the PVC, walk the calipers through the QRS onset and note that the PVC is only about 50 ms premature, there can be little doubt it is His refractory at this point.

We may now ask how a His refractory PVC changed retrograde conduction without going over the His bundle? There must be an accessory pathway. It is not a conventional AV pathway since the PVC would only influence the tachycardia by going over the AP via the atrium and atrial activation was not changed. It must be a concealed (conducting only retrogradely) nodoventricular or nodofascicular AP that enters the AV node via the NVAP and interferes with retrograde conduction but otherwise does not perturb the circuit. This excellent access to the circuit from the RV apical region suggests that the RV is part of the circuit and we are dealing with NVRT or nodofascicular reentrant tachycardia (NFRT) (**Figure 6.3E, left panel**).

Having said this, it is conceptually possible that the NVAP is a bystander pathway that gets into an AVN reentry circuit via its good access and affects retrograde conduction—that is, AVNRT with a bystander concealed NVAP (**Figure 6.3E, right panel**). I believe we are at our limits of understanding to confidently distinguish the latter two.

Nonetheless, we can say that there is no doubt that anterograde conduction is via a slow pathway and that there is a concealed nodoventricular AP present that is probably but not necessarily the essential retrograde limb of the circuit.

The tracings were adapted with compliments of Dr. Reginald Ho.

Figure 6.3E

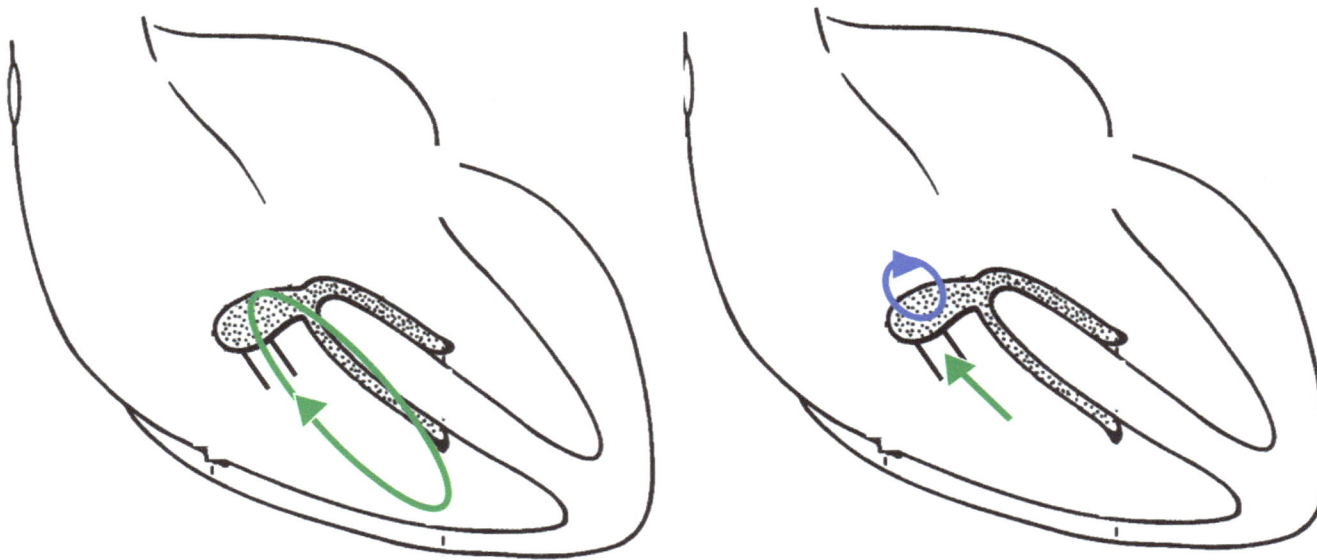

Problem 6.4

The patient is a 54-year-old woman with recurrent WCT of LBBB morphology and no other cardiac issues.

In **Figure 6.4A**, a PVC from the RV has been programmed into the cardiac cycle during a WCT. The initial tachycardia has a LBBB-type morphology, acceptable although not entirely typical for LBBB aberrancy. The tachycardia after the PVC has a relatively typical RBBB pattern. The PVC has a relatively narrow QRS and is very late coupled (hardly premature), hence, in all likelihood, fused. Of course, an RV PVC would tend to "normalize" the QRS of LBBB or that of right-sided preexcitation. P waves are not seen.

Figure 6.4A

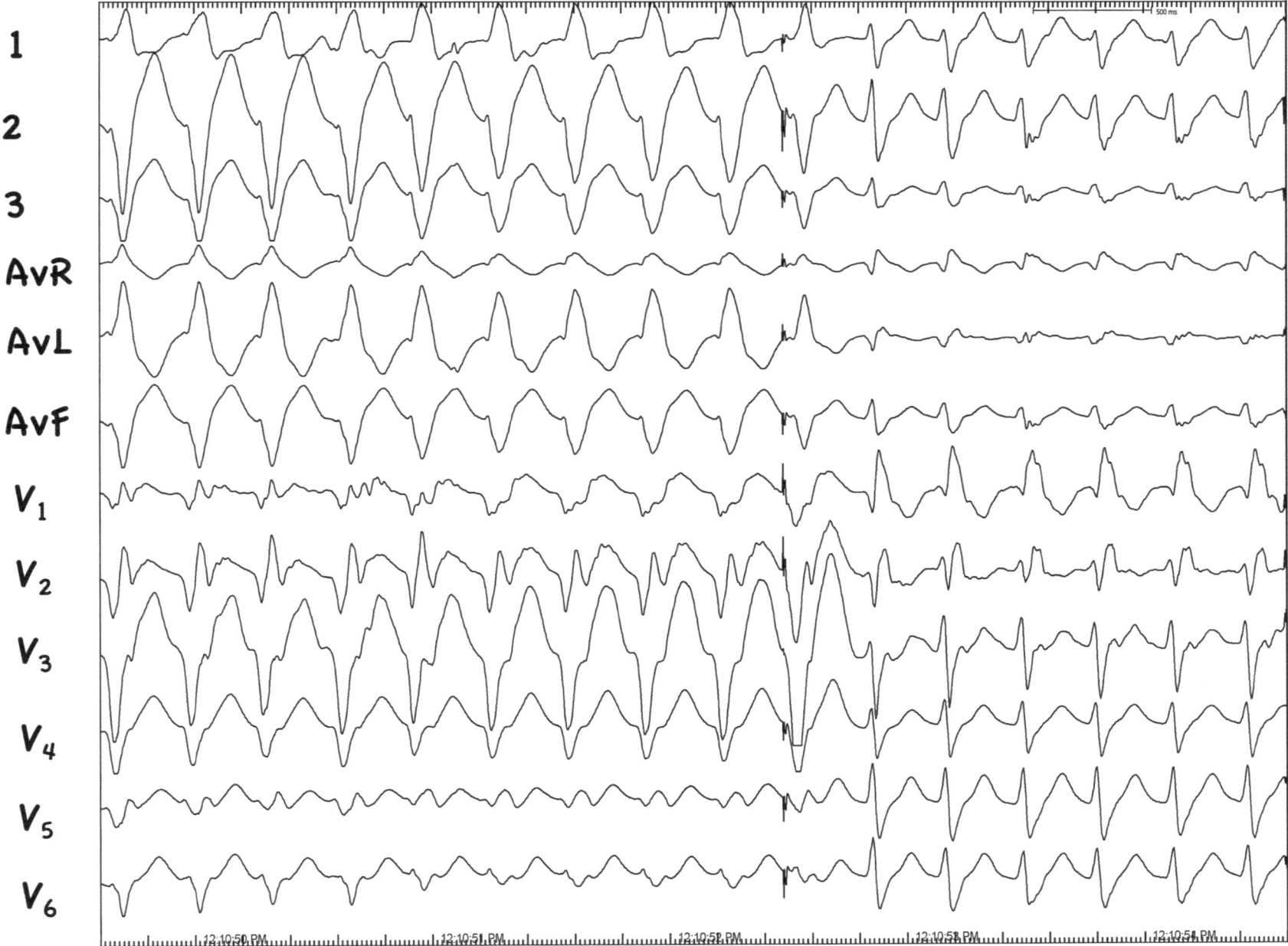

At this point, we need to know if the tachycardia is reset and the relative CLs of each of the RBBB and LBBB type of tachycardia (**Figure 6.4B**).

It is now apparent that the CL of the tachycardia has not changed at all and the tachycardia has not been reset, i.e., the QRS is right "on time" after the PVC. *This of course helps since the odds are now enormously in favor of "one" tachycardia on the tracing.*

If we assume we are dealing with an SVT (the RBBB side has a typical RBBB aberration pattern), we have limited diagnostic possibilities. The first possibility is an SVT with and without a bystander AP. This is less likely (not impossible) in our patient, in whom preexcitation has never been observed.

Figure 6.4B

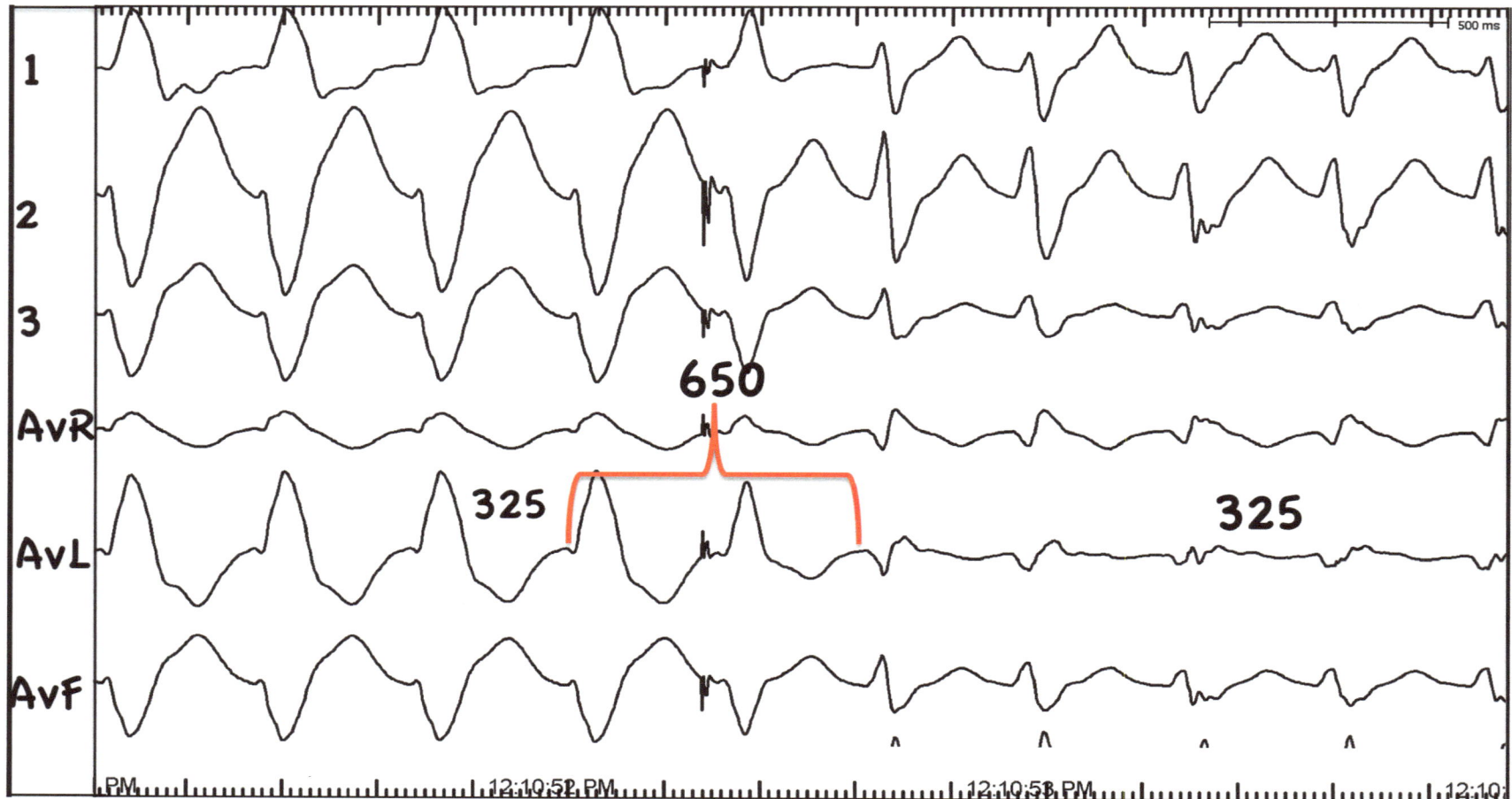

The second possibility is LBBB resolving and transforming to RBBB aberration, the latter by transeptal conduction "peeling back" refractoriness or "preexciting" the LBBB allowing it more time to recover excitability. This latter would fit well specifically with AT or AVNRT since the tachycardia CL is oblivious to the presence or absence of each bundle with either of these diagnoses.

The intracardiac recordings (**Figure 6.4C**) verify the diagnosis of typical AVNRT.

Figure 6.4C

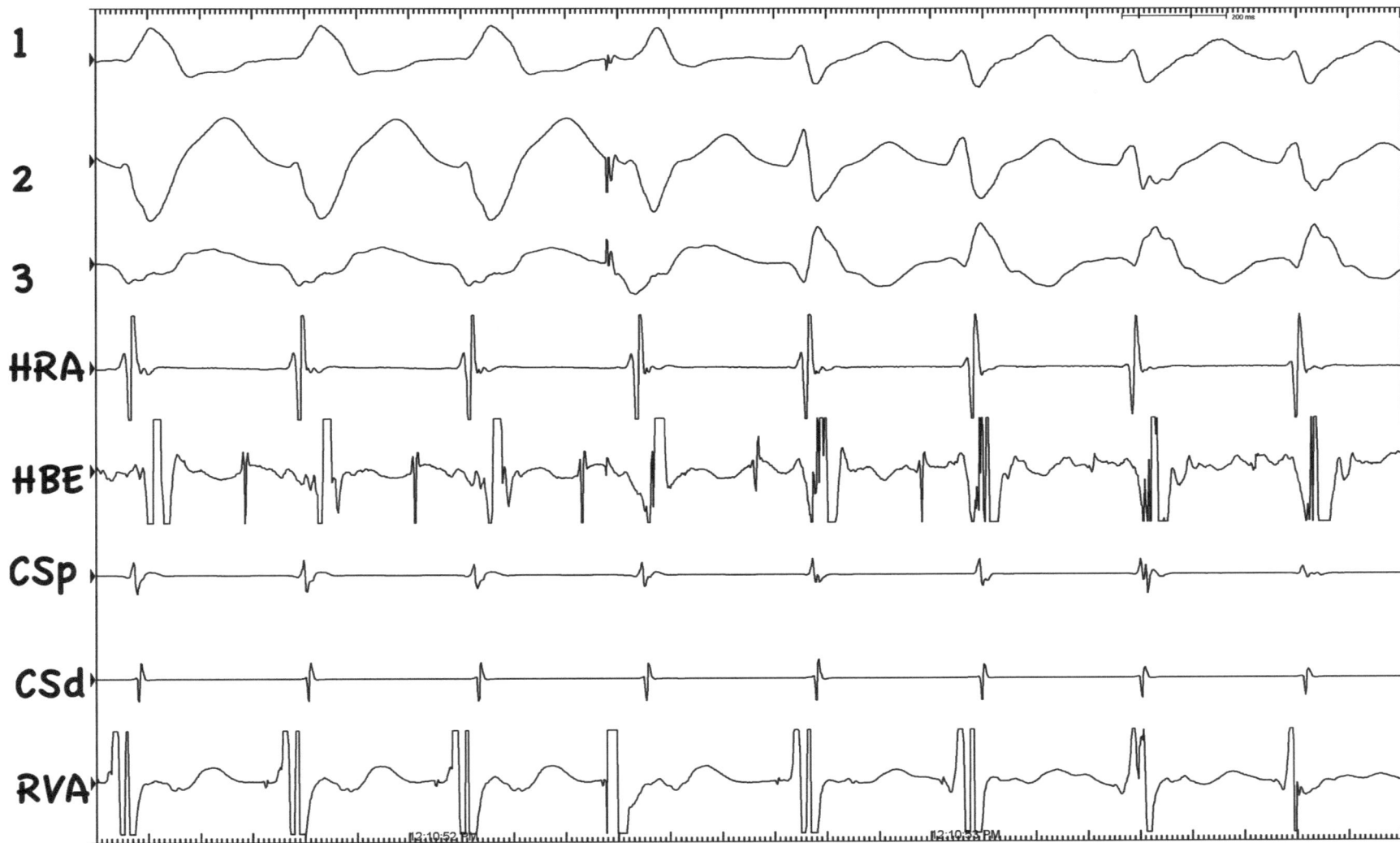

Problem 6.5

The tracing in **Figure 6.5A** is recorded from a young individual with no structural heart disease with a normal baseline ECG. It can be described as a generally regular WCT with a LBBB pattern quite acceptable for LBBB aberrancy. The differential diagnosis is:

1. SVT with LBBB aberrancy
2. VT (right ventricular exit site)
3. Preexcited tachycardia

Although not entirely unequivocal, there is a deflection in the ST segment that is probably atrial activity. This is not helpful, since AV association can be seen with any of our potential diagnoses. The termination of the tachycardia is a little confused by ectopic activity but the tachycardia ends with a P wave, so we can reasonably eliminate AT from our candidate diagnoses.

Figure 6.5A

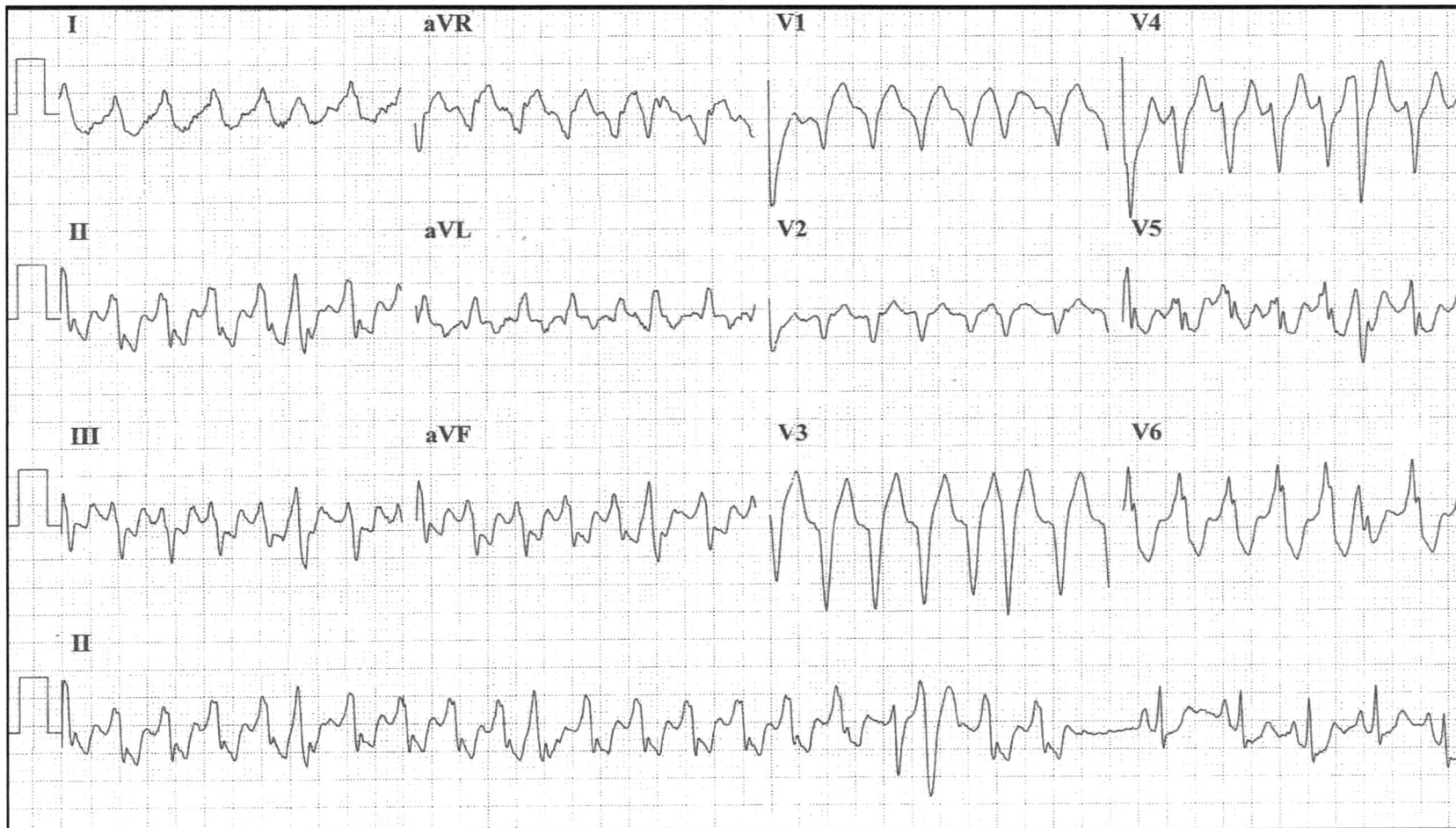

I am drawn to the irregularity caused by the ectopic beats, and one brief segment is magnified in **Figure 6.5B**. Putative P waves are indicated by the **blue arrow**. The PVCs are also LBBB type, slightly different than the WCT beats. They are late coupled and approximately 100 ms premature to the next destined QRS (**red arrows**). *The key observation is that the following destined QRS is advanced or "reset" by the PVC.* We note that the interval surrounding the PVC is 630 ms, when it should be approximately 710 ms, if the PVC did not alter the prevailing rhythm. This is a very late-coupled PVC, and it is most probably fused with the WCT beat. Thus, we have "reset" and fusion, the hallmarks of macroreentry.

Figure 6.5B

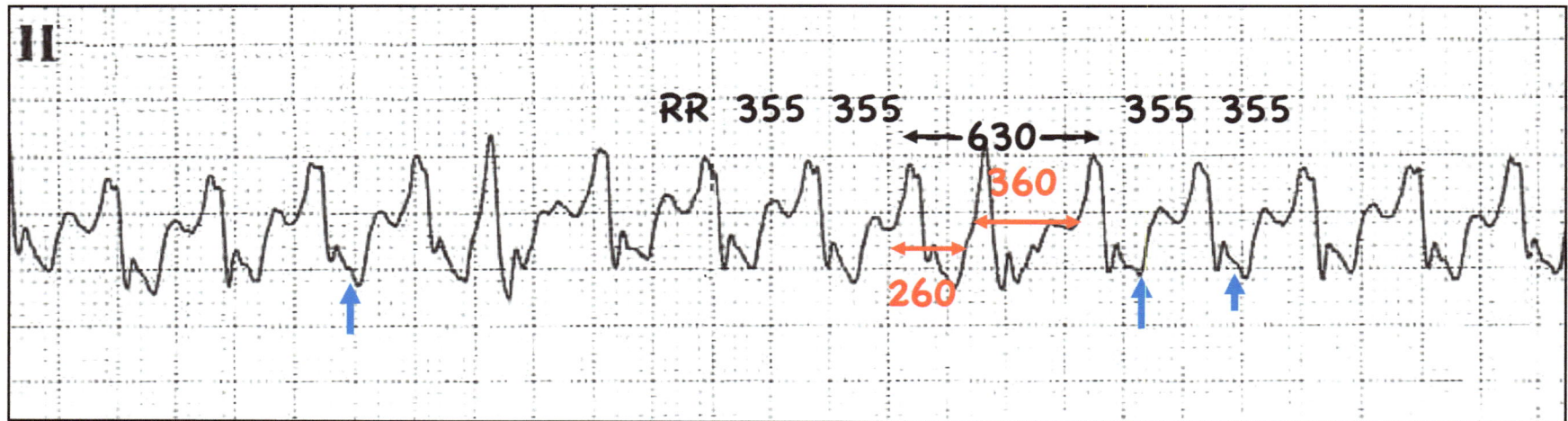

We further note that the post PVC interval is 360 ms or approximately 1 cycle. Our RV PVC got into the circuit and advanced the next cycle by exactly one CL. This is analogous to thinking of it as the "PPI = TCL" after entrainment. *The amount of reset of the return cycle paralleled the degree of prematurity of the PVC suggesting that little to no decrement occurred in the circuit as a result of prematurity.*

If we bypass some of our EP jargon in the last paragraph, it is easy to appreciate that our RV PVC got into the circuit readily to advance the next expected beat in proportion to its prematurity. *We therefore conclude that the RV must be part of the circuit.*

I don't think we can take this any further. We have, of course, ruled out AVNRT and AT, which would not be affected by a late-coupled PVC. The most likely mechanism for an individual with no structural heart disease, based on prevalence of arrhythmia mechanism, would be orthodromic AVRT (the RV would be *in the circuit* for a right-sided AP or a left-sided AP with LBBB) but theoretically, one could not rule out VT (RV origin or BBR) or antidromic AVRT over a right AP. This individual did not wish to have EP study.

Problem 6.6

The tracing **Figure 6.6A** shows a PAC from the HRA programmed into a regular WCT with LBBB morphology. A believable P wave is seen in the ST segment throughout, and the HRA electrogram is probably not necessary for this exercise if you wish to have an initial try at it omitting the HRA.

The differential diagnoses for this tachycardia include the "usual suspects": realistically VT preexcited tachycardia and SVT with LBBB aberrancy.

Figure 6.6A

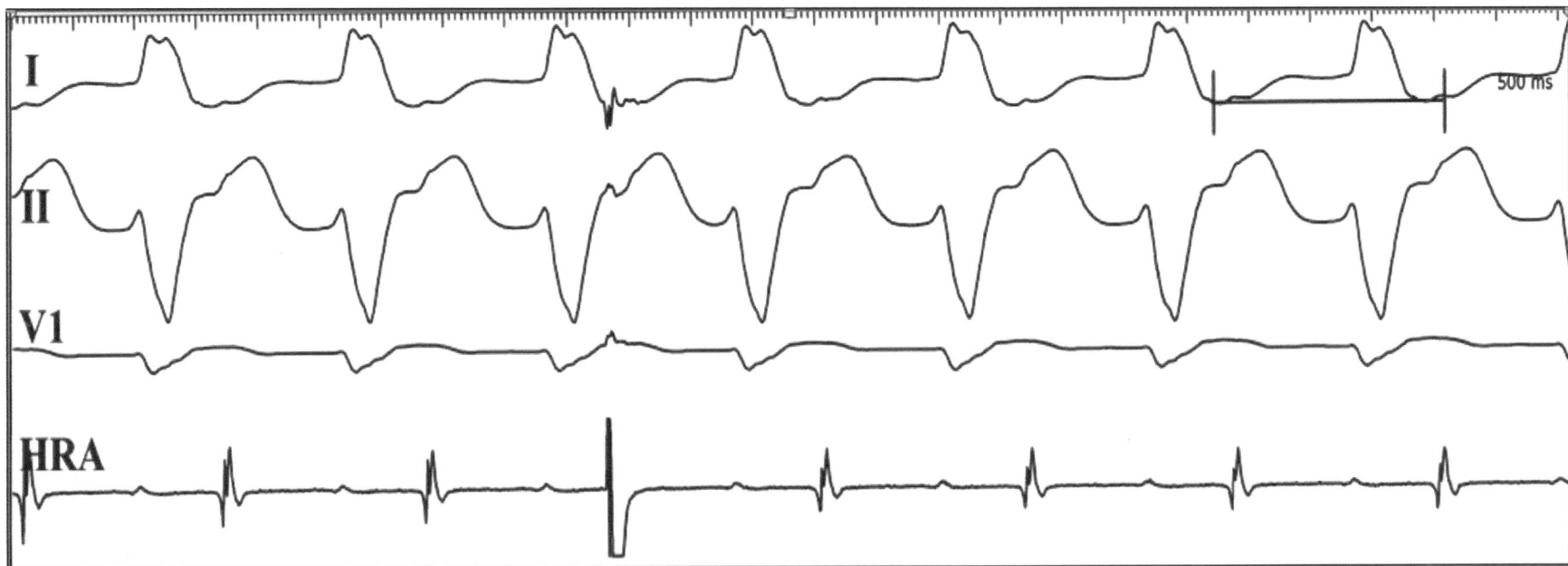

After initial observations, the *critical task examining the ectopic beat is to see how it affects the tachycardia*; the measurements are provided in **Figure 6.6B**. We observe that a minimally premature PAC advances (resets) the subsequent QRS. This informs us that the PAC from the HRA has excellent access into the tachycardia mechanism, ruling out VT categorically.

Figure 6.6B

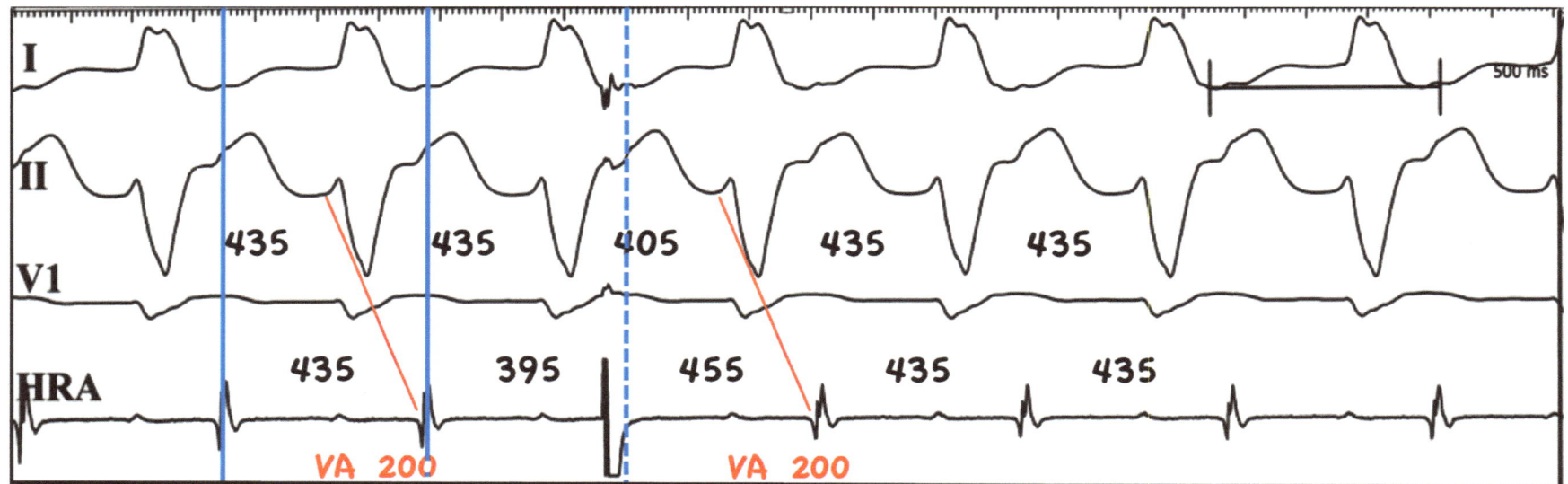

This PAC is so late that in all probability, it collides with the atrial activation of the previous beat resulting in atrial *fusion*. I have provided a **dashed blue line** to show the expected arrival of the next atrial beat in absence of the PAC and note that the PAC is only about 40 ms premature. We now have atrial fusion and resetting of the subsequent beat which means *macroreentry* with rare exceptions. *Furthermore, the atrium has good access to the circuit and must be part of the circuit (excluding mechanisms such as AVNR, VT, JT, or NVRT).* Of our 3 original candidates in the differential diagnosis, we are left now with SVT, either preexcited or with bundle branch block aberration.

We next note that the first VA after the QRS is advanced remains at 200 ms, i.e., the same as prior to the reset. Thus, the A exactly follows the advanced V (i.e., is "linked" to it) making AT very unlikely.

Because we have fusion and reset and have ruled out AT and VT, we are left with AVRT with the QRS either preexcited or aberrant. Do we have enough information to answer this last question? We will need to see the other electrograms to establish this without doubt, but we can say that the HRA PAC that is only 40 ms premature to the atrial rhythm is unlikely to advance ventricular activation via the normal AV conduction system. This suggests that it must be conducting over an accessory pathway.

With more leads available in **Figure 6.6C**, we see that the His A (**arrow**) has just depolarized prior to arrival of the PAC, so the atrial septal tissue must be refractory. Therefore our WCT must utilize an AP for anterograde conduction. Theoretically, the retrograde limb with this central activation system may be a septal AP but AVRT from one pathway to another is much less common than antidromic tachycardia (down an AP, up the normal AVCS) making antidromic tachycardia the much higher probability option. This was found to be the case.

Figre 6.6C

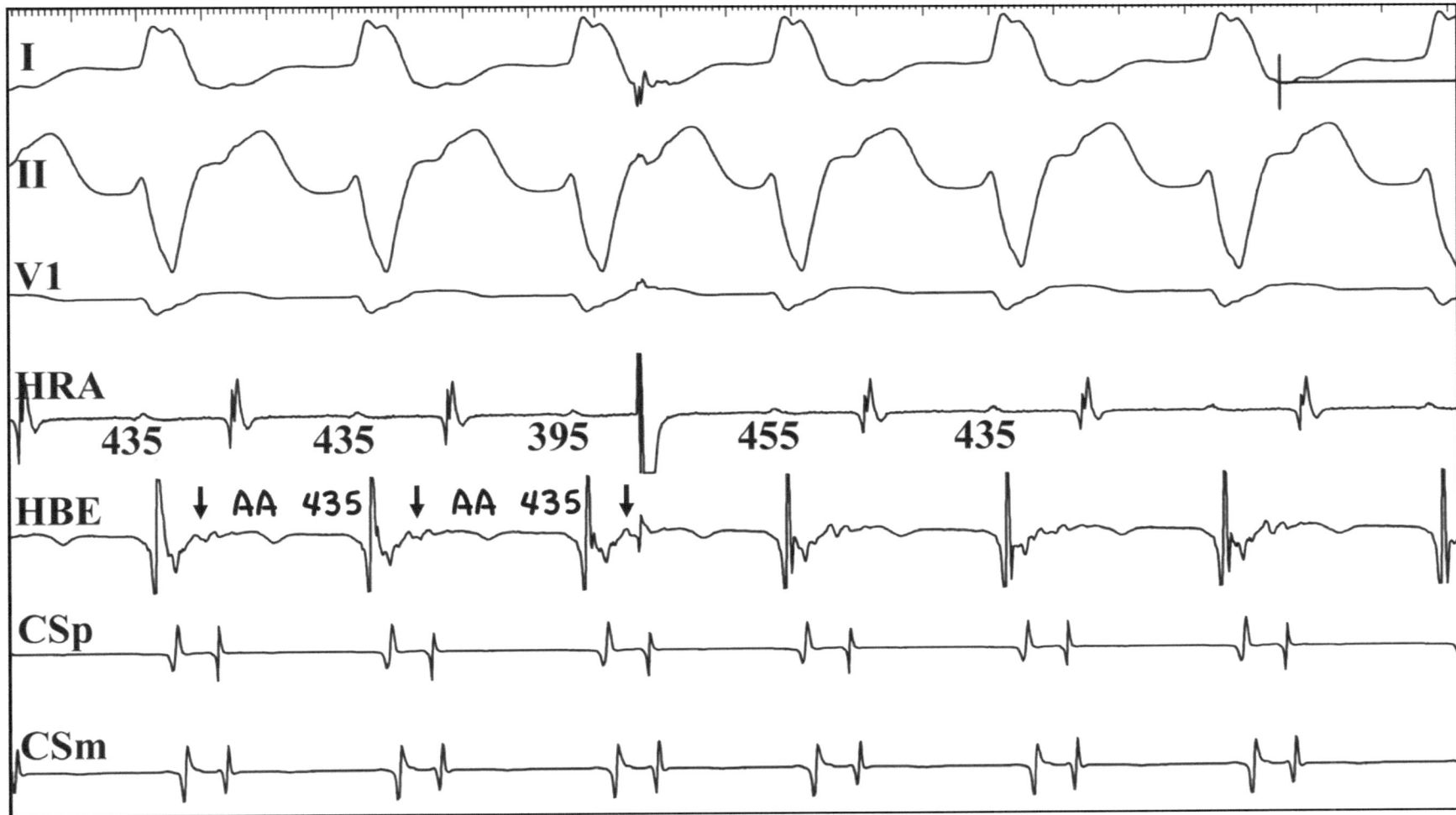

Problem 6.7

The WCT in **Figure 6.7A** terminates spontaneously. AV dissociation is readily apparent from our initial overview, which confines our diagnostic problem to VT, AVNRT, NVRT, or JT. A His deflection is present in front of each QRS, but this doesn't help at this point as it may be anterograde or retrograde and conceivably present with all our possible diagnoses. It is time to bring out the calipers, sweep the tracing for irregularities and make a few measurements (**Figure 6.7B**).

Figure 6.7A

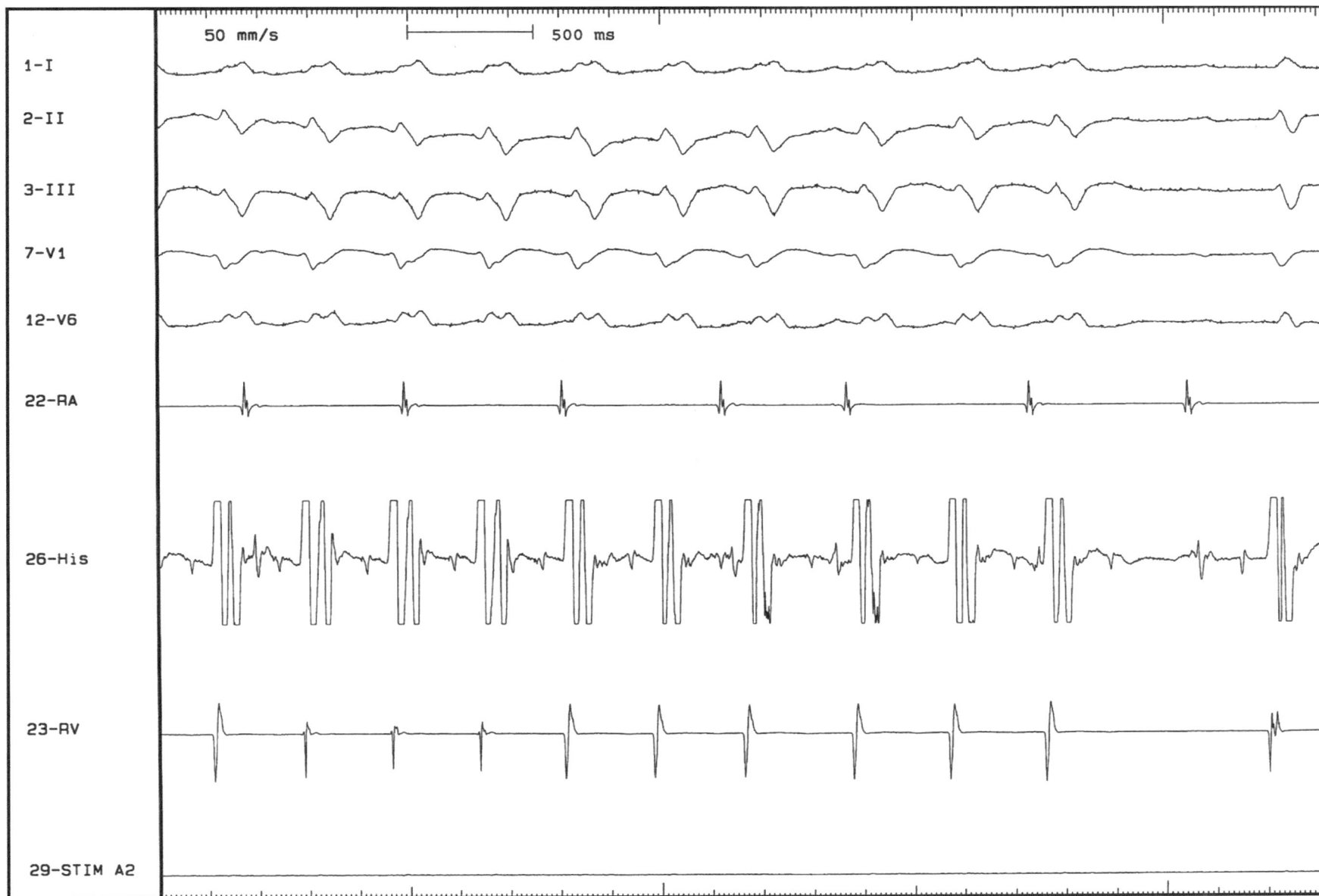

Figure 6.7B

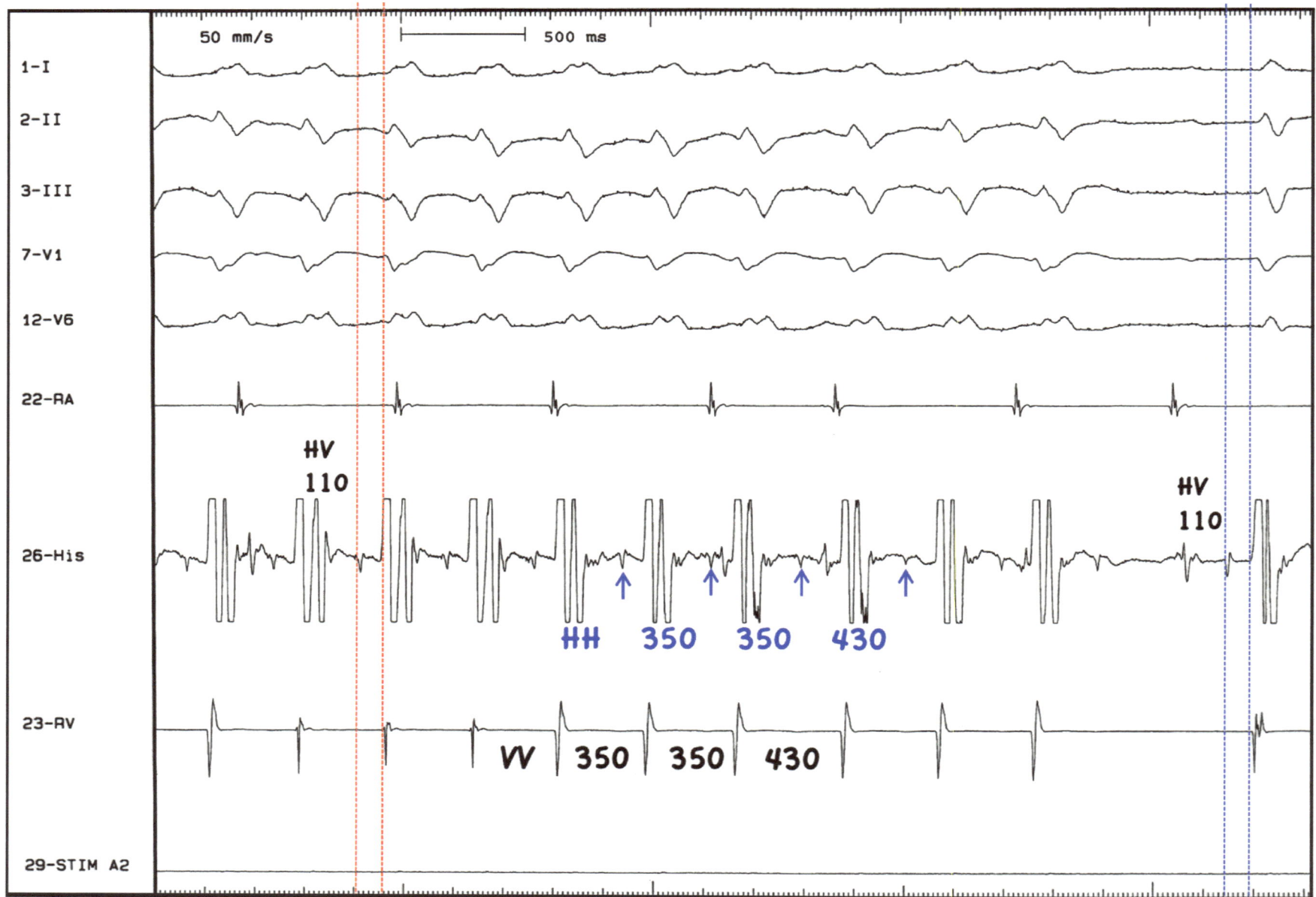

The one sinus beat available shows left-axis deviation, an HV of 110 ms, and early ventricular activation at the RV apical EGM. The long HV raises our antennae for VT related to BBR.

Interestingly, the HV during WCT is also 110 with early ventricular activation again at the RV apex. The QRS is compatible with a LBBB pattern and the breakout of the WCT at the RV apex is the same as that during sinus rhythm. The CL of the WCT is quite regular, 350 ms, but we have been given a gift of one long cycle of 430 ms. The **first** EGM to delay is the RV apex with the His following subsequently. This *excludes* AVNRT and JT, since the delay initially evident in the RV could not be caused by a change in AVNRT or JT, which would delay the H first. We

have thus simplified our problem, since it has to be VT, with the remote theoretical possibility of NVRT still on the table.

Is it BBR VT? We note that the prolongation of the HV interval *preceded* the prolongation of the VV interval, i.e., the HV predicted the HH. Thus, conduction delay between the His recording and the exit from the RBB (RBB delay) may well have caused prolongation of the CL with the RBB as part of the circuit. Absolute proof of this can be provided by ablating the RBB and stopping tachycardia, but for all practical purposes, this can only be BBR.

The circuit is shown schematically in **Figure 6.7C** where the asterisk (★) indicates the conduction delay in the RBB.

Figure 6.7C

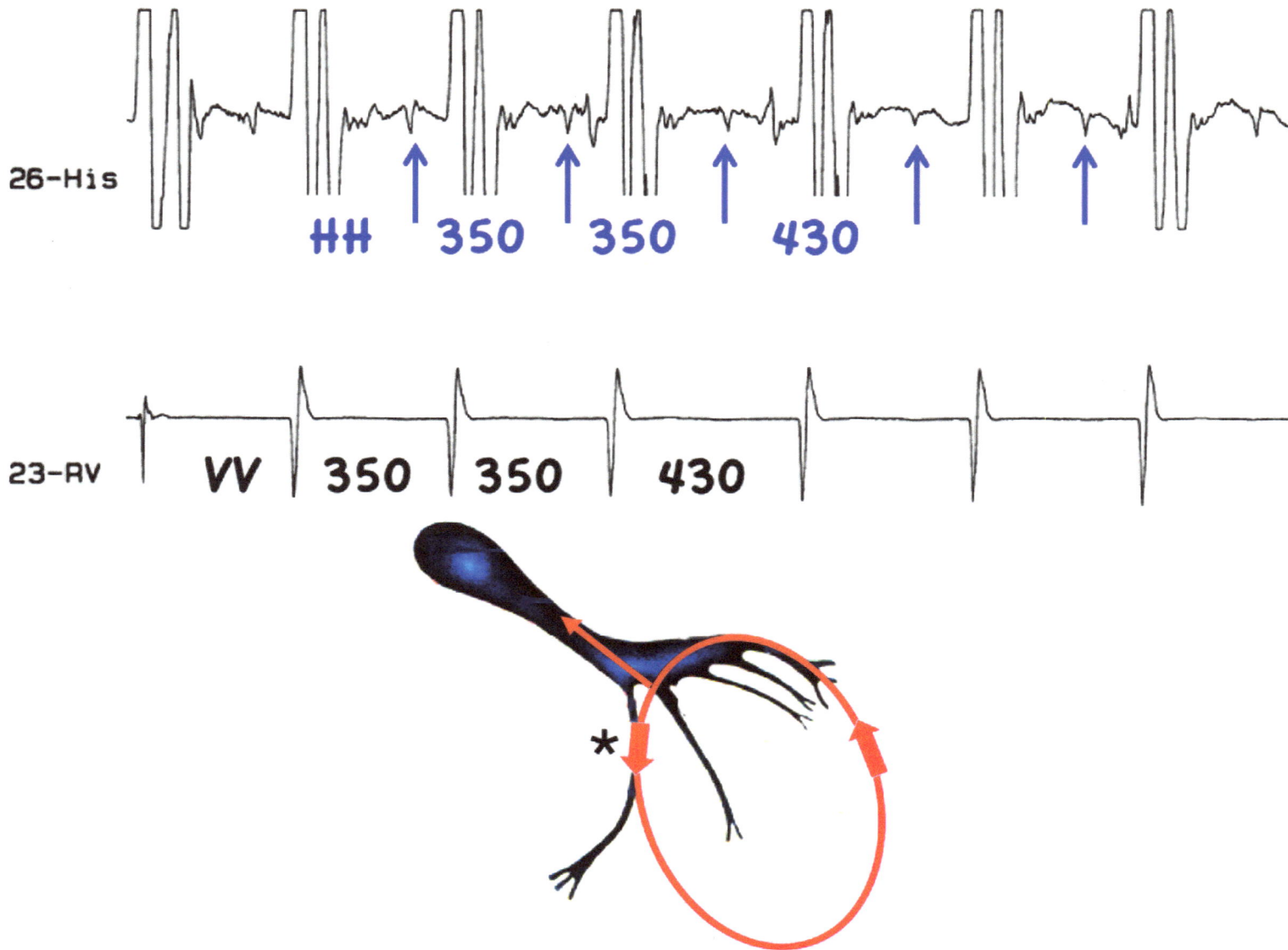

Chapter 7

Exploration of the "Sidelines"

Problem 7.1

My long-standing friend and teaching partner, Eric Prystowsky, might call a case like this a "gotcha."

As you go through **Figure 7.1A**, you may understand what he means by that.

Figure 7.1A

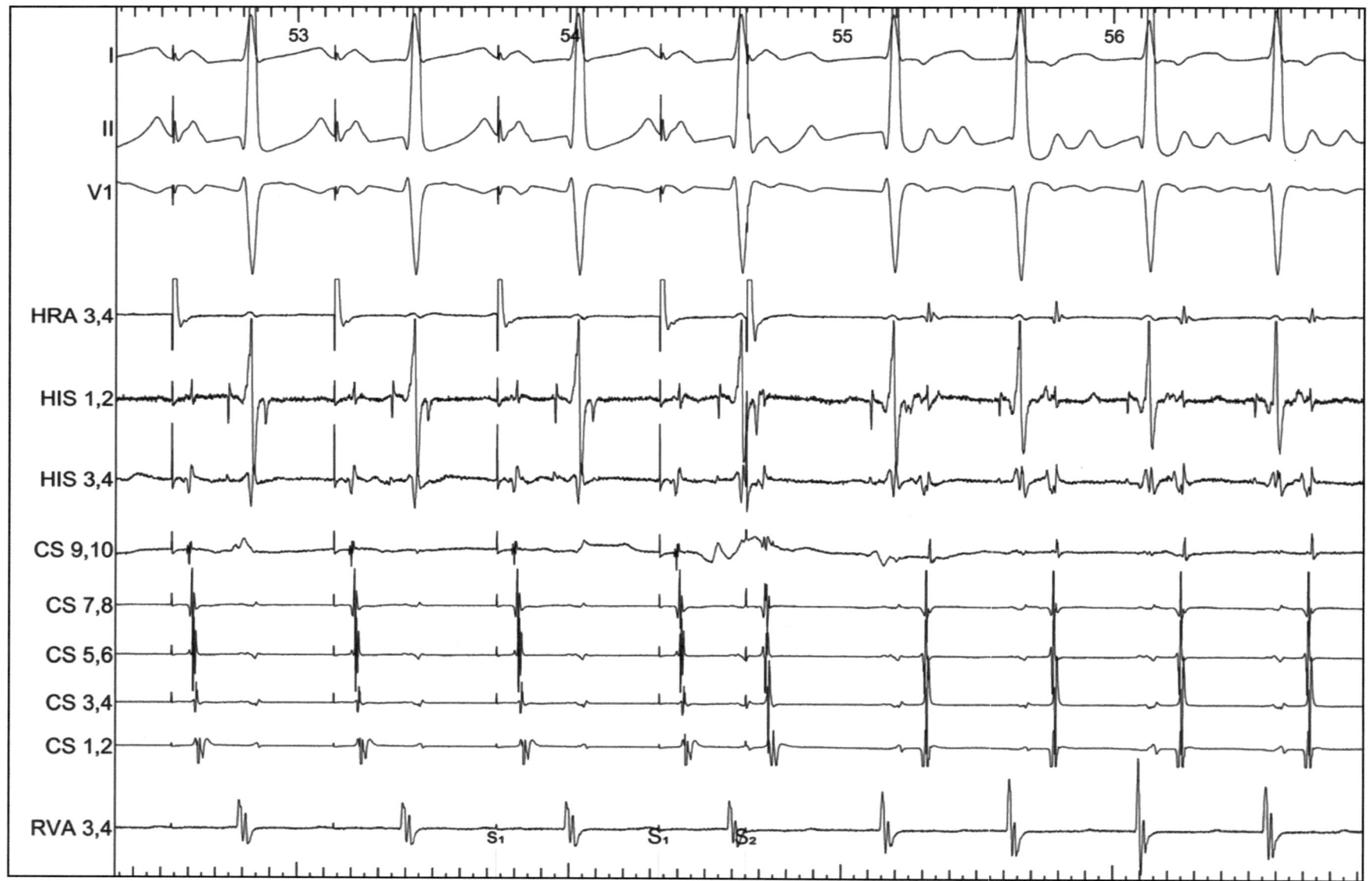

The problem in **Figure 7.1A** is obviously to determine the mechanism of the SVT, with the usual culprits being AT, AVNRT, and AVRT. Looking at the annotated **Figure 7.1B**, we appreciate 3 evident zones from left to right.

Figure 7.1B

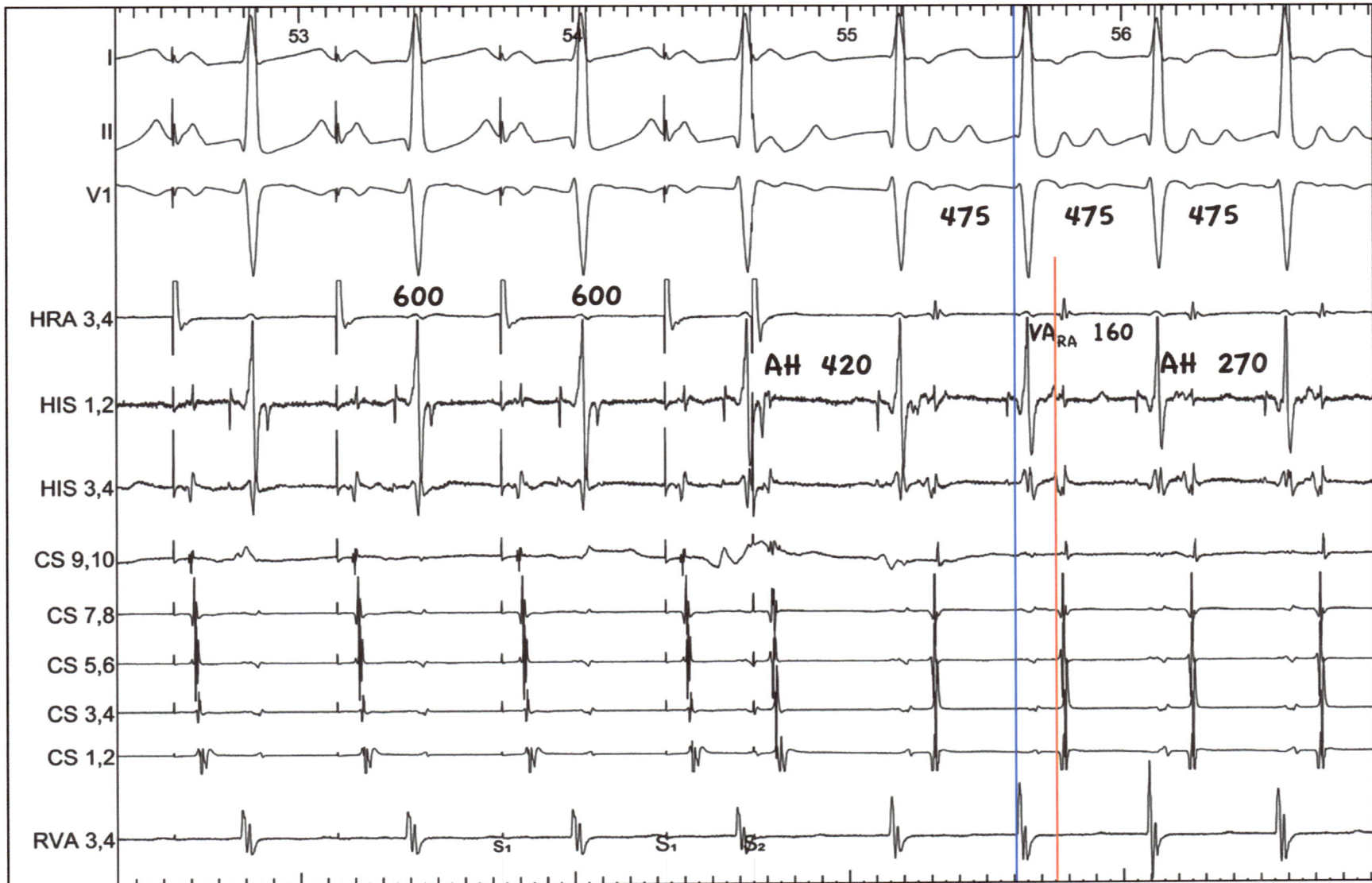

Starting with zone 1, we see atrial pacing at a CL of 600 ms, and the drive is "clean" or unobstructed with ectopy or artifact. An atrial extrastimulus starts zone 2, the transition zone. We observe a huge "jump" or prolongation of the AH interval. This can only be a slow AVN pathway, discounting the much less likely possibility of AV block with emergence of SVT initiated by a junctional escape. This doesn't really help us, as a slow pathway can be the antegrade limb of AVRT or be manifest with AT.

Looking now at zone 3 or the SVT, we move our calipers and make the measurements you see annotated. We see that the first VA interval is essentially the same as the ongoing tachycardia. This essentially rules out AT, since it would be coincidental if the *first A of the SVT* were to fall into place at the VA of the tachycardia (the VA seems "linked"). It is still not clear whether we are dealing with AVNRT or AVRT. To facilitate visually "lining up" the events, we draw lines at the onset of QRS (**blue**) and front of the earliest A (**red**).

We have a problem now, since the VA intervals at *all* the sites are virtually identical! This can mean only one of 2 things: the first possibility is that there is more than one retrograde route and we are looking at fusion of 2 or more retrograde atrial routes. Alternatively, we could be mistaken in where the catheters are actually positioned.

In **Figure 7.1C**, I have compressed the time to make it more comparable to looking at a standard ECG. Compressing is one of those little "tools" that help you see things that actually seem *less* clear the faster the sweep speed (such as P waves or T waves). The negative P wave in lead 1 (**red arrow**) now stands out *if one looks at the ECG*. Its onset actually precedes the earliest rapid atrial EGM and this can only be atrial activation from left to right, most compatible with a left lateral AP as the predominant and probably exclusive source of atrial activation. That was indeed the case, and the left AP was ablated. The CS catheter was not distal enough and also probably "off" the AV ring, suggested by the very far-field ventricular EGMs, with the EGMs misleadingly late.

Figure 7.1C

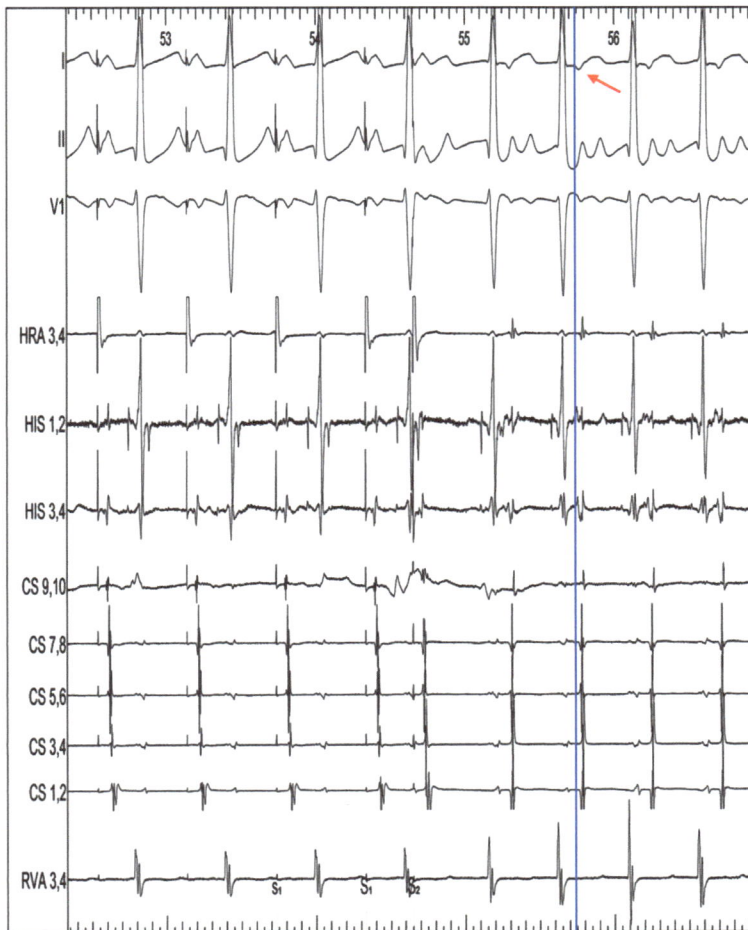

The observed AVRT in this example utilized a slow AVN pathway. AVRT over the fast pathway was not observed prior to or during the study. This raises the possibility of an alternate strategy, namely ablating the slow AVN pathway, a strategy that may be appropriate under certain circumstances. Of course, both would have to be ablated if AVNRT were inducible or a clinical tachycardia.

A tracing often has an interesting zone that acts as a magnet to get attention, be it a run of WCT, a long pause, or a striking change in the tracing. This brief example exemplifies the importance of not abandoning the usual systematic plan and undercutting the "checklist," not forgetting the ECG and the other "sidelines." My old friend and brilliant teaching colleague, the late Mark Josephson, always began his discussions of such cases by admonishing the trainee to always look on the "outside" first—that is, the ECG. Not bad advice!

Problem 7.2

There is no glaring atrial activity during this regular SVT, but there is a hint of a terminal "glitch" just after the QRS in some of the leads such as V_1 (**Figure 7.2A**). V_1 and the inferior leads are generally the most useful for identifying P wave activity, but all leads should be examined.

Figure 7.2A

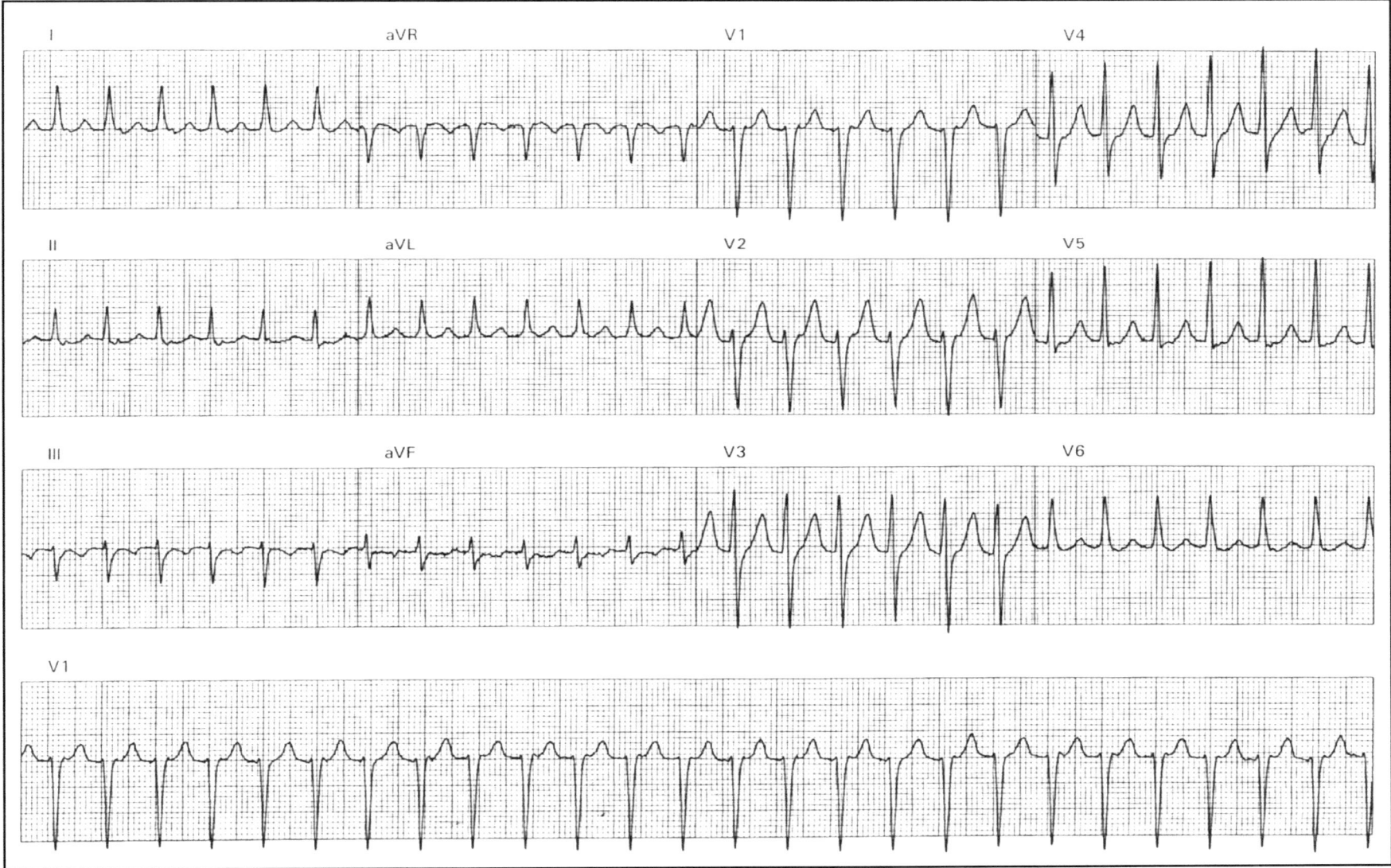

It is time to enlarge an area of interest (**Figure 7.2B**). We are fortunate that the tracing is quite "clean," free of significant arti–fact. We now appreciate the terminal glitch a little better but note further that it is not always there (**red arrows**). This strongly supports the veracity of our "candidate" P wave and further shows that the *tachycardia continues without an associated P wave*. At this point, we have ruled out AVRT and AT as mechanisms. We can now reframe our problem as "SVT that doesn't require atrial participation," a relatively short list that includes AVNRT, NVRT, and JT.

Figure 7.2B

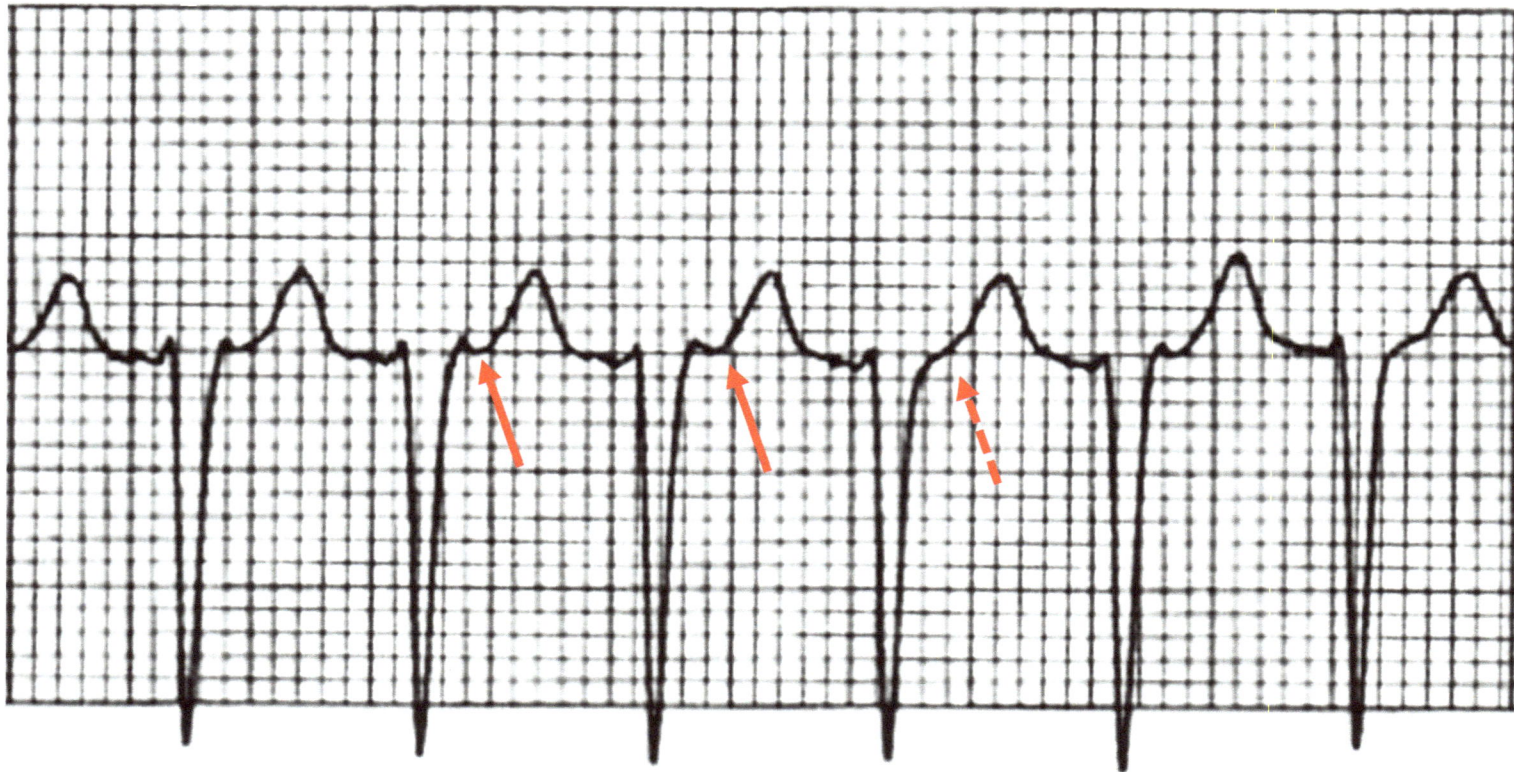

V 1

Our impression is substantiated by the intracardiac recording showing SVT continuing oblivious to VA block (**Figure 7.2C**). The atrial activation is also central with earliest A in the septal region.

Figure 7.2C

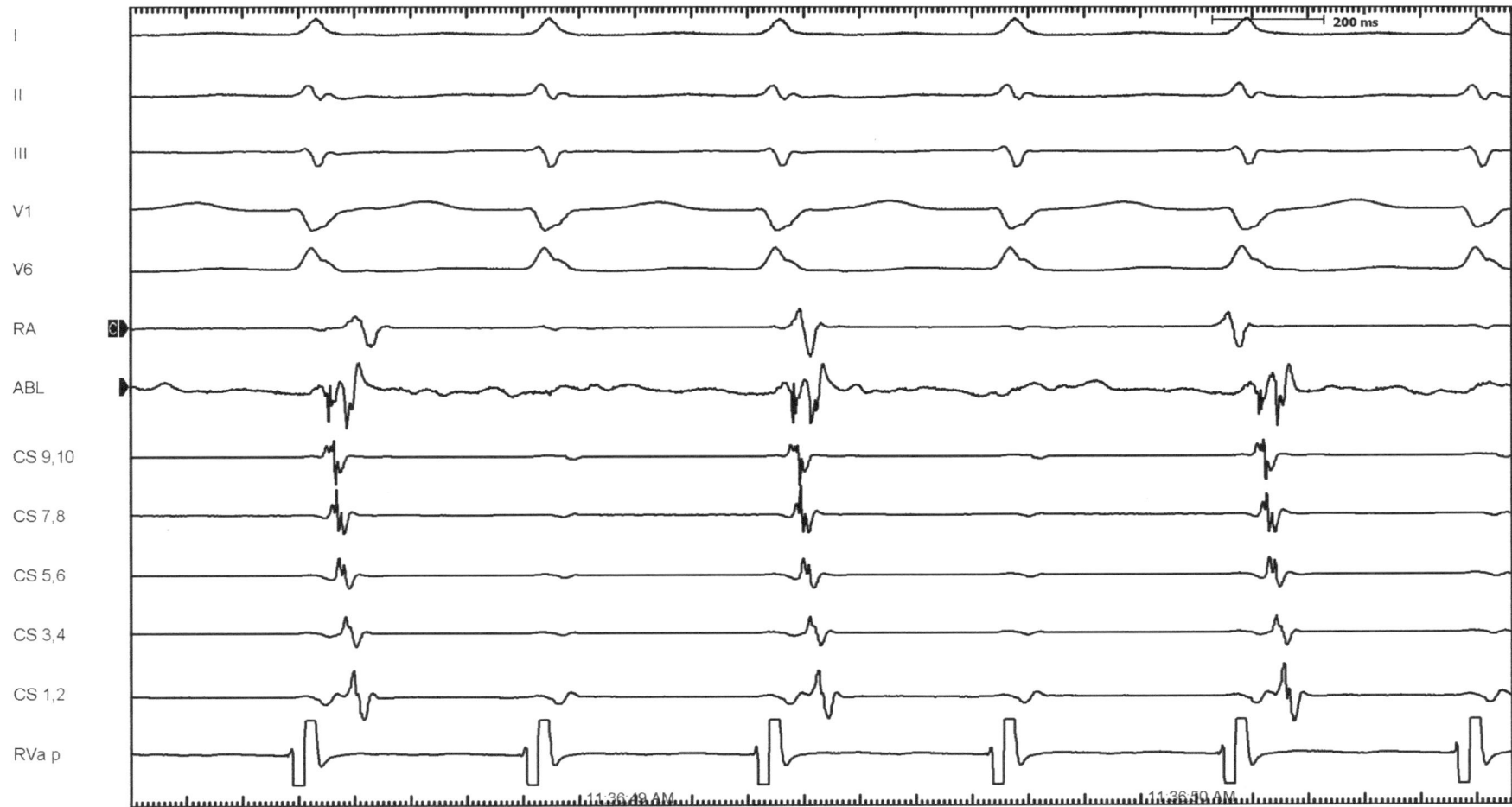

The most likely diagnosis by far on the basis of probability is AVNRT, but a maneuver is now required (**Figure 7.2D**), and a late-coupled PVC is inserted into the cardiac cycle during SVT at a time when the His should be refractory. This unequivocally advances the next ventricular cycle, proving that there is another route for the PVC to get to the tachycardia mechanism other than the normal retrograde His route. This can only be retrograde conduction over a NFAP or NVAP.

Figure 7.2D

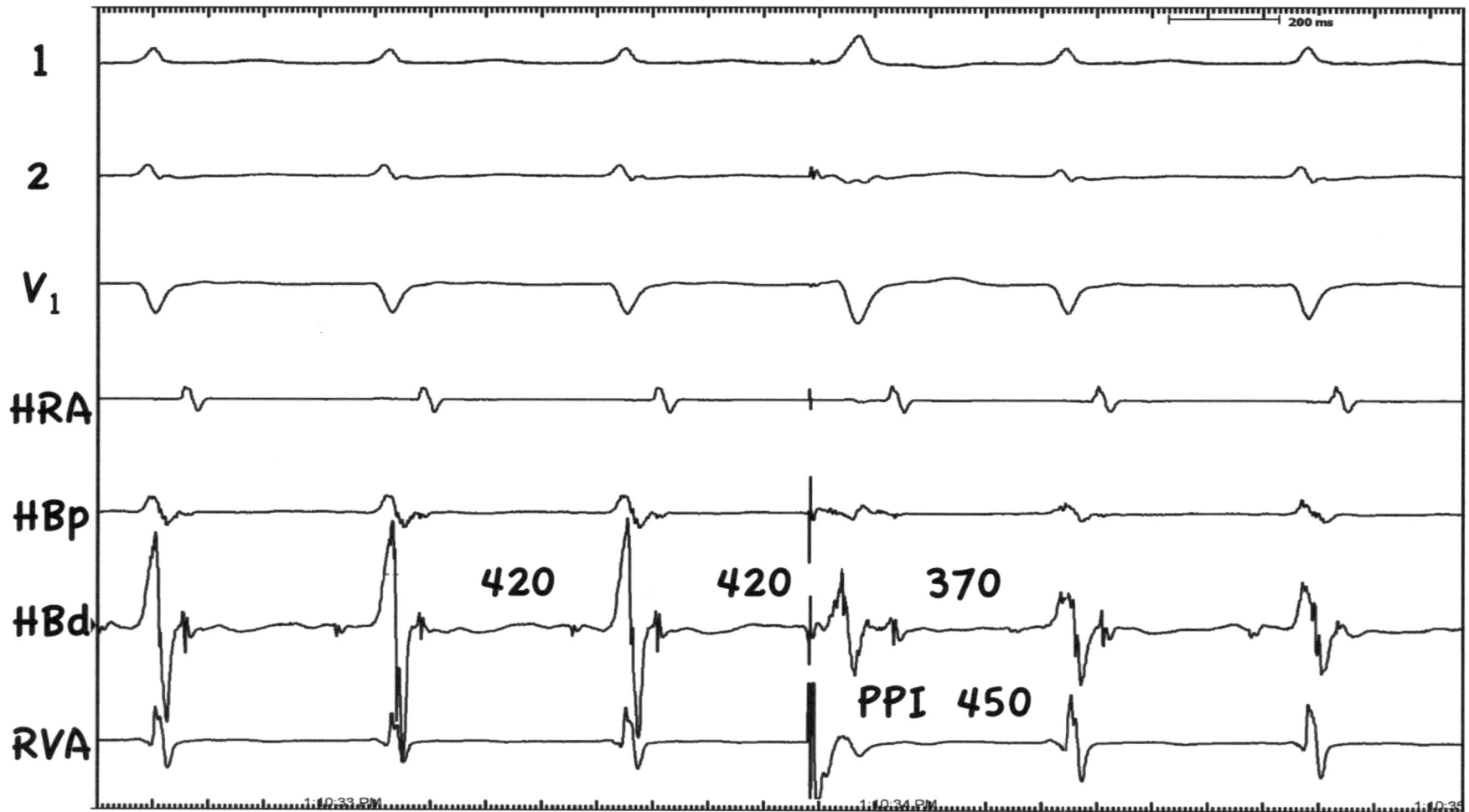

Recall that the PVC that fuses with the tachycardia QRS and resets the tachycardia is essentially equivalent to entrainment for one cycle, so entrainment diagnostic criteria (Michaud criteria) apply. Thus, the PPI–TCL at the RV electrogram is only 30 ms, far shorter than that usually seen for AVNRT (> 115 ms), verifying that the RV is essentially "in" the circuit. This is what you would expect with NV or NF reentry.

As a final very interesting observation, you may have noted that the A after the PVC is **NOT** advanced even though the subsequent QRS **IS** advanced. This would not happen with an atrioventricular AP, since reset of the next QRS in that case could only follow advancement or delay of the A. In our case, the PVC did NOT affect retrograde conduction, although it obviously must have gotten into the anterograde limb to advance the next QRS. One can imagine the morphological architecture that would allow this, although in truth it can only be guessed at.

Case provided with the compliments of Dr. J. Leitch.

Problem 7.3

The tracing of **Figure 7.3A** shows a WCT interrupted by a PAC. We begin by looking at the beats after sinus rhythm resumed and observe that the QRS is relatively normal. Importantly, we note at best a rudimentary His bundle EGM, so that we would not necessarily expect to see a His during the WCT. That is, the absence of a His deflection will not be diagnostically useful during the WCT.

Figure 7.3A

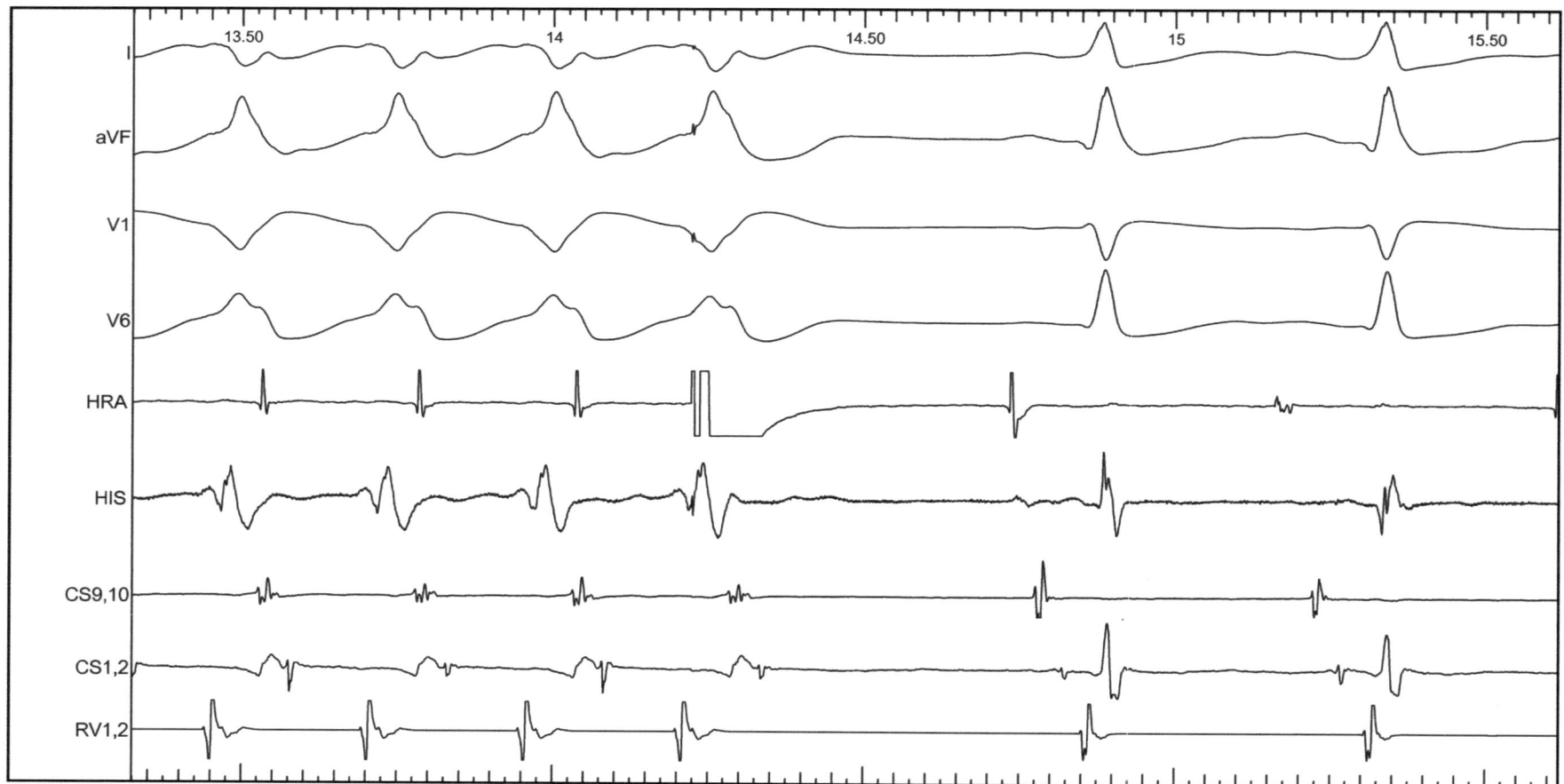

We then direct our attention to the WCT. The QRS morphology is LBBB type and is potentially compatible with VT, aberrancy, or preexcitation. The RV apex (RV apical EGM) activates very early, at the onset of the QRS (**Figure 7.3B, red line**). This eliminates a conventional AV accessory pathway, which would result in initial ventricular activation at the base of the ventricle.

The atrial leads available are limited with the His A not visible and the HRA position is unknown but probably not "high" (onset of the P wave in sinus rhythm is well ahead of the RA EGM). Thus, the atrial activation may be central, but this is not clearly evident in the leads available.

Figure 7.3B

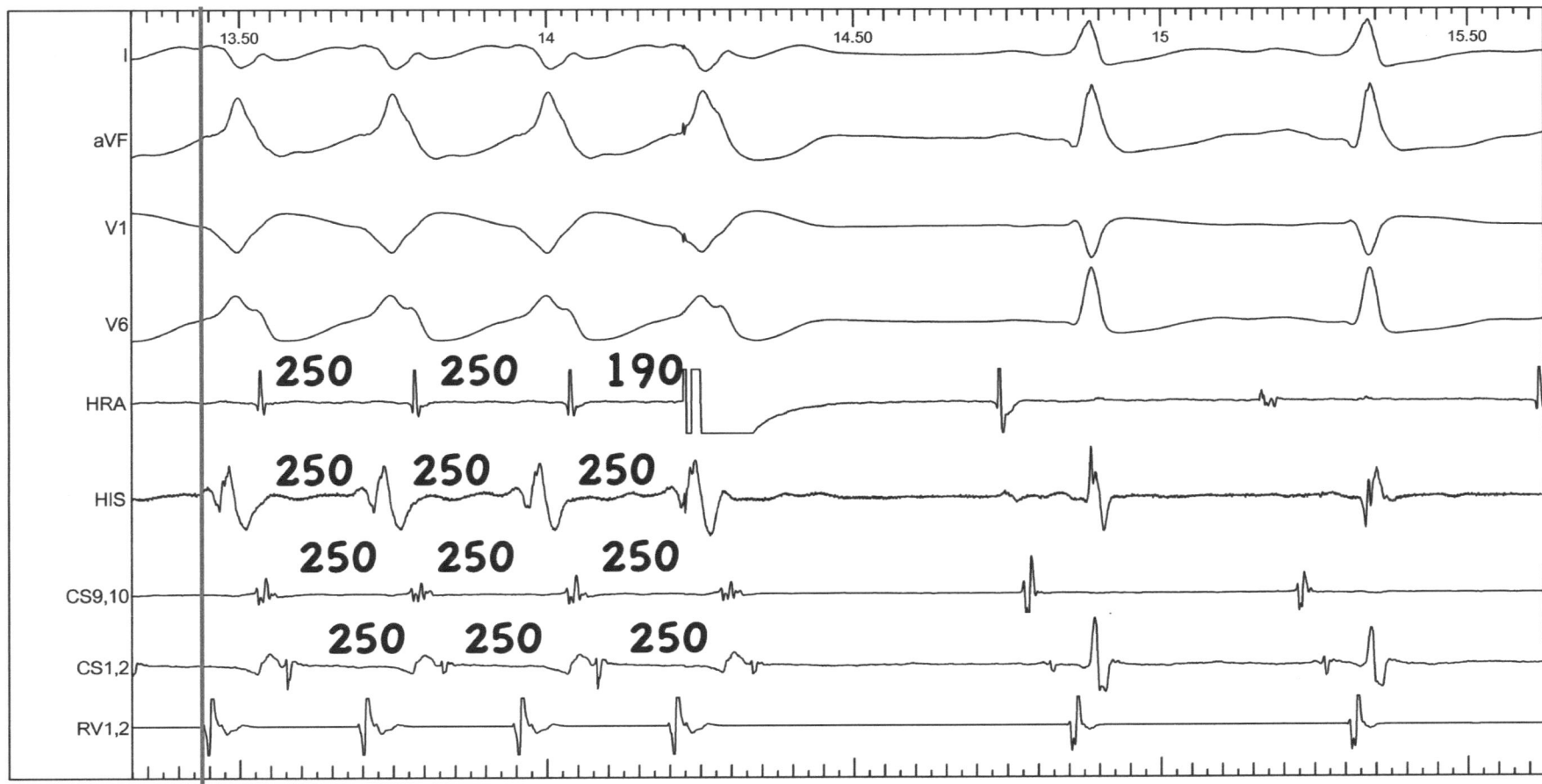

The CL of the WCT is 250 ms and the RA PAC that interrupts it is coupled at 190 ms. The **critical observation** at this point is noting that CS atrial EGMs are "on time" and are not advanced by the prematurity of the RA EGM. This tells us that the arrhythmia is caused by macro reentry since we have **fusion** of atrial activation, which is associated with **reset**, in this case, termination of tachycardia. The RA PAC *could not* influence a point-source AT if atrial activation were already underway when the PAC activation reaches it. That is, it could not go "upstream" against the orthodromic wave already in motion. This could theoretically be any macroreentrant tachycardia involving the atrium (AT or AV reentry) but *not* focal AT. It is not VT, which could not be terminated with a PAC that doesn't reach the ventricle.

Finally, we note that the RA PAC would have arrived at the atrial septum (as approximated by CS 9–10, i.e., the proximal CS) when the septum was refractory, having been depolarized by the previous atrial wave. Thus, the PAC reached a **refractory** AVN and could NOT have influenced the change via the AV node, proving the participation of an AP during WCT.

To summarize at this point, we began with a differential diagnosis for our WCT including VT, SVT with aberrancy, SVT with anterograde conduction over an accessory pathway. VT was readily ruled out by termination with a PAC that didn't reach the ventricle.

Any AT was essentially ruled out because it would be too coincidental to have AV block simultaneously with a termination in the atrium. Ruling out VT and AT essentially leaves us with an AV reentrant tachycardia.

The anterograde limb of the tachycardia must be an AP since termination occurred with a PAC arriving at the atrial septum (i.e., the AV node) when this latter was refractory.

The AP could only be atriofascicular, since earliest ventricular activity was noted at the RV apex. The retrograde atrial limb of the circuit is unknown from this tracing (i.e., AVN or another AP) but it is fair to say that antidromic tachycardia (anterogradely over an AP, retrogradely over the AVN) is much more likely than the very uncommon AP-to-AP circuit. In this case it was indeed antidromic with anterograde conduction over the atriofascicular AP and retrograde conduction over the normal AV conduction system.

In the schematic illustrating the mechanism of the tracing (**Figure 7.3C**), the wave front of the paced atrial beat is **purple**, the orthodromic wave of the tachycardia is **green**, and the atriofascicular pathway is **red**.

Figure 7.3C

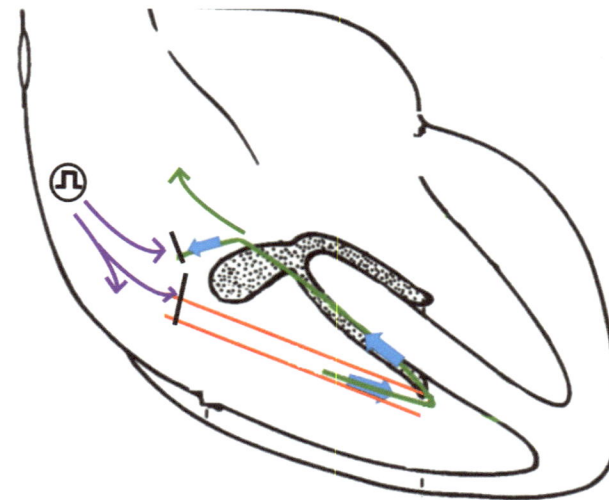

Based on a tracing provided with the compliments of Dr. Raja Selvaraj.

Problem 7.4

The tracing in **Figure 7.4A** can be summarized as spontaneous termination of a WCT. Note that the coronary sinus EGMs are recorded unipolar in this tracing, although this has no bearing on the interpretation.

Figure 7.4A

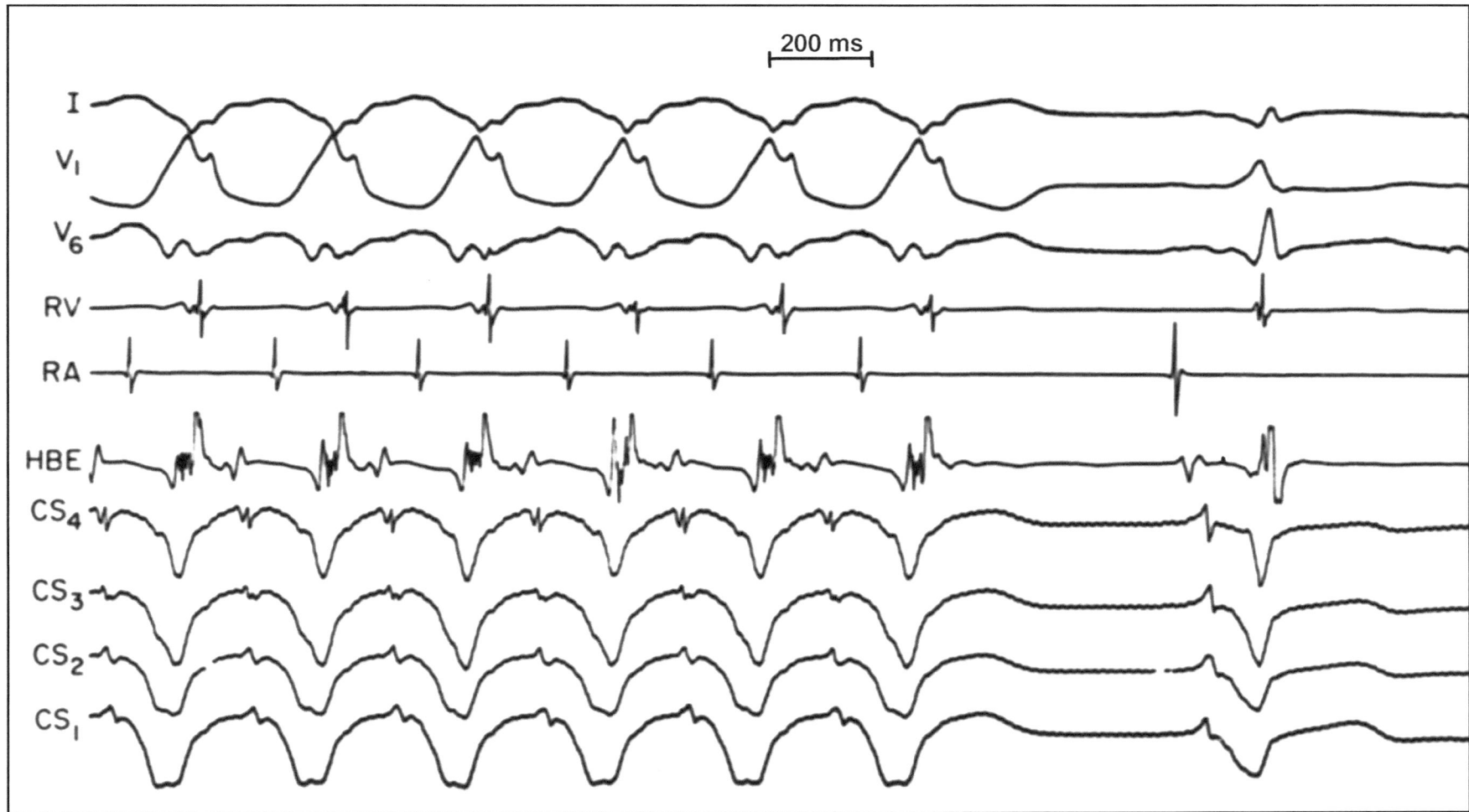

Many of us might be attracted to the "interesting" part of the tracing and ignore the normal sinus beat (i.e., the "sidelines") after termination. The normal beat is preexcited with a left lateral AP pattern (**Figure 7.4B**). The delta wave is negative in lead 1, and the HV is essentially 0 (**dashed red line**). In addition, earliest ventricular activation as provided by the unipolar CS leads is at the distal CS (CS poles 1 and 2).

Figure 7.4B

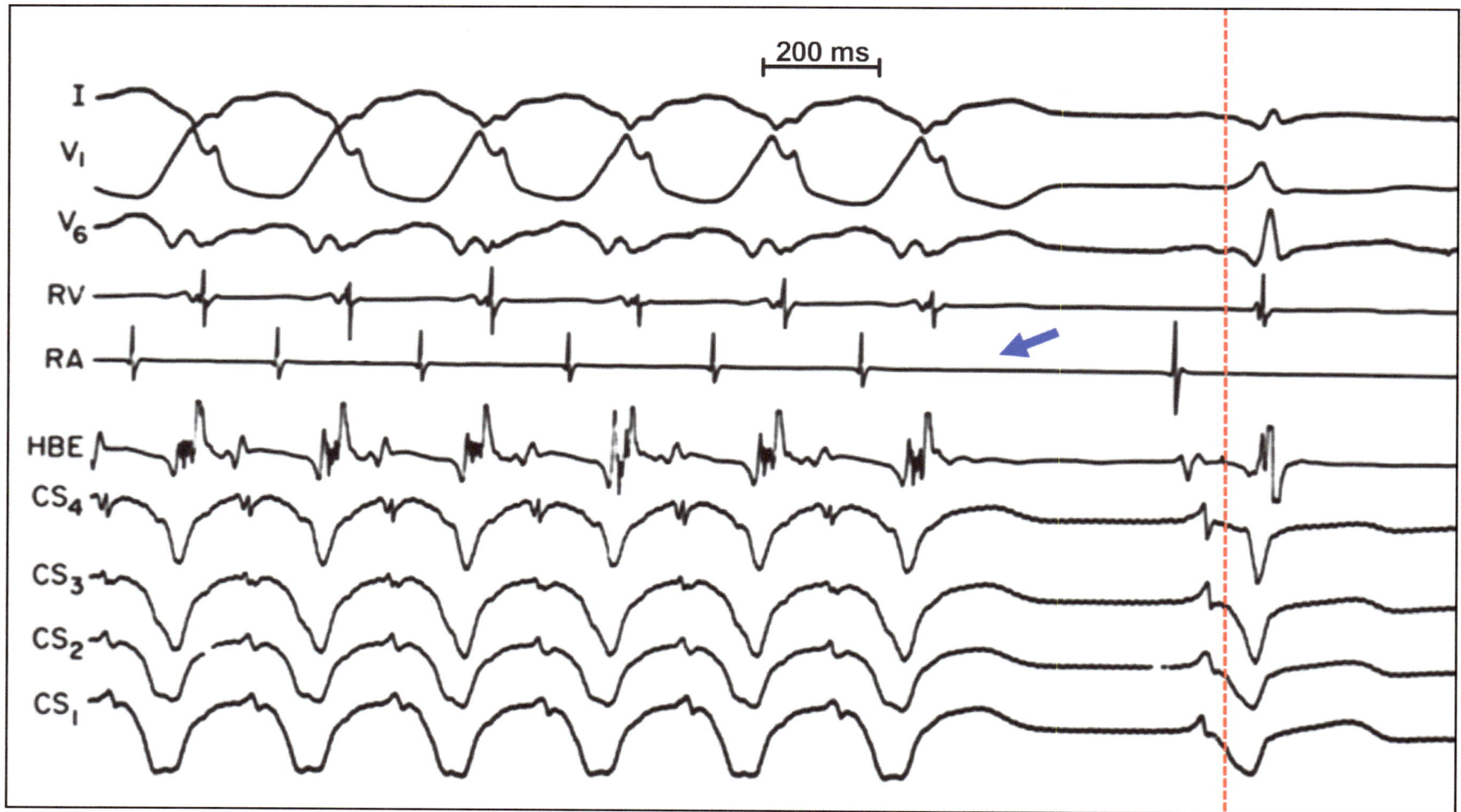

Moving to the WCT, one now recognizes that the QRS is fully preexcited over the same left lateral AP. The retrograde activation sequence is central, most probably over the normal AVCS since statistically, antidromic AVRT is considerably more likely than pathway-to-pathway reentry.

Focusing on the termination, we note that tachycardia terminated *without* atrial activation (**blue arrow**). This in itself essentially rules out VT since one would have to postulate spontaneous termination of VT with *coincidental* VA block occurring at exactly that instant.

Problem 7.5

Figure 7.5A is a Holter record and shows WCT with an apparent P wave in the ST segment that terminates spontaneously, with the last event being a P wave. Sinus rhythm resumes after a couple of accelerated junctional beats. Without seeing AV dissociation or how the recorded leads translate to standard ECG leads, the differential diagnosis for this tachycardia remains open. One might at this point *look at the "sidelines"* of the major area of interest and notice the "mini" ECG display recorded over a longer span that encompasses the WCT displayed. Is this useful?

Figure 7.5A

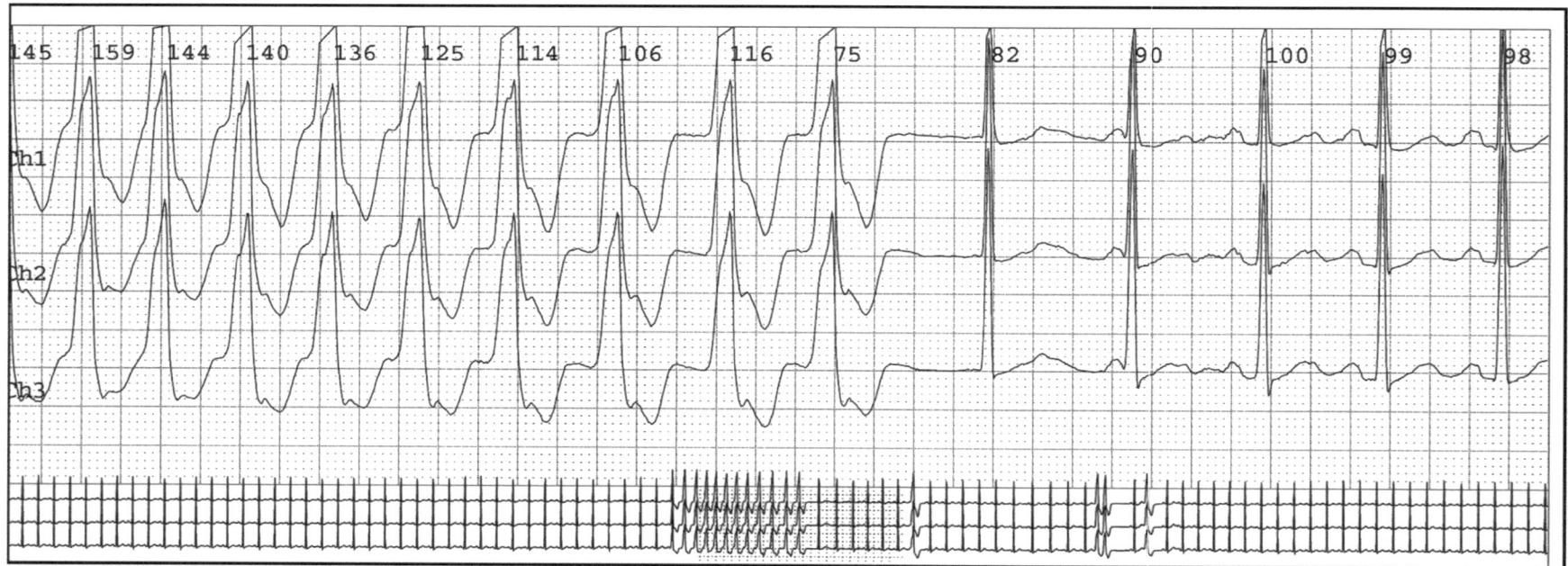

I have merely enlarged the area of the mini display in **Figure 7.5B** to show a few ectopic beats recorded. It becomes clear that the ectopic beats are NOT preceded by any atrial activity and are clearly PVCs. Since these PVCs have the identical QRS morphology as the WCT, the latter can only be VT.

It is often useful to look for single ectopic beats occurring at other parts of the record, and in this instance, it made the diagnosis. Alternately, the mini display also shows the onset of the WCT, which would of course demonstrate that the WCT begins with a ventricular event, hence VT.

Figure 7.5B

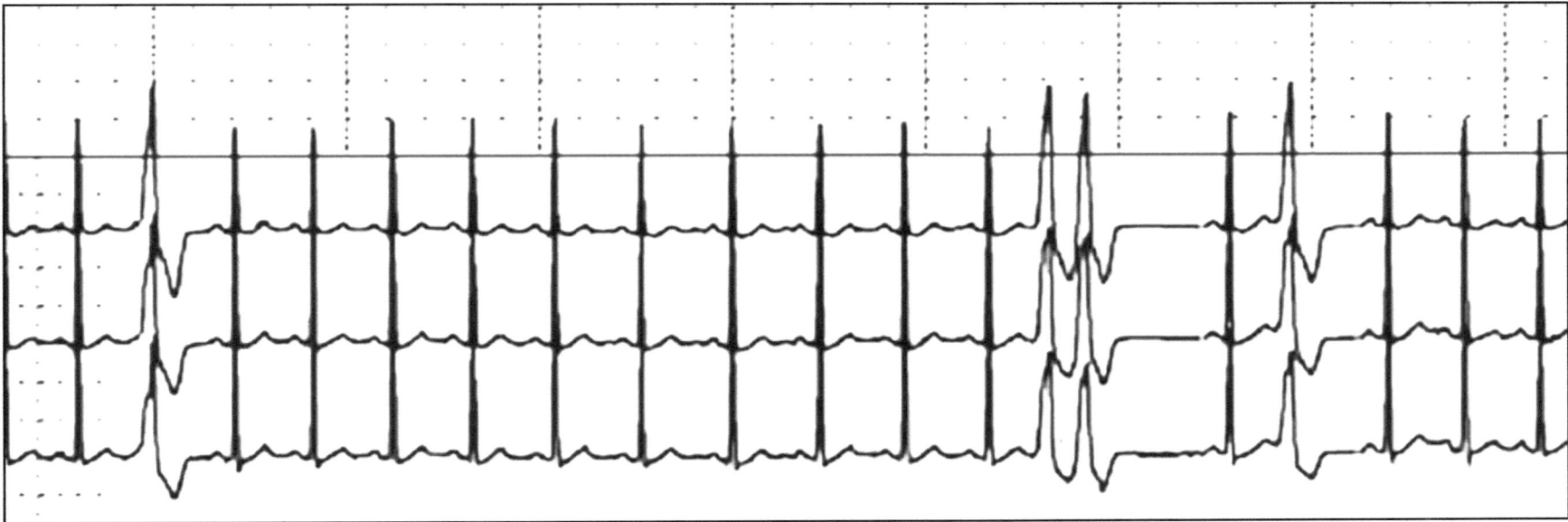

Problem 7.6

This is nequivocally atrial fibrillation (**Figure 7.6A**), and the challenge is to diagnose the wide complexes. We start with the first of 3 beats that are normal QRS and are preceded by a clear His deflection. The WC beats are of LBBB morphology, totally irregular, and reasonably compatible with AVN conduction with LBBB during AF.

Figure 7.6A

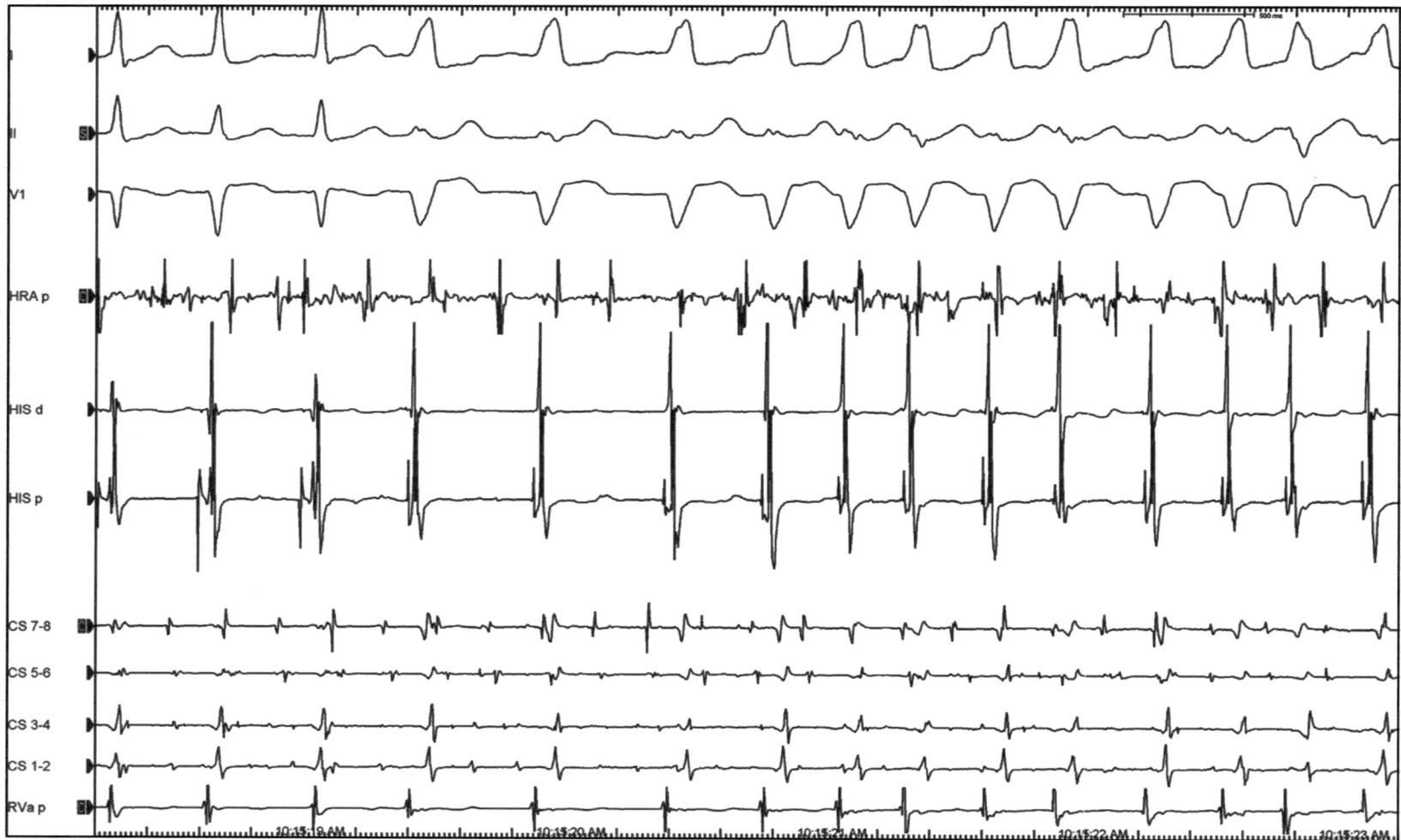

We magnify the area of interest, **Figure 7.6B**, and are drawn to a His deflection associated with each WC beat. The HV is < 0. This can only be ventricular or preexcited. A highly irregular ventricular rhythm of similar CL to the normal ones in the context of AF is unlikely to be VT, leaving us with a diagnosis of preexcitation. We now observe the ventricular activation sequence and note that the RV apical EGM is virtually simultaneous with the onset of the QRS, a situation not compatible with a conventional AV accessory pathway, where earliest ventricular activation is expected at the base of the heart and relatively late at the RV apex (**Figure 7.6C**). This early RV apical activation is the "signature" of the atriofascicular AP inserting from the atrium into the RBBB terminus region.

Figure 7.6B

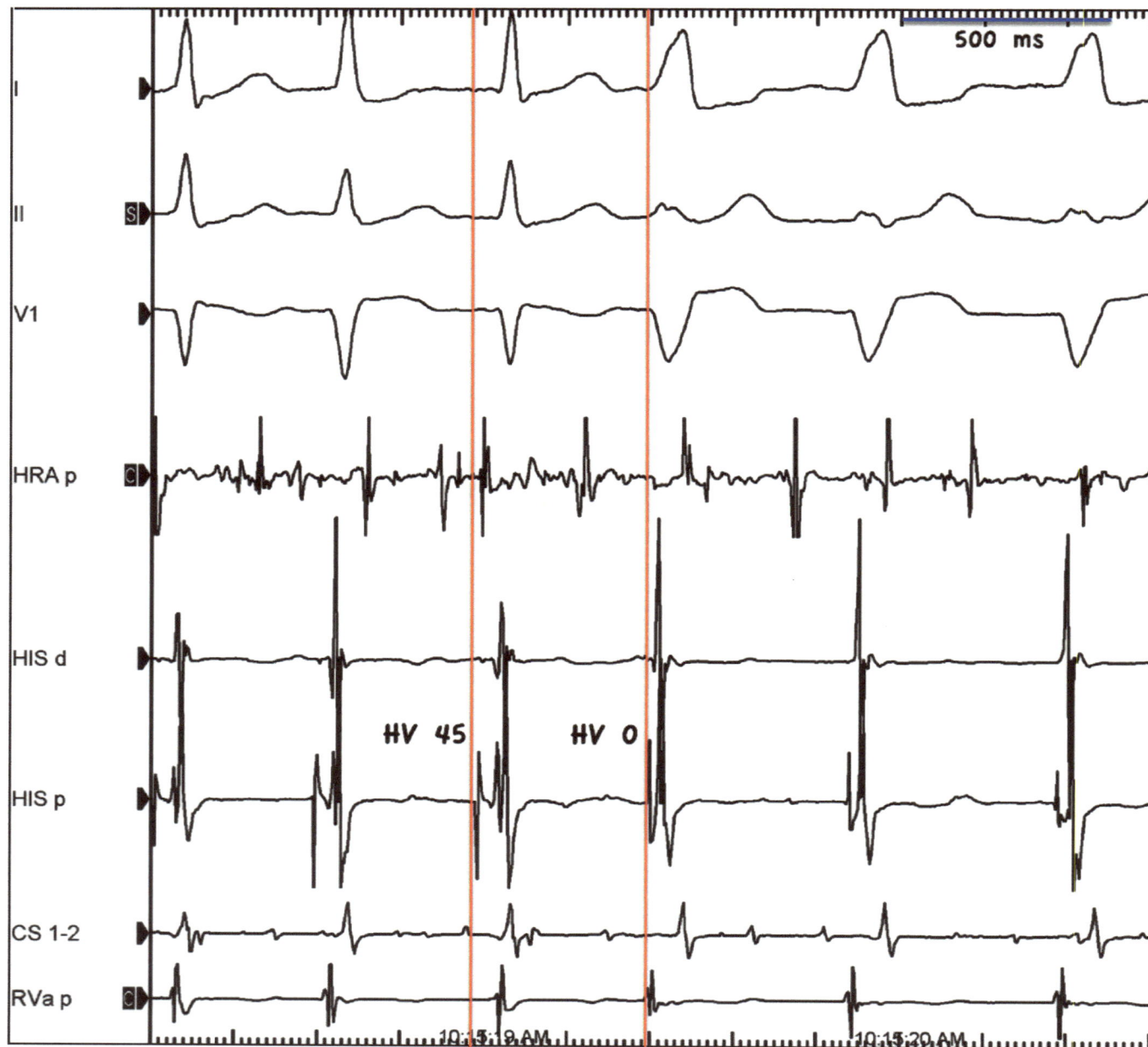

Figure 7.6C

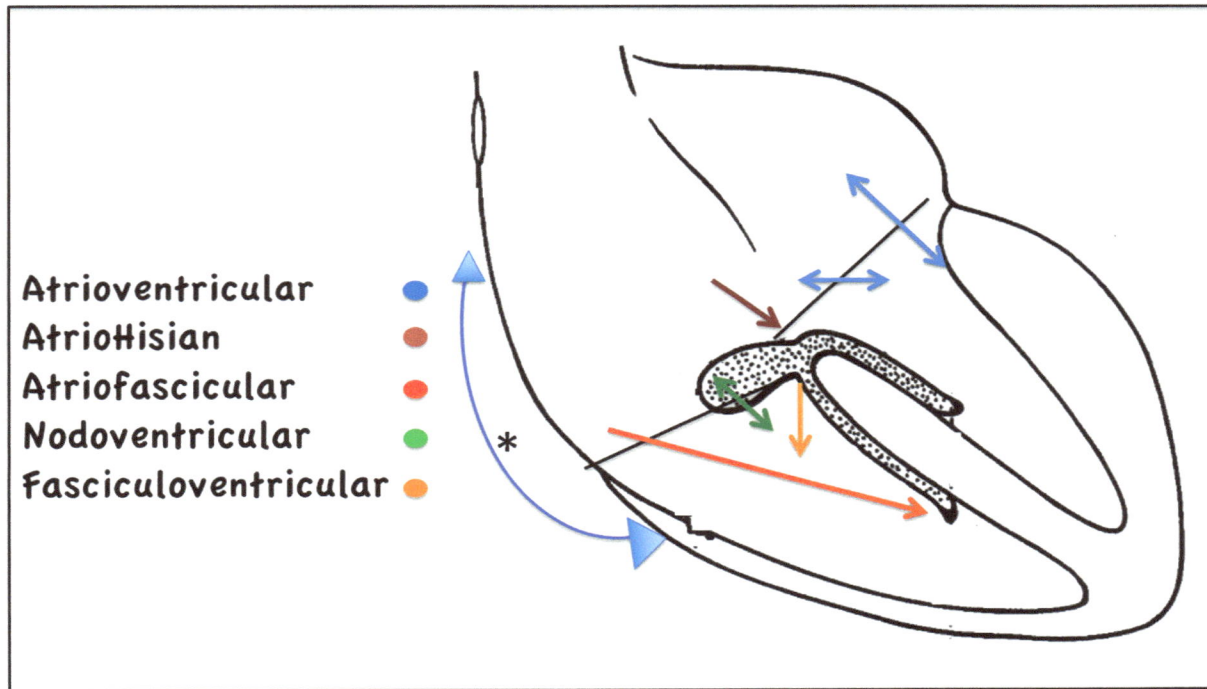

Atrioventricular ●
AtrioHisian ●
Atriofascicular ●
Nodoventricular ●
Fasciculoventricular ●

On a final note, one might ask why the HV relationship during WC beats is constant. One might expect a differing relationship (variable fusion) depending on relative conduction from the atria through the AV node versus the AP. A clue to this is provided by the clear His recording that *reverses polarity* after transition from the narrow QRS to the WC beats. The His inscribed during WC beats is actually a retrograde His. The rapid conduction from the pathway insertion site to the His suggests a direct connection of this pathway to the RBBB,

hence suggesting an "atriofascicular" AP as opposed to an atrioventricular AP.

Figure 7.6C schematically summarizes the different types of accessory connections, most reasonably named by their origin and insertion sites (hence, "atrioventricular," etc.).

The asterisk (★) refers to an uncommon atrioventricular AP (**light blue**), a long pathway that actually may originate well away from the AV ring in the higher atrium and similarly may end in the ventricle away from the AV ring as illustrated.

Problem 7.7

An overview of this tracing (**Figure 7.7A**) suggests SVT with the P wave virtually simultaneous with the QRS ("P on QRS"), and a reflexive look at this suggests AVNRT (as it did to the referring physician). However, the main point of this tracing is to emphasize the hazard of coming to a hasty conclusion.

Figure 7.7A

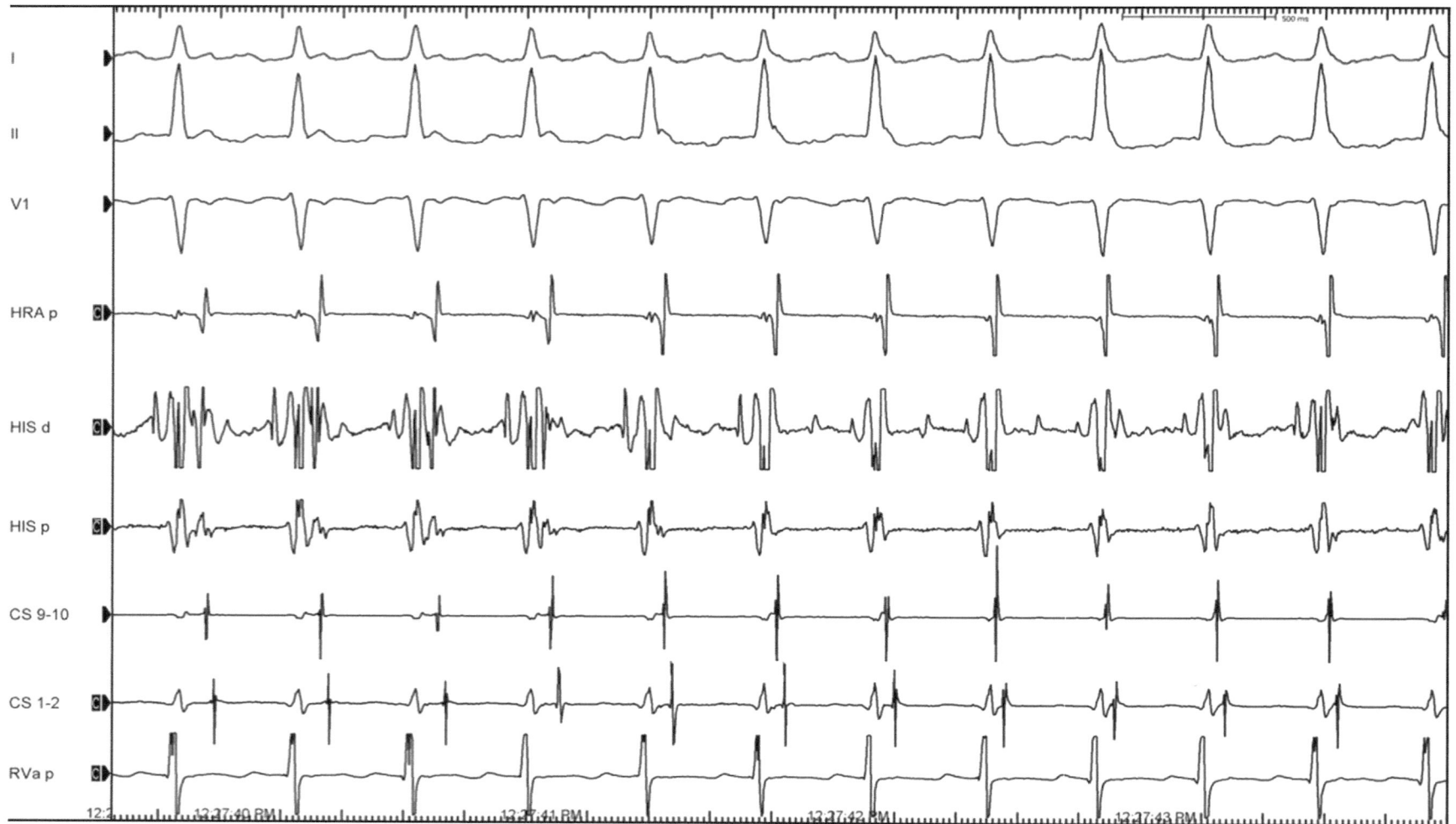

The differential diagnosis of a "P on QRS" SVT is in the "Regular Supraventricular Tachycardia with Very Short QRS to P" section in Chapter 8 and a more methodical look at the tracing leads one to the correct diagnosis (**Figure 7.7B**).

Figure 7.7B

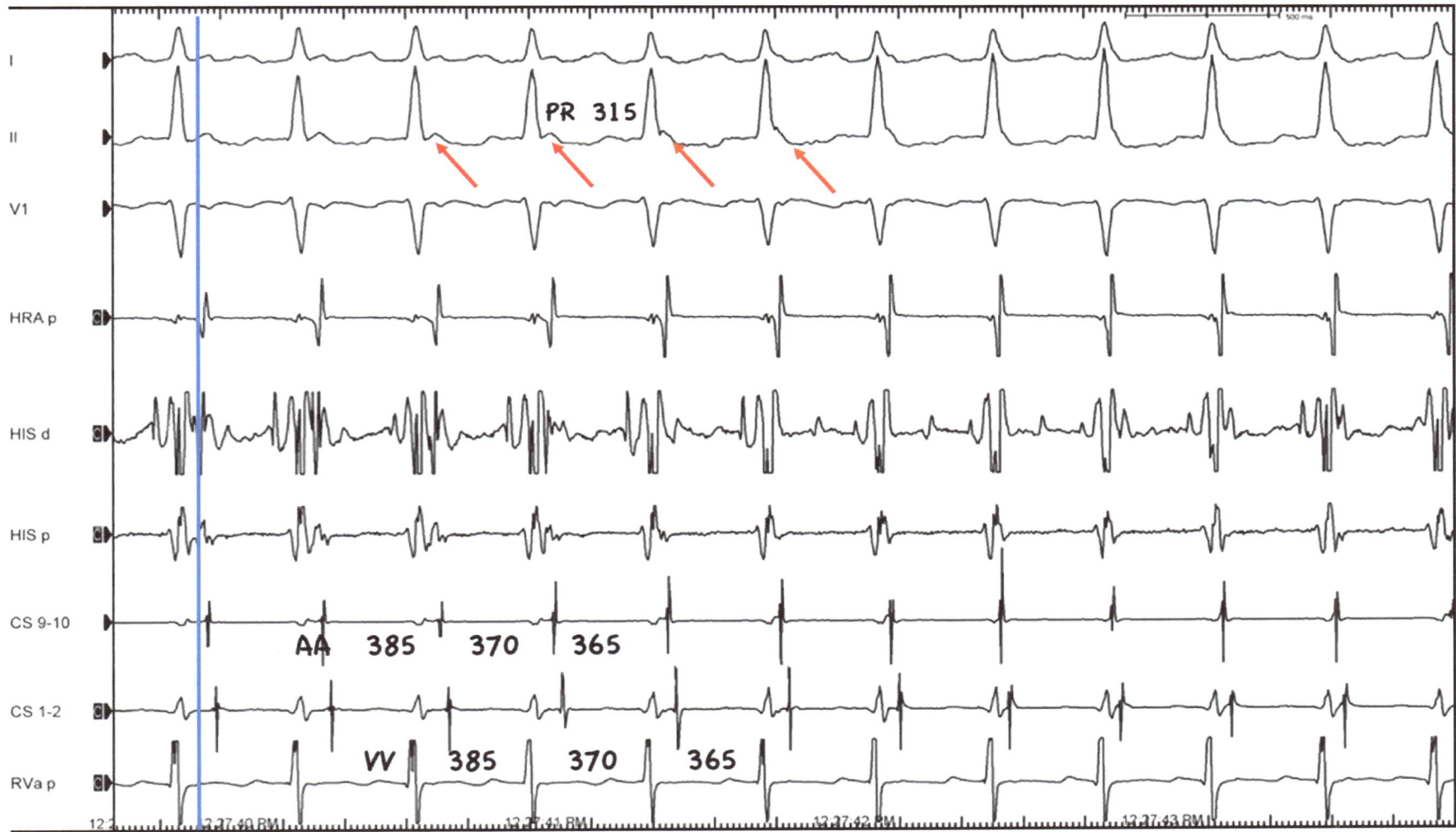

We now observe that the P and QRS relationship is changing slightly. The P wave is evident on the ECG during the first few cycles. The variable AV relationship is related to slight variability the atrial CL, and the V merely follows the A. The P wave is positive in leads 1 and 2, incompatible with AVNRT, which should have "low to high" atrial activation. The atrial EGMs show atrial activation at the HRA (**blue line**) nearly simultaneous with the HBE atrial EGM, suggesting a right atrial source of activation.

This is a right AT with slow AVN pathway conduction. We are fortunate enough in this tracing to have some variability in atrial CL to make it obvious. However, you might imagine an AT with no variability in CL, such as the last 5 cycles of this tracing. Many of us have been fooled by this type of tachycardia at some point, myself included!

Chapter 8

Explanatory Notes and Tables of Differential Diagnosis

The "KEY" Elements of Tracing Analysis

Analysis of a tracing be it ECG or EGM begins with an overview and identification of the key elements one needs to make a diagnosis. These include:

1. QRS morphology and ventricular activation sequence
2. P-wave identification and atrial activation sequence
3. His bundle location
4. AV relationship

The "tools" of analysis are then put to use.

Cycle Length Variability ("Wobble")

Looking for CL variation during a tachycardia can be extremely productive. A simple but important principle is that the cause of a CL change CANNOT be downstream from the observed change. For example, if the P–P interval prolongs suddenly and prolongs the tachycardia CL, it cannot be VT!

"Zone" Analysis of a Complex Tracing

A complex ECG is often read from left to right, but it can be very useful to look at the recording and divide it into zones. For example, a tracing showing two different tachycardias can be divided into6 three zones: tachycardia 1, tachycardia 2, and a transition zone, each to be considered separately. *It is often productive to start with the zone that is easiest or clearest to understand and then build from there.*

It is also often productive to *enlarge* zones of interest to clarify subtle observations or make finer measurements.

Supraventricular Tachycardias

Regular Supraventricular Tachycardia
1. AT
2. AVNRT
3. AVRT
4. JT
5. AFl
6. Sinus tachycardia
7. VT with narrow QRS

Regular Supraventricular Tachycardia with VA Block (Fewer Ps than QRSs)
1. AVNRT
2. JT
3. Nodoventricular or nodofascicular reentry
4. VT with narrow QRS

Regular Supraventricular Tachycardia with Very Short QRS to P (< than 100 ms approximately, "P on QRS")
1. AVNRT
2. AT with slow pathway conduction
3. Junctional tachycardia
4. Nodoventricular or nodofascicular reentry
5. VT with narrow QRS

Irregular Supraventricular Tachycardia (AF Mimickers)
1. AFl with variable block
2. SVT with ectopy
3. Alternation between more than one anterograde AVN pathway or retrograde AVN pathway or both (i.e., multiple anterograde and/or retrograde AVN pathways).
4. Alternation between more than one anterograde AVN pathway or retrograde AP or both.
5. Non–reentrant AVN tachycardia (2-for-1 AV conduction)
6. Alternation between more than one tachycardia mechanism sharing part of a circuit (i.e., AVNRT and AVRT)

Wide QRS Tachycardia

1. Supraventricular tachycardia with aberrant conduction (bundle branch block)
2. Preexcited tachycardia
3. Ventricular tachycardia
4. Artifact
5. Paced rhythm
6. "Pseudo" tachycardia related to marked ST elevation (for example, sinus tachycardia with the elevated ST segment merging with the QRS giving appearance of a "wide" QRS)

Preexcited Tachycardia: 2 Broad Categories

1. The accessory pathway is a "bystander," that is, it is not directly related to the mechanism of the tachycardia. The most common examples would be AFl or atrial fibrillation, where the arrhythmia mechanism would not be altered by the presence or absence of preexcitation. Clearly, the clinical manifestation of the arrhythmia nonetheless may be profoundly altered. A potential diagnostic clue to bystander status, in addition to the continuation of tachycardia unchanged in the absence of preexcitation, is the potential *presence of fusion* for anterograde conduction. If anterograde conduction is conducting exclusively over a single AP, the tachycardia will always be maximally preexcited, such as you would expect with antidromic tachycardia with anterograde conduction over a single AP and retrograde conduction over the normal AVCS.

2. The AP is part of the tachycardia mechanism. This is generally as the anterograde limb of a macroreentrant circuit.

If the His bundle EGM is not visible, or the HV interval is < 40 ms* during tachycardia, yet we are certain that the His bundle catheter is positioned where the HBE should be recorded and was clearly identifiable prior to the tachycardia induction and after its termination, this can only be one of two things:

1. Preexcitation
2. Ventricular rhythm

---

* The lower limit of normal HV conduction time has not been accurately and precisely quantified, and there is undoubtedly some overlap between the lower range and abnormal HV. Nonetheless, 40 ms is arguably a reasonable number.

Sudden Shortening of the PR Interval

1. Intermittent conduction over an accessory pathway ("intermittent preexcitation")
2. Junctional extrasystole
3. PAC
4. PVC
5. Shortening of the PR interval by resolution of delay in the AV node or His–Purkinje system, often after pause or rate slowing
6. Shift to a fast AVN pathway in a patient with dual AVN pathways

Of all these possibilities, the most common would probably be late-coupled PVCs that interrupt the PR interval.

Termination of a WCT with a Narrow QRS Complex at Same CL

1. AVRT with spontaneous resolution of functional bundle branch block (ipsilateral to the AP) on the last cycle
2. Spontaneous termination of VT with a supraventricular (AV nodal or AV) echo beat after the last VT QRS
3. A capture beat terminating VT

This phenomenon is, with rare exceptions, related to spontaneous resolution of functional bundle branch block during SVT, where the affected bundle branch is part of the circuit. For example, normalization of LBBB aberration in orthodromic AVRT over a left lateral AV pathway would result in shortening of the VA interval, which arrives prematurely in the AV node and may well block. A fortuitous atrial capture beat following the VT termination at the CL of VT is theoretically possible but very unlikely. This is because VT almost universally results in concealed retrograde penetration of the AV node even in the absence of VA conduction, and this would delay the arrival of the capture beat. Additionally, one would have to postulate that a relatively late-coupled capture beat at CL of VT would terminate VT without apparent fusion (essentially impossible) or that the VT terminated and a capture beat at the CL of VT fortuitously arrived.

Tachycardia with Both RV and LV "in" the Circuit (See Problem 2.2)

1. Bundle branch reentry
2. AV tachycardia with ipsilateral bundle branch block
3. NV tachycardia with ipsilateral bundle branch block
4. AP to AP reentry (one to each ventricle)

Concept of Reset and Fusion

This diagram explains the concept of "fusion and reset," one of the most useful and important concepts in understanding arrhythmia mechanisms. The image on the left in **Figure 8.1A** depicts a focal source of arrhythmia, for example, an automatic focus in the ventricle. A PVC may well summate or "fuse" with the QRS of the tachycardia but will NOT be able to get into the focus because it is colliding with the wave emanating from the focus.

Figure 8.1A

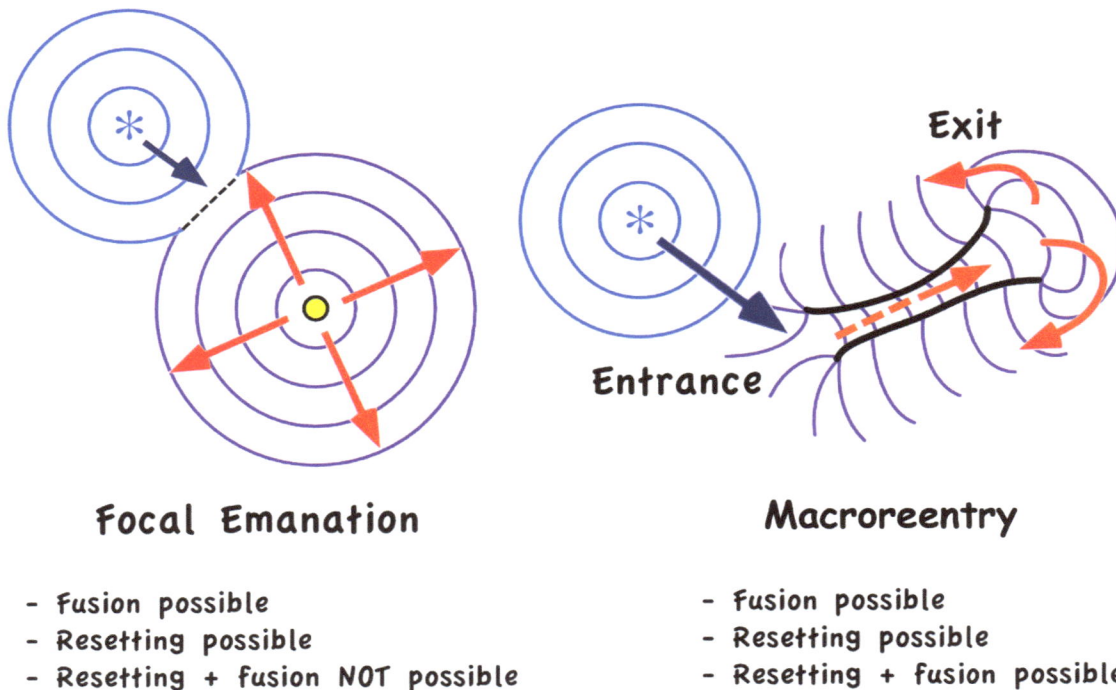

Focal Emanation

- Fusion possible
- Resetting possible
- Resetting + fusion NOT possible

Macroreentry

- Fusion possible
- Resetting possible
- Resetting + fusion possible

If we move to the right diagram, one sees that the wave from the PVC is able to get into the "excitable gap" or "entrance" to get into a critical slow conduction zone to affect it (advance, delay), which then proceeds to come out the other end to "reset"

the timing. It may even terminate the arrhythmia. The fundamental reason for this stems from the **separate entrance and exit to the critical part of the circuit**. With very few exceptions (can you think of any?), this means macroreentry.

Figure 8.1A is based on one provided by Dr. John Miller, a master electrophysiologist and teacher.

Index